TH BIG BOOK of 15 MINUTE WORKOUTS

01 SEP 2015

26 AUG 2016

ST THOMAS
Tel. (01792)
655570

KT-489-059

WITHDRAWN
SWANSEA LIBRARIES

6000167158

The information in this book is meant to supplement, not replace, proper exercise training.
All forms of exercise pose some inherent risks. The editors and publisher advise readers to take full responsibility
for their safety and know their limits. Before practicing the exercises in this book, be sure that your equipment is well-maintained,
and do not take risks beyond your level of experience, aptitude, training, and fitness.
The exercise and dietary programs in this book are not intended as a substitute for any exercise routine or dietary regimen
that may have been prescribed by your doctor. As with all exercise and dietary programs,
you should get your doctor's approval before beginning.

Mention of specific companies, organizations, or authorities in this book does not imply endorsement by the author or publisher,
nor does mention of specific companies, organizations, or authorities imply that they endorse this book, its author, or the publisher.

Internet addresses and telephone numbers given in this book were accurate at the time it went to press.

© 2011 by Rodale Inc.

All rights reserved. No part of this publication may be reproduced or transmitted in any form or by any means, electronic or mechanical,
including photocopying, recording, or any other information storage and retrieval system, without the written permission of the publisher.

Rodale books may be purchased for business or promotional use or for special sales. For information, please write to:
Special Markets Department, Rodale Inc., 733 Third Avenue, New York, NY 10017.

Men's Health is a registered trademark of Rodale Inc.

Printed in the United States of America

Rodale Inc. makes every effort to use acid-free ⊗, recycled paper ♲.

Book design by Laura White
with George Karabotsos, design director of *Men's Health* Books

Photo editor: Mark Haddad

All photography by Beth Bischoff

Cover stylist: Kathy Kalafut
Cover hairstylist: Giovanni Giuntoli at Maxine Tall Management for Redken
Cover makeup: Lynn LaMorte

Library of Congress Cataloging-in-Publication Data is on file with the publisher.

ISBN-13: 978-1-60961-800-1 hardcover
ISBN-13: 978-1-60961-735-6 paperback

Trade paperback and direct-mail hardcover editions published simultaneously in September 2011.

Distributed to the trade by Macmillan

2 4 6 8 10 9 7 5 3 1 hardcover

2 4 6 8 10 9 7 5 3 1 paperback

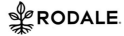

RODALE.

We inspire and enable people to improve their lives and the world around them.
www.rodalebooks.com

Contents

Acknowledgments

It takes a small army to create a big book. And this Big Book was no exception. I can't possibly give sufficient thanks to all those who helped move this project from a simple idea to a big, thick book filled to the brim with really cool, superfast workouts. But I'll try, first by sharing my appreciation for *Men's Health* magazine Editor-in-Chief David Zinczenko and the entire *Men's Health* staff for creating such a successful brand that inspires men to live healthier lives. It's my hope that this book helps to forward that mission.

My heartfelt thanks go to Fitness Editor Adam Campbell, author of the book that launched this series, *The Big Book of Exercises*; and to my editor on this book, Jeff Csatari, for the opportunity and for his calm, unflappable guidance from start to finish.

Stephen Perrine and the entire *Men's Health* Books team, including Debbie McHugh, Ursula Cary, and Erin Williams for catching my mistakes.

Book group Design Director George Karabotsos, and the talented designer on this book, Laura White. Photographer Beth Bischoff for the beautiful chapter openers and workout pictures; assistants Geoffrey Goodridge and Esteban Aladro; and models Sidney Wilson, Kyle Fields, Todd Trofimuk, Andy Speer, and Currin Wilkerson for holding those barbell squats for so long.

Executive Vice President and Publisher Karen Rinaldi, Chris

Krogermeier, Sara Cox, and everyone else at Rodale Books who were so enthusiastic and helpful.

For sharing their invaluable expertise in health, fitness, and nutrition, I thank Sean Armstead; Craig Ballantyne, CSCS; Joan Salge Blake, RD; Traver Boehm; Kurt Brett; Mike Brungardt; Jay Cardiello; Michael A. Clark, DPT; Hannah Davis; Amy Dixon; Gregory Florez; Martin Gibala, PhD; Tony Gentilcore; Bill Hartman, PT, CSCS; Carter Hays; Tom Holland; Katrina Hodgson; William Kraemer, PhD; Christopher Knight, PhD; Jim Liston, CSCS; Ashley Ntansah; Scott Mazzetti, PhD; Mike Mejia, MS, CSCS; Scott H. Mendelson; C.J. Murphy; Stuart Phillips, PhD; Wayne Phillips, PhD; Lauren Piskin; Carrie Rezabek; Craig Rasmussen, CSCS; David Raye; Robert dos Remedios, CSCS; Juan Carlos Santana, CSCS; Jonas Sahratian; Jyotsna Sahni, MD; Michelle M. Seibel, MD; Tina Schmidt-McNulty; Tara Stiles; Patrick Striet, CSCS; Jason Talanian, PhD; Mark Verstegen; Diane Vives; Wayne Westcott, PhD, CSCS; Jordan Yuam, NCEP; Valerie Waters; and Victoria Zdrok, PhD.

And of course, my family. Dave, none of this happens without your undying support; daughter Juniper for hugs and smiles, and Mom and Dad for always lending a helping hand. Thank you.

— *Selene Yeager*

Introduction:
The 15-Minute Secret

Why 15 Minutes Is All You Need to
Add Lean Muscle, Shed That Gut,
Build Endurance, and Gain Tremendous Confidence.

I don't have time to

work out. Does that sound familiar? Sure it does. We've all said it at one time or another. Lack of time is the number-one reason men, in survey after survey, give for why they don't exercise.

Look, time is a guy's most precious commodity these days—because he has so little "free time" to do what he wants. You, too, no doubt. You work 50 to 60 hours a week. You need to shop for food and wash your underwear. Maybe you have a family or a big social life. You have investments to monitor, you volunteer at a homeless shelter, your old man needs help fixing the backyard fence. And there are tweets to post! When are you going to find an hour or so to run to the gym three or four times a week?

The 15-Minute Secret

You probably can't. But you don't have to. You don't need an hour to get in shape. Heck, you don't even need a half hour if you exercise strategically. All you need to build the body you want is 15 minutes. According to a recent study published in the *European Journal of Applied Physiology*, 15 minutes of resistance training *was just as effective* as 35 minutes was in elevating resting energy expenditure for up to 72 hours after the exercise. That means you can burn calories and build muscle in half the time you thought possible. And you'll actually have a much better chance of slimming down with those quick workouts than lengthy gym sessions. A study in the *International Journal of Sports Medicine* found that volunteers who were trying to lose weight had a much better chance of sticking to an exercise plan if their workouts were cut to 15 minutes.

It makes sense. You can always find 15 minutes to spare, right? (If you need help, see "Free Minutes!" on page x for simple ways to squeeze time into a busy day.) Fifteen minutes for something so important to your health as exercise is totally doable with a little effort. That's why we've created this book and a superfast fitness program composed entirely of 15-minute workouts. Now, just because we're slashing workout time by half or more doesn't mean you're getting any less effective of a workout. Most of these workouts are designed as time-efficient circuits. You activate just as many muscle fibers—maybe even more—and you accomplish that a lot

quicker, without a lot of down time, so you're actually adding an aerobic component to strength-training. Every second of exercise will count a little more than it ever has before. Instead of working out longer, you'll be working out smarter and faster so you can get on with the rest of your life.

What's more, you'll never get bored with the workouts in this book simply because there are so many to try. You'll find total-body workouts using barbells, dumbbells, kettlebells, sandbags, even exercise bands. No access to equipment? That's okay. You can choose from a dozen metabolic workouts that use only your own bodyweight for resistance. There are workouts that target specific body parts—your chest, your legs, your core. You'll find 15-minute programs customized to your particular body type, and high-intensity interval training workouts that crank up your metabolism fast and keep it elevated for hours so you continue burning calories long after you've hit the shower. There are workouts to prevent and heal aches and pains. There are even workouts that'll help you be stronger, sexier, and last longer in bed. And because research has proven that combining a nutrition plan with an exercise program is more effective than diet or exercise alone, we've created a weight-loss and nutrition chapter—complete with delicious recipes—that'll deliver fast results. Everything in the book, even the recipes, are choreographed to be quick and efficient. That means you'll be ready to eat in 15 minutes or less, too!

After paging through this book, you'll quickly recognize that the vast majority of the photographs show resistance or weight-lifting exercises. We go heavy on muscle-building because of the importance of muscle to a man's overall health. It's not simply for performance or vanity. Recent research shows that diminished muscle mass and strength are empirically linked to declines in the immune system, the onset of heart disease and type 2 diabetes, as well as weaker bones, stiffer joints, and slumping postures. Muscle mass has also been shown to play a strategic role in protein metabolism, which is particularly important in responding to stress. Decreased muscle mass also correlates with a decline in your body's metabolic rate—the rate at which your body burns calories. Muscle burns more calories at rest than fat does. As you get older, your body naturally loses muscle mass. If you don't do anything about it (read: strength train) and you continue to eat as much as you did in your 20s, you will, without a doubt, put on weight.

You can see why the *Men's Health Big Book of 15-Minute Workouts* can be such an important tool for good health and longevity. By keeping workouts brief, you are more likely to do them regularly. By making workouts mostly about building muscle, you automatically burn more calories; strengthen your heart, bones and joints; and fortify your body against the diseases and illnesses that plague men who don't make the time to take care of themselves.

Your time has come to improve your life, for life!

It takes just 15 minutes to start—right now.

The 15-Minute Secret

Free Minutes!

15 WAYS TO FIND 15 MINUTES FOR EXERCISE EVERY DAY! (DITCH THE STUFF THAT'S WASTING YOUR PRECIOUS TIME.)

1. FLIP OFF FACEBOOK. On average, Americans now spend a whopping 7 hours a month on Facebook, according to Neilsen. Let's do the math: Seven hours a month works out to 105 minutes each week, or hmmm, guess what, exactly 15 minutes every single day. You don't have to banish FB from your life entirely, but limit it to two short sessions a day, like once in the morning over coffee and later in the evening. Then log out and stay off.

2. SAY "NO!" We know. Guys think they can do it all and you hate to say "no." But we think you'll really like it once you try it. Next time someone (not your big boss) asks you to do something you really don't want or need to do, say, "I'm sorry. No. I just can't," and feel the freedom—and all that free time—wash over you.

3. PLAN YOUR PEAKS. We all have certain times of the day when we are most focused and productive. Schedule your biggest tasks for that time (for many people it's in the morning, say 9 a.m.). You'll get it done more quickly and efficiently than if you wait to tackle it during a natural low point (like midafternoon).

4. DO ONE THING AT A TIME. We all pride ourselves as being supreme multi-taskers, but trying to do too many things at once means getting nothing done. Sit down with your to-do list. Pick an item, and do it and only it. You'll be shocked at how quickly each tasks gets done when you give it your full energy and attention.

5. RECORD YOUR SHOWS. A typical hour-long TV show contains just 40 to 42 minutes of real content —the rest is commercials. Watch two shows and that's 40 to 45 minutes you could have spent doing something else. It's well worth investing in a digital TV recorder, so you can watch just what you want when you want, and free up hours (and at the end of the year, days) to pursue more healthy activities, like 15-minute workouts.

6. LEAVE WELL ENOUGH ALONE. Is it really all that important that your hubcaps be spotless? Stop wasting precious time with a bottle of Armor All, buffing every little imperfection out of your bucket seats, and aim for adequate instead.

7. BE DECISIVE! You can easily waste hours choosing what home sound system is best or which brand of sneakers to buy (it's called analysis paralysis). At some point, you need to stop waffling and move forward. Set a time limit, say 45 minutes, for comparison shopping, weighing pros and cons, etc., then make a decision and go forth.

8. BUY TIME. Yes, you actually can buy more hours in the day by paying for services that suck up tons of time. Before you pooh-pooh the idea of hiring a laundry or cleaning service, sit down and do a little math. What is an hour of your time worth? How do you spend your disposable income? When you consider that you might be blowing a few hundred bucks on restaurant meals and golf accessories you don't really need while you slave away all your spare time mowing the back 40, it's time to reconsider your expenditures. Hire a landscaping service to do the heavy duty stuff a few times a month and buy yourself hours every week.

9. INK IT IN YOUR CALENDAR. Amazing how you find time for everything on your calendar, right? That's because it's there in black and white demanding your attention (and time). Block out your workouts as you would work appointments and you won't miss a one.

10. USE AN EGG TIMER. Certain activities are black holes for time. All the little things you plan to do for just a few minutes—surfing the Web; playing games on your phone; "window shopping" all the new apps for your iPhone or iPad—can suck away hours if you're not careful. Keep an egg timer on your desk. When you sit down, set it for 15 or 20 minutes. Then, shut down when the bell rings.

11. TOUCH IT ONCE. When a paper comes across your desk (or in the mail), touch it once and deal with it immediately. Piling up stacks of paper not only creates distracting clutter, you also waste time revisiting it again (and again) or worse, losing something important. (Try it with email too.)

12. MAKE A CALL. IMing and emailing can be great time savers. But sometimes it takes 15 messages to accomplish what you could do in a 40-second phone call. As soon as it starts getting complicated, pick up the phone.

13. PUT THINGS IN THEIR PLACES. I used to waste minutes (hours...days) looking for my keys. At any given time they could be anywhere, and I mean anywhere— coat pockets, drawers, messenger bags, the clothes dryer, my car, and, my personal favorite, hanging from the door lock. Finally, I bought a 75-cent hook, hung it by the phone as my desig- nated key spot, and I have not lost my keys since. Try this trick with anything you lose regularly. It works.

14. SET OUT YOUR STUFF. This one is repeated more often than *It's a Wonderful Life* at Christmas, but it works. Setting out your exercise clothes at night makes it far more likely that you will get up and get moving for a morning workout, instead of hitting snooze (or worse, skipping the whole affair entirely) because it's too daunting to get out and start rummaging around for your workout gear.

15. GET UP 15 MINUTES EARLIER. Ridiculously simple, right? Yep, and it works. Vow to get up and work out at 5 a.m. every day and you'll never do it. But even the most nocturnal of night owls can set their alarm (and roll out of the sack) a mere 15 minutes earlier in the morning. Even if you don't use that extra time for your workout, it gets you out the door and to your office earlier than usual, so you get more done earlier in the day. So you're more likely to feel entitled to take that 15 minutes for yourself later in the day.

Chapter 1:
The Genius of the 15-Minute Workout

Why Less Is More When It Comes to Exercising
for Fitness, Strength, and Health.

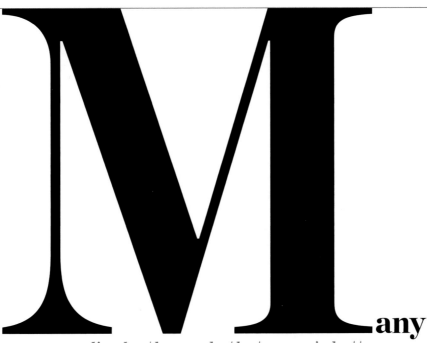

Many men live by the credo that more is better. If 1 tablespoon of cough syrup will ease your cold symptoms, well then 2 will work even faster. What's better then a cheeseburger? A double cheeseburger with extra pickles. And so it seems for exercise as well. If 45 minutes in the gym will trim that belly, then 2 hours must transform us into, well, *Men's Health* cover models.

But take a look at the cardio junkies next time you're at the gym. You know the ones who are slogging out endless miles on the treadmill or elliptical trainer. If you watch them over time, you'll notice something startling: Their bodies don't change. At all. Not one iota. Most of them are just as soft when they step off the treadmill for the 1,000th time as they were when they first hopped aboard. That's because they're stuck in the old thinking that if you do hours and hours

The Genius of the 15-Minute Workout

of cardio, you'll burn pounds and pounds of fat. Wrong. Cutting-edge science all points in the opposite direction: If you want to scorch calories, burn fat, and get faster and stronger, go harder, not longer.

The more, more, more mind set is more than a waste of time; it keeps many people from doing anything. Since we think we have to do a ton to get results, sometimes we don't exercise at all. It's a mentality that sets us up for failure before we even start. As it turns out, it is far more important to know what kind of exercise to do rather than how long to do it for. Because much of what we think is going to make us thin or keep us fit actually does neither. In a study published in the *International Journal of Sports Nutrition and Exercise Metabolism* researchers asked a group of volunteers to do 45 minutes of steady, moderate cardio exercise (like a brisk elliptical workout) 5 days a week for 12 weeks and compared their results to another group that did no exercise. The result? At the end of the study, the exercisers had experienced no change in their body composition, same as their couch-potato peers. Depressing? Not at all. The good news is that you have permission to stop wasting your time. You can finally free yourself from marathon gym sessions. Instead, exercise scientists now say you can shed fat, firm flabby spots, boost your heart health, and fend off a host of ills, both mental and physical, not by doing more, but by doing less. You can do this in as little as 15 minutes if you do the right program.

Brief Workouts, Big Rewards

That's exactly what you get with the *Men's Health Big Book of 15-Minute Workouts*: A scientifically proven shortcut to building muscle and losing weight. We've pooled all our expertise and pored through the latest research to create what we call our Superfast Workout Program. At the heart of it is resistance training, which has been proven to be the quickest way to burn fat and build a lean, hard body. When you lift weights, microscopic tears occur in your muscle fibers, which sounds like a bad thing, but it's actually the first step in shedding blubber and building strength. This fiber breakdown speeds up a process called muscle protein synthesis that uses amino acids to repair and reinforce those fibers—i.e., you're building muscle. That helps you lose weight in a few ways. One, all that lifting and rebuilding burns calories not just while you're exercising, but also long after you're done. Two, muscle is metabolically more active than fat, meaning that it burns more calories just to sustain itself. The more muscle you have on your frame, the more calories you are burning even when that frame is lounging on the sofa! Finally, being stronger makes you more active. Research shows that people become more spontaneously active when they start lifting weights because they're stronger and have more energy. The only downside to all this might be having to buy a smaller belt for your trousers.

A pound of muscle takes up 20 percent less space than a pound of fat. So you'll be leaner all over.

The best part: You can get all these body-building benefits in no time—just 15 minutes is all it takes. That's right, we've condensed the reps and removed all the sitting around and waiting between moves for a supereffective and superfast workout. It's not only time-efficient, but it also increases your energy expenditure both during and after exercising. Researchers from Southern Illinois University recently found that one set of 10 reps of 9 exercises (which took less than 15 minutes to complete, by the way) raised resting energy expenditure (the number of calories you burn when you're just sitting around) by just as much as three sets, which took the volunteers 35 minutes to do. Fifteen or 35? Take your pick.

Finally, to speed your results, if weight loss is your goal, we've added cardio to the mix. Not the 45-minutes-to-an-hour-a-day variety that may barely budge the scale, but the superfast fat burn variety, known in scientific circles as high-intensity interval training (or HIIT). While the government keeps upping the ante on its cardio exercise recommendation—up a half hour, from 60 minutes a day to 90 minutes a day for weight loss—a large and growing body of research is pointing in the opposite direction—that HIIT is drastically superior to regular cardio workouts in improving cardiovascular functioning, improving insulin sensitivity, and, of course,

burning calories. What determines whether or not you shed fat is not the duration of your workouts, but the intensity. In other words, it'll take many hours to walk away from that extra weight. But you can sprint it off in no time.

Superfast exercise builds up lactic acid in your muscles because you're working harder and faster than your body can clear it, which triggers a release of human growth hormone, a powerful natural elixir that promotes fat loss and muscle building and will crank your metabolism to Maserati intensity. And it works fast. Just 30 seconds of sprinting on a stationary bike is enough to send your level of the growth hormone soaring by 530 percent. Another important benefit of interval training: Your metabolism stays elevated for up to 24 hours after a high-intensity workout.

All that fat burning translates into a leaner you in half the workout time. In a study of 18 volunteers, Australian researchers found that those who performed superfast workouts that included 8-second full-on sprints followed by 12 seconds of recovery 3 days a week lost about 5 ½ pounds while those in a similar group who pedaled for twice as long at an average pace actually gained a pound of fat over the same period. Even better, the exercisers who were heavier at the start shed the most, with two losing about 18 pounds each. Even better, the weight you lose is pure fat. In one study by Laval University, researchers found that even when HIIT exercisers burned half as many calories during their actual

The Genius of the 15-Minute Workout

workout sessions, they still lost nine times more fat after 15 weeks of working out than their traditional long-cardio-bout peers did after 20 weeks.

The benefits don't stop at weight loss. HIIT workouts also help you get fitter faster (so you have more energy for everything you love to do). In a striking head-to-head showdown, Canadian researchers found that a group of exercisers who cranked out short stationary bike workouts that included a series of 30-second sprints 3 days a week improved their fitness by about 30 percent—nearly identical to the improvements made by a similar group of exercisers who pedaled for 90 minutes to 2 hours at a lesser intensity.

Interval training is also the ticket for the fast path to good health. Researchers in Norway reported that interval training was far more effective at reducing blood pressure, controlling blood sugar, and improving cholesterol than traditional one-speed workouts.

When you stop and think about how your body works, all this seemingly counterintuitive science suddenly makes a lot of sense. Our bodies are built to adapt to the work we demand of them. When you get up and go out the door for a leisurely jog, you're asking your slow-twitch (endurance) muscle fibers to wake up and get to work, but all of those fast-twitch (speed and power) muscle fibers go largely untapped. Over time, many of the neurons that once served fast-twitch fibers will get rewired to serve their slower counterparts. Others

will die off. Turning up the intensity of your workouts not only gives you firmer, more sculpted muscle tone by tapping into all of those unused fibers, but also speeds up your fitness gains, says HIIT-training researcher Martin Gibala, PhD, professor of kinesiology at McMaster University. "High-intensity exercise kind of shocks your system. Your body thinks, 'He's making me do some really hard work,' so it increases your total exercise capacity—your ability to use oxygen and burn fat—in a fraction of the time than if you'd exercised less intensely," he says. In fact, according to neuromuscular researcher Christopher Knight, PhD, of the University of Delaware in Newark, there's an almost immediate effect when you tap into your fast-twitch fibers with strength training and/or high-speed intervals. "We've found that you can increase your fast-twitch firing rates after just 1 week of training," he says.

That's the superfast secret. You combine 15-minute resistance training workouts with 15-minute HIIT workouts over the course of a week to lose the most weight. Scientists already know that combining cardio and resistance training works faster and better than either alone. When Pennsylvania State University researchers put overweight people on a diet and then had them do cardio, resistance training and cardio, or no exercise at all, they found that though each group lost roughly 21 pounds, the lifters dropped 6 more pounds, or—40 percent more—of fat. That's right, nearly every ounce they lost was in the form of fat, while the other two groups dropped precious metabolism-revving muscle as well. Now you get to reap all of these rewards in a fraction of the time you ever thought possible.

But the 15-minute secret doesn't just give you the shortest, most effective workout on the planet. You'll also:

1. Trade Fat for Muscle

Whether you want to be ready to go shirtless on your beach vacation or are just looking to boost a flat butt, 15 minutes is all it takes. Premier strength-training researcher Wayne Westcott, PhD, CSCS, instructor in the exercise science department at Quincy College in Quincy, Massachusetts, confirms that when you choose your exercises wisely, a handful of moves—just four in some cases—of moves is all you need to change your body composition. "Navy research shows you can get tremendous overall improve-ment—losing 4 pounds of fat and adding 2 pounds of muscle in 8 weeks—by doing just four exercises that work every major muscle," he says. The four key moves: squat, chest press, row, and ab curl, done a few times each. That's 15 minutes for a total-body transformation.

2. Burn More Calories

Even better, the calorie-burning benefits of even the shortest strength training bout keep coming long after you've left the gym. That study from Southern Illinois University is worth repeating: Researchers found that when volunteers did just one set of nine exercises, or about 11 minutes of strength training, 3 days a week, they increased their resting metabolic rate (the number of calories burned when they were just hanging out) and fat burning enough to keep unwanted weight at bay. And then even more great things will happen.

3. Stay Young

Unless you do something to stop it, your body loses muscle as you move through adulthood, says Tina Schmidt-McNulty, fitness center exercise specialist at Purdue University Calumet Fitness Center. When you consider that muscle is your body's biggest calorie burner—burning five times as many calories per pound as fat—it's like "taking your foot off the gas pedal of your metabolism right as you enter adulthood," explains Schmidt-McNulty. That metabolism meltdown can lead to a creeping weight gain of 1 to 2 pounds per year.

More and more research is pointing to how important strength training is for middle-age and older men. One of the most recent studies, in the *Scandinavian Journal of Medicine & Science in Sports*, analyzed 96 untrained men ages 40 to 67 who had been randomly assigned to one of four fitness programs: strength training, endurance training, both strength and endurance training, or no training program at all. After 21 weeks, only the strength-training-only group showed significant changes in strength and muscle fiber composition in the legs. While the group that did both strength and endurance training showed strength

The Genius of the 15-Minute Workout

gains, there was no significant change in their muscle fibers. The endurance-only group showed neither strength nor muscle improvement. The researchers say the results suggest that strength training is the most effective way to prevent age-related muscle atrophy.

4. Look Sharper in Your Clothes

Even if the scale doesn't take a wild downhill ride, that lean muscle tissue minus the fat will let you tuck in your shirt with ease (and pride). How's that? Because 1 pound of fat takes up 20 percent more space on your body than 1 pound of muscle. Strength training—just 15 minutes a shot—is all it takes to keep your youthful muscle (and waistline) for life.

5. Sleep Better

High-intensity exercise helps you sleep like a baby, which in turn helps you lose weight. Australian researchers recently reported that exercisers who did total-body strength training for 8 weeks enjoyed a 23 percent improvement in their sleep quality. Even better, they were able to fall asleep faster and sleep longer than they had before they started exercising. That's important because poor sleep wrecks your waistline.
In fact, Stanford University scientists have found that body weight rises proportionately as hours of sleep drop below 7½ a night, likely because sleep deprivation triggers the release of the hunger hormone ghrelin and the fat-storage hormone cortisol.

6. Strengthen Your Bones

Resistance training is second to none for building bones. Though men don't lose bone at the rapid rate women do, they're still not immune from the ravaging effects of osteoporosis in their old age. That's why you need to make all the deposits to the bone bank you can while you can. A study of 124 men and women published in the journal *Osteoporosis* recently reported that high-intensity exercise like that found in our Superfast Workouts increased bone density in high-risk spots like the spine, hips, and legs in just 40 weeks. By contrast, those doing low-intensity exercise actually lost bone mineral density over the same time.

7. Be More Flexible

Flexibility is the first thing to go, because your muscles shorten over time. Left unchecked, you can lose a full 50 percent of your flexibility over adulthood, which means waving a long-distance goodbye to your toes…from your knees. Using those muscles through a full range of motion, like you will in these 15-minute workouts, will keep all your limbs limber. In a study published in the *International Journal of Sports Medicine*, scientists reported that men and women doing just three full-body workouts a week for 16 weeks increased the range of motion in their hips and shoulders and also improved their sit and reach test scores by 11 percent. You'll find specific stretching and strengthening workouts in this book for even greater flexible benefits.

8. Prevent Heart Attacks

Regular resistance training strengthens your most important muscle—the heart—and improves the health of your entire cardiovascular system. In a study published in the *Journal of Applied Physiology*, scientists reported that volunteers who strength trained just 3 days a week for 8 weeks lowered their systolic blood pressure (the top number) by an average of 9 points and their diastolic blood pressure (the bottom number) by an average of 8 points. That's enough to slash your risk of stroke by 40 percent and bring down your risk of heart attack by 15 percent.

9. Make Your Job Less of a Pain

It doesn't take long to make a difference in how you feel and perform at work. Just about 2 minutes. In a study presented at the World Congress on Exercise Is Medicine, 198 office workers were asked to do a single 2-minute stretching exercise, 12 minutes of exercise per day, or no exercise at all. It turned out that those who did the 2-minute exercise (a lateral arm raise using elastic tubing) reduced neck and shoulder pain just as much as the group that exercised for six times as long.

10. Avoid Diabetes

Muscle is simply good medicine. A 2003 study from the University of Sydney, in Australia, reported that resistance training could improve insulin sensitivity, which means fewer blood sugar spikes and crashes as well as fewer of the binge-eating episodes that low blood sugar can trigger. Similar research from the University of Massachusetts showed that men who added two total-body weight workouts a week to their existing aerobic exercise program had insulin levels 25 percent lower after a high-carboyhdrate meal than did men who did only aerobics.

Research also shows that resistance training is particularly good for burning visceral fat, the kind deep in your belly that smothers your internal organs and raises your risk for metabolic syndrome, also known as pre-diabetes. Even if you already have diabetes, it's not too late to benefit. Austrian scientists have found that men and women with type 2 diabetes who started strength training were able to significantly lower their blood sugar levels and improve their condition.

11. Prevent Cancer

Resistance training fends off cancer-causing free radicals, according to a study from the University of Florida. Researchers there found that people who did resistance-training workouts 3 days a week for 6 months had significantly less oxidative cell damage than their non-lifting peers. High-intensity exercise, like the kind found in our HIIT workouts, also has been shown to protect against breast cancer.

12. Think Faster

Canadian researchers found that after a year of just once-weekly strength training boosted brain power among volunteers

The Genius of the 15-Minute Workout

by nearly 13 percent. Other research has reported that strength training improves short- and long-term memory, verbal reasoning, and attention span. Now that's a mind-muscle connection!

13. Stress Out Less

Survival of the fittest is especially true when it comes to handling stress. Scientists at A&M University discovered that the fittest people have significantly lower levels of stress hormones than their couch-potato counterparts. Also, scientists at the Medical College of Georgia have found that blood pressure levels return to normal faster after a stressful situation in people with more lean muscle tissue compared to those with less.

14. Be Happier

Pushups and pullups may work as well as Paxil for improving your mood. Researchers from the University of Sydney recently reported that people who lifted weights on a regular basis were far less likely to suffer symptoms of major depression. Short bouts of cardio may be equally powerful. Scientists from Bowling Green State University reported that as little as 10 minutes of cycling improved the mood of 21 men and women, compared to a similar group who did nothing during that time.

15. Have More Time

That's the real reason you picked up this book, isn't it? You know that if you can get all the benefits of exercising for just a 15-minute time commitment, you are less likely to blow off a workout. You'll be more likely to stick with an exercise program for life—because you'll have so much more time to spend living!

Start Now!

So if the 15-minute secret is so great, why aren't more people using it? Because they don't know how to make it work for them. But, armed with these new findings, we've set our minds to creating the most comprehensive guide possible to unleash the magic of the 15-minute secret. And even we were amazed by how the Superfast Workout Plan can be adapted to every kind of exercise to meet every conceivable workout goal.

The Superfast Workouts are the most versatile you'll find. You don't even need to step foot in a gym (unless you want to). You'll find dozens of workouts you can do right in your living room. You can swim, bike, jump rope, elliptical train, and even power walk for your HIIT workouts. You'll even find Superfast Workouts to help you perform better on the tennis court or in road races, if that happens to be your weekend passion. Following the schedule that we provide on page 19, you'll choose three Superfast Resistance-Training Workouts and one HIIT workout each week. You'll find at least two versions of most strength-training workouts because it's important to switch up your exercises as often as possible to keep your results coming. "Your body adapts to meet the specific challenges you place on it," says strength-training researcher Wayne

Phillips, PhD, founding partner in the STRIVE Wellness Corporation. "If you constantly challenge it in different ways, it will continue adapting and you'll be less likely to hit a plateau. You're also less likely to become bored with your workouts." That's why we built more than 80 different 15-minute workouts into this book for you, to surprise your muscles with new and different challenges.

Which workouts should you choose? If you're looking for a major makeover, you probably want to start with the total-body workouts, which you do 3 times a week for 3 or 4 weeks. If you're looking to work on a specific part of your body, there's a wide array to choose from and you can alternate between them, choosing say, the Six-Pack Abs Workout and the Deltoid Definer Workout during the week. The HIIT workout you choose depends on what kind of cardio you like to do. Just page through Chapter 10, so you can plan which ones you want to do ahead of time.

Suffer from tight hamstrings, back pain, or job stress? Whatever your special needs, you'll find specialty workouts that will address your most common body (mental or physical) woes. On the 2 open days when you're not doing a resistance-training workout, you can select one of these.

There you have it. It takes almost no time. You can do it anywhere with your favorite equipment or none at all. No more excuses standing between you and your best body ever. Flip the page and let's get started.

◼

Chapter 2:
All of Your
15-Minute-Workout
Questions Answered

Everything You Need to Know to Get the Most Out of the
Superfast Workouts in This Book.

When people

first hear about the 15-minute secret, they have questions. Lots of questions. You're kidding, right? How does it work? How much should I lift? How hard should I go? What equipment do I need?

In many ways, the same rules apply that you'd use for longer workouts. But there are some specific guidelines that will help you reap maximum rewards from your short workouts. That's why this chapter provides the 411—the short-workout basic principles and philosophies and the answers to all of your questions. We want you armed with all the info you need to feel prepared in the gym, at home, anywhere you exercise. If your buddies say, "Fifteen minutes? Baloney!" You can just smile, finish your workout, and enjoy all that free time you have left in your day.

All of Your 15-Minute-Workout Questions Answered

Fifteen minutes is half the standard recommendation of 30 minutes a day. How can it work?

Great question. Because it's actually not half the standard recommendation. In fact, these 15 minutes exceed the standard exercise recommendation. It's true. What most people don't realize is that the 30 minutes a day the Centers for Disease Control and Prevention (CDC) recommends is for moderate exercise, such as brisk walking or washing your car. If you do moderate exercise only, you need to do 150 minutes a week, or about 30 minutes a day, 5 days a week to get benefits. But if you work out more vigorously, using the 15-minute secret, those official exercise recommendations are slashed in half to 75 minutes a week, or about 10 to 15 minutes a day. And in the end, those faster workouts work better. Remember: In a study by Australian researchers, exercisers who did 20-minute workouts that included high-intensity sprints 3 days a week shed fat pounds while their peers who did 40 minutes of cardio actually gained weight.

Do I need to use a stopwatch?

No. To make the program easy, we've designed every workout to take 15 minutes or less. Now, if you take longer rest periods, your workout may extend a few minutes longer, but our goal in this book is to give you the most effective and efficient workout possible in just 15 minutes. On days when you have more time, go ahead and do two or more circuits or double up on the workouts. That's cool, too. But you don't have to do that, and, in fact, trying to overreach might derail your progress altogether. A study in the *International Journal of Sports Medicine* found that people had a much better chance of sticking with an exercise routine if it was limited to just 15 minutes.

What should I eat before a workout?

You don't need to have any special foods before your superfast workouts. In fact, because the workouts can be intense, especially the HIIT routines, it's best not to have a belly full of food. If it's been more than 3 hours since you've eaten, you might want to have a small snack, like half a banana or a handful of trail mix, just to raise your blood sugar and give you an energy boost 30 to 45 minutes before you plan on exercising.

How quickly will I see results?

Depending on which workouts you do, anywhere from 2 to 4 weeks. Since men tend to carry less weight in their lower bodies, if you do our workouts that emphasize lifts for the legs, you'll start to see new muscle in as little as 2 weeks.

How much weight should I lift?

The short answer: enough to feel heavy. This is especially important if you're new to weights. Studies show that novice lifters tend to err on the too-light side when they strength train. In a study where novice weight lifters were allowed to select the weight of their choice for their exercise session, not a single volunteer chose one that was heavy enough to stimulate muscle growth. So, when you're starting out, choose a weight that feels heavy and makes you work. Use it to master proper technique for the exercise. Once you've got that down, there's a better way to figure out the proper weight that will lead to strength and muscle gains: Choose the heaviest weight that allows you to complete all of the prescribed repetitions with good form. Good form means no cheating, no using momentum to help you lift the weight. It'll take a little experimentation to find your weight. Let's take as an example a barbell bench press. You probably have a good idea of the weight you can bang out 10 reps with. Add 10 or 20 pounds more to the barbell and solicit the help of a spotter. The weight is appropriate if you can do 8 or 9 reps with perfect form, but on the 9th or 10th rep, you start to struggle or push it up more slowly. If you struggle earlier in the set or lose form by arching your back, the weight is too heavy. Take some weight off the bar until you find your ideal 10-rep weight. Then adjust accordingly for each particular exercise's prescribed repetitions.

How many times do I do each exercise?

Each workout description includes a "start here" paragraph that explains how to do the program, either as straight sets or in circuit fashion. (Most of the workouts are designed as efficient circuits. More on that later.) And the step-by-step instructions for each exercise tell you how many repetitions to do.

Do I need to lift superslow?

Nope. In fact, you'll make greater gains if you speed things up a bit and lift a little faster. "By picking up the pace, you recruit more of your unused fast-twitch muscle fibers, which take a lot of energy to move," explains resistance-training researcher Scott Mazzetti, PhD, of Salisbury University in Salisbury, Maryland. Mazzetti and his co-workers found that when volunteers performed springy, split-second reps during their strength-training sessions, they recruited more muscle and increased their calorie burn by about 28 percent—that adds up to 72 extra calories, or the amount you'd burn walking a mile, over the course of a full-body workout. Ramping up your repetition rate also revs up your metabolism by as much as 5 percent for hours afterward.

Do I stop between the exercises?

In general, no. Most of the superfast workouts are done circuit style, which means you do a series of exercises in succession without resting between exercises, before starting from the top and completing the circuit again. There's an important strategy behind this: Because you never let your heart rate come down between moves, you get a calorie-burning cardio workout as well as a muscle-firming strength challenge. Circuits are an extremely efficient way to exercise, which is why they make up the bulk of the workouts in this book. But don't worry, your body will also be getting rest, it's just active rest. Many of these workouts are ordered so the exercises alternate between upper- and lower-body exercises. So, for example you would do a squat followed by a chest press followed by a hip bridge followed by a dumbbell row and so forth, with little or no rest between them. That way your upper body gets a break while your lower body works.

Can I do all my superfast workouts on consecutive days or should I spread them out?

Spread them out. You'll be doing three resistance-training workouts per week. Those should be on alternate days, with a day of recovery between them. One day a week will be reserved for the HIIT workout of your choosing and 1 day is for complete rest.

Scientists at the University of Texas Medical Branch in Galveston have generated a tall body of research that confirms that every-other-day lifting works wonders. In short, they found that muscle protein synthesis, which is what happens as your muscles are being repaired, is elevated for 48 hours after a resistance-training bout. So if you hit the kettlebells Tuesday at 10 a.m., your body remains in muscle toning, elevated metabolism mode until 2 days later, when muscle synthesis returns to normal.

What about cardio? Shouldn't I be doing that four times a week to lose weight?

High-intensity interval training workouts are actually much better than traditional cardio for losing weight.

But the truth is, even on your superfast resistance-training days, you'll be raising your heart rate. We now know that weight training and the sprint-type training characteristic of HIIT strengthen your heart and lungs, lower blood pressure, control cholesterol, and shape up your cardiovascular system as well as, if not better than, classic aerobic exercise. So nearly any workout you choose in this book will count as cardio.

And don't worry, you'll still be burning plenty of fat, even though you're working well above the "fat burning" zone. Vigorous exercise may burn more stored carbs while you're doing it, but it burns far more fat in the long run. Hard efforts trigger the release of hormones like epinephrine, that stimulate fat release from your fat cells. "Your body also responds to hard efforts by building more mitochondria [cellular components that produce energy] and producing more fat-burning enzymes, so you become better at burning fat, not just glycogen [stored carbs] during exercise," says HIIT researcher Martin Gibala, PhD, professor of kinesiology at McMaster University.

Should I join a gym?

You can. But you don't need to. You can do many of the 15-minute workouts in your living room with minimal (sometimes no) equipment. And for a couple hundred bucks, you can put together the perfect home gym. But there's no question that belonging to a good gym opens up a world of workout possibilities that would likely not exist at home. There also are some people (I am one) who simply work out harder and longer and give just a bit more in a gym environment. Many men are also inspired by being surrounded by kindred spirits. Whether it's due to a sense of competition with other males or teamlike camaraderie, some men are motivated by exercise with others. One recent UK study found that exercising in a group can double the amount of endorphins your body releases compared with working out alone.

My advice: Start immediately. Do the workouts you can with what you've got and see how it goes. If you're happy, but don't feel like you have quite enough equipment to get the job done, check out "What Gear Do I Need" on pages 16 and 17 and gear up if you need to. If it really isn't working for you, it's time to check out the local fitness clubs.

Do I need a spotter?

Not often. Most of the workouts in this book involve bodyweight exercises or lightweight dumbbells that won't get you into trouble. However, anytime you are using heavier weights or lifting a barbell over your head or chest (think bench press), it's a good safety measure to ask a friend for a spot. Accidents happen.

How do I know if I'm working my muscles hard enough?

If you have the breath to ask, you may not be. Seriously, for strength workouts, use the guidelines under "How Much Weight Should I Lift?" The final repetition

or two should be very tough. You should need to work hard to complete it with proper form and not be able to easily do more. For your HIIT workouts, simply use the talk test, which measures how many words you can spit out while you're cranking out your efforts. Researchers have found it to be a very accurate way to judge exercise intensity without a heart rate monitor or other equipment. Those same researchers recommend using the Pledge of Allegiance as your guide. It works like this:

- **Low-intensity activity (warmup):** You should be able to comfortably say the entire pledge—all 31 words—breathing at the usual pauses.
- **Moderate aerobic activity:** While working at this level you should be able to easily recite four to six words of the pledge at a time. You shouldn't have to strain to get the words out of your mouth. You'll be working at this intensity during most of the resistance-training circuits.
- **High-intensity activity (intervals):** This is an all-out effort (what your should be making during the hardest parts of your HIIT workouts). When cranking it at this intensity, you should be able to speak only a word or two between breaths. (You'll know you're fully recovered from these efforts when you can say the whole pledge comfortably.)

If I work out after lunch, should I eat a recovery meal afterward?

You don't have to scarf something immediately, as you would if you had skipped the preworkout lunch. The idea

All of Your 15-Minute-Workout Questions Answered

that you need to eat a fast-acting recovery meal or shake as soon as possible after training is rooted in research on endurance athletes who were doing 2½-hour workouts. Your 15-minute superfast workout won't deplete your glycogen stores. Besides, you ate lunch, so your body isn't running on empty.

Should I stretch before I exercise?

It's not necessary to "stretch" per se, because when most people think of stretching they mean static stretching—the bend-over-and-touch-your-toes kind. But it is important to warm up your muscles at least briefly to prevent injury and improve performance. You can do that even without adding much time to a short 15-minute workout simply by running in place or cranking out 20 jumping jacks and some mountain climbers. Another great approach is dynamic or active stretching, which is simply doing moves that flex your muscles while you are actively moving. Try this routine recommended by Eric Cressey, CSCS, a Massachusetts-based trainer who works with professional and Olympic athletes. He calls it the Microwave because it can warm up your entire body in just 45 seconds. Do 6 reps on each side of your body.

1. Walking High-Knee Hug (*stretches your glutes and hip flexors*) Stand with your feet apart. Raise your left knee toward your chest, grasping it with both hands below the kneecap. Pull it to the middle of your chest as you stand tall. Release it and step into the offset lunge.

2. Offset Lunge (*stretches the groin and legs*) Step forward with your left leg toward about 11 o'clock. Slowly lower your body until your left thigh is parallel to the floor. (Your right knee should nearly touch the floor.) Keeping your lower back straight, bend forward and touch both hands to the floor just inside your left foot. You are now in position for dynamic stretch #3.

3. Overhead Reach (*targets the middle back and stretches the chest and activates the core*) Keeping your left hand on the floor, reach overhead with your right arm as you rotate your torso upward. Both arms should form a straight line. Bring your right hand back down to the floor so that you're in the offset lunge position again.

4. Hip Lift (*stretches your hamstrings*) Keeping your hands on the floor rock your hips back and straighten both legs. Step forward with your right leg and stand straight up.

Now repeat this sequence but use the opposite leg or arm for each move.

What gear do I need?

Many of the exercises are bodyweight moves. Others require fitness equipment. Here's a rundown of the gear required to do many of the superfast workouts in this book.

DUMBBELLS: Hand weights are a must have. Many of the superfast workouts use them. With a few sets of dumbbells, you can work every body part; they don't take up much space, and they're relatively cheap (about a dollar a pound, but shop around). What's more, dumbbells allow you to exercise through a greater range of motion than exercise machines do or even barbells, for that matter. For the best results, invest in three sets: light (2 pounds—for shoulder exercises—to 15 pounds), medium (20 to 35) and heavy (40 plus). Another good option is an "all in one" adjustable set like PowerBlocks, which takes up less space.

BENCH: Technically, you don't need a bench. You can use a stability ball, chair, or even the floor for many traditional bench moves. But a bench does make it easier to lift a heavier weight with proper form, so an exercise bench is worth the investment if you're going to be working out at home. Look for one that is adjustable, so you can perform exercises on both an incline and a decline. You can find adjustable benches at most sporting goods stores.

BARBELL AND WEIGHT PLATES: Go to the gym and you'll see the standard 7-foot Olympic barbell. It weighs in at about 45 pounds and is great for squats, lunges, deadlifts, and a variety of lower body exercises. You can buy shorter, lighter barbells for home use if you find you like them.

KETTLEBELL: These weighted balls with handles originated in Russia decades ago, but have recently been getting a lot of love here in the States. Because the kettlebell's weight is off-center (hanging beyond your hand), it makes traditional dumbbell moves more difficult because your body's stabilizing muscles must work overtime to control your movement. The handle also allows you to perform a variety of explosive and swinging movements. These exercises build strength and endurance in your back, legs, shoulders, and core. You'll find two kettlebell workouts starting on page 256. Like dumbbells, kettlebells come in a wide range of weights. Or you can invest in an adjustable set like the 20-pound Weider PowerBell. It comes with a 5-pound handle and adjustable 2.5-pound plates that allow you to have seven different weights in one bell.

MEDICINE BALL: I love medicine balls. With them, you can tone your abs and strengthen your core without doing a single crunch. They're also second to none for sports-specific training. You'll find a wide array of medicine balls in all sizes, weights, and materials at PerformBetter.com. For the biggest bang for your buck, look for one that is rubberized and bounces so you can toss it against the wall or floor. Check out pages 272 and 278 for full medicine ball workouts.

STABILITY BALL: Also known as a Swiss ball or a physioball, this large inflated exercise ball is the perfect addition to any home gym. As the name implies, stability balls are ideal for balance training, and they make great core-toning tools. In a study of 41 exercisers, researchers at Occidental College in Los Angeles found that muscle activity

33

Percentage of men who say that they have no time to get back in shape because of their jobs.

All of Your 15-Minute-Workout Questions Answered

spiked in the upper abs, lower abs, and obliques by 31 percent, 38 percent, and 24 percent, respectively, when crunches were performed on the ball instead of flat on the floor. You also can use one instead of a bench for chest presses and seated exercises. These days, you can buy stability balls in nearly every big-box store, such as Target and Wal-Mart, and even in some supermarkets. PerformBetter.com offers heavy-duty balls if you're looking for extra durability.

EXERCISE BAND: If you travel a lot, pick up a few exercise bands. They're feather light, dirt cheap (less than 20 bucks), and put a complete gym in your carry-on bag. In fact, few workout tools beat the efficiency of the multitasking resistance band. You can step on the middle and grab the ends for arm curls, hold the ends at your shoulders for squats, and choke up on the band and perform some upright rows without even changing position. You also can tie the ends together and use it as a large band to perform assorted hip, leg, and glute moves. Exercise bands come in a variety of thicknesses giving more or less resistance. A good brand is Thera-Band, which offers latex-free bands. Or try Superbands, extra-strong, long resistance bands for heavy-duty use. You can also buy a band utility strap that allows you to easily affix the band to doorjambs and poles.

FOAM ROLLER: You can't beat these pressed foam cylinders for a self-massage that will keep you in the game. Roll your achy body parts along one and say, "Ah." (You'll find a terrific 15-minute foam roller workout on page 344.) Either 6 by 18 inches or 6 by 36 inches is fine. Find them at sporting goods stores or order them online.

JUMP ROPE: Really, any jump rope will do. But for the best jumping experience, go with a beaded jump rope, which lays short pieces of plastic tubing along a thin rope. The beading adds heft to the rope, so the rope maintains a wide U-shape to jump through and makes it easier to maintain momentum.

BOSU BALANCE TRAINER: Half stability ball, half wobble board, the Bosu trainer, which looks like half of a stability ball on a platform, helps build strength and coordination. With the ball side up, you can do crunches, squats, even plyometric hops. Then flip it over and do pushups, or try standing on it for advanced balance work.

STEP OR BOX: A step, like the Reebok aerobic step, gives you a sturdy platform for stepups, elevated pushups, and plyometric jumping moves. For a higher, more rugged platform, you also can invest in an adjustable squat box (elitefts.com). It provides a stable, no-slip surface to lift from, and you can quickly raise and lower the height of this box for stepups, split squats, and any number of upper- and lower-body moves and jumps.

15

Percentage by which your endurance improves when you exercise to music, according to the *Journal of Sports & Exercise Psychology.*

How to Use This Book
Your guide to a leaner, fitter, stronger you—in half the time!

Pick three superfast resistance-training workouts a week: Choose from any of the 15-minute workouts in the book. Schedule them into your week so that your muscles have a day to rest and recover in between workouts. One option is the Monday-Wednesday-Friday schedule shown below. You can do the same workout on all 3 days (although you should start to mix them up after 3 weeks so it doesn't get too easy for your body) or you can do three different 15-minute workouts, one on each of those days. You can pick from total-body workouts and those that target specific muscle groups, workouts that prepare you for a particular sport, and workouts that help you prevent back pain. Note that if you have time-specific goals (such as a beach vacation or an upcoming class reunion), you should do one of our total-body workouts on all 3 days for fastest results. But once you've achieved that goal (and high school is once again ancient history), you can switch over to another workout. With this book, you can keep on personalizing workouts to meet your ever-changing fitness needs.

Rest and recover: The day after each hard workout should be spent either resting or doing a specialty, non-resistance-training 15-minute workout or a stretching workout of your own. Or you can just do some light cardio, such as a quick jog or bike ride. We recommend doing something light but it's optional, totally your call.

Pick one HIIT workout: Once a week, say on a Saturday, you will commit to doing one of our challenging HIIT workouts, your secret weapon for burning fat and losing weight.

Take off at least 1 day a week: That's it! Now you'll have tons of time to do everything else you love!

Sample Week on the 15-Minute Exercise Plan

Monday	Tuesday	Wednesday	Thursday	Friday	Saturday	Sunday
Your Body Is Your Barbell Workout	Rest, brisk walk, light cardio, or specialty workout (optional)	**The Classic Powerlifter**	Rest, stretch, light cardio, or other non-resistance workout (optional)	**The Sandbag Workout**	**Outdoor HIIT Workout**	Use all the time you saved for something completely indulgent!

Chapter 3:
The Superfast Weight-Loss System

Eating Healthy Doesn't Have to
Complicate Your Life—Or Slow You Down.

There are more

than 350 individual exercises packed between the covers of this book. But none of them is as important to maintaining your health, weight, and fitness as your diet. You're probably eager to get to sweating, so skip ahead if you like, but come back in 15 minutes and read this chapter because it's a simple fact that a good diet and regular exercise work better together than exercise does alone.

You can find dozens of studies to back up what makes logical sense: Diet and exercise pack a powerful health punch. Here's a study that says a lot: Several years ago, Pennsylvania State University researchers took a group of overweight people and split them into two groups. The people in one were told to eat whole grains as their only form of bread, pasta, and rice. The other group was told to avoid whole-grain products and to keep eating the refined grains they were used to. Both groups

The Superfast Weight-Loss System

were encouraged to do moderate exercise regularly. After 12 weeks, the exercisers who ate whole grains had lost a significantly larger percentage of belly fat than the exercisers who ate refined grains. With the exercise level the same among both groups, a healthier diet made all the difference. And not just for weight loss. The whole-grain group enjoyed an average 38 percent decrease in their levels of C-reactive protein, a warning signal of heart disease and diabetes, while the refined-grain group saw no change.

To power workouts and boost calorie burn, you need to eat purposefully, not mindlessly. That's why we developed the Superfast Weight-Loss System, a plan that is grounded in eating lean, healthy protein, which your body uses to form muscle, as well as special fat-burning foods to complement the workouts in this book. Whether you want to lose weight or not, this is a healthy nutrition plan that you can maintain for life.

Trim Carbs, Pump Protein

The Superfast Weight-Loss System is based on the scientific fact that when people diet, often much of the weight they lose comes from muscle instead of fat. So, how does one lose weight without losing the all-important calorie-burning muscle? The answer: reduce the intake of certain carbs, eat more protein, and do resistance training for exercise.

Study after study shows that for building lean muscle while burning off flab, you can't beat the power of protein.

In a study published in *Nutrition Metabolism*, dieters who increased their protein intake to 30 percent of their diet ate nearly 450 fewer calories a day and lost about 11 pounds over 12 weeks without employing any other dietary measures.

Strength training takes that protein and molds it into lean muscle. In a study of 48 volunteers at the University of Illinois, researchers showed that those who combined a resistance-training plan with a high-protein diet lost 22 pounds (and only 1 pound of muscle), while a group eating a high-carb diet that was identical in calorie count lost 15 pounds, 2 of which were muscle.

Other research shows how reducing carbohydrates can impact weight loss. A groundbreaking study by exercise scientists at the University of Connecticut placed overweight volunteers on a reduced-carbohydrate diet like the one in this book and a 3-day-a-week weight-lifting program. The group shed 22 pounds, nearly 2 pounds a week during the study, and here's the best part: It was almost exclusively (97 percent) from fat.

Just as the workouts in this book are designed to be quick and efficient, so too is the Superfast Weight-Loss System. And by that, we don't just mean fast results, but also that it takes little time and effort to follow. Chapter 11 has recipes for delicious meals you can make in 15 minutes or less, guidelines for a kitchen makeover, and a list of the best foods for burning fat. But first, let's tweak some of the eating habits that may be keeping you from achieving the body you want.

37

Percentage of an average 20- to 49-year-old man's daily sugar intake that comes from snacks.

Everything You Need to Know About the Superfast Weight-Loss System

HOW TO BUY THE BEST BREAD

Check the ingredient list:

- Is the first ingredient a whole grain?
- Does each slice have 2 or more grams of fiber?
- Do "inulin" or "poly-dextrose" show up?

The first two answers should be yes, the third, no. With whole grain, no nutrients are stripped away. That means you're eating natural fiber, not inulin or poly-dextrose, two additives used to artificially boost fiber.

With the Superfast Weight-Loss System, you eat more, not less, but what you eat will trigger your body to burn stored fat. At the same time, you'll enjoy more protein from sources like eggs, cheese, beef, poultry, and fish and savor a fair share of delicious natural fats. Research shows that this helps people better control blood sugar, hunger, and cravings. The end result: You'll lose weight faster and more easily than ever. And you won't feel deprived, which is what derails most dieters' efforts.

What to Eat

This plan is incredibly simple: Eat any combination of the foods from three categories: high-quality proteins, low-starch vegetables, and natural fats (see the table on page 27). Snack on nuts and seeds or low-calorie fruits. Drink lots of water. Eat this way until you feel satisfied—who has time to count calories?—and you'll automatically burn off fat. Fast workouts, fast weight loss, fast results. That's what this book is all about: speed.

The Guidelines

Put high-quality protein on your plate.
Do this at every single meal. Protein helps you incinerate pounds on nearly every weight-loss front. For one, just eating it burns energy. About 25 percent of the protein calories in your food are burned off in digestion, absorption, and chemical changes in your body caused by digestion, so protein has less of a caloric impact than most foods. And protein is nature's appetite suppressant because it takes longer to digest than most carbs do. As mentioned earlier, protein also preserves your hard-earned, metabolism-revving muscle tissue while you're losing fat. A recent study in *Medicine and Science in Sports and Exercise* found that a weight-loss diet with 35 percent of its calories from protein preserved muscle mass in

The Superfast Weight-Loss System

STOP SPEED EATING

People who eat rapidly until they are full are 3 times more likely to be overweight than slow eaters, according to a Japanese study of 3,000 adults.

athletes, while a diet with just 15 percent protein led to an average loss of 3½ pounds of muscle in just 2 weeks.

It's particularly important to start the day with a protein-packed morning meal. A Purdue University study found that eating lean protein (such as Canadian bacon, egg whites, or low-fat yogurt) at breakfast keeps you satisfied for longer than it would if you were to consume it at other times of the day. Protein sticks with you, so you won't be tempted by the box of doughnuts someone left by the coffee maker. "Try to get at least 1 ounce (30 grams) of protein at breakfast," recommends Joan Salge Blake, RD, a clinical associate professor of nutrition at Boston University. Remember, eating protein stimulates muscle growth. In fact, every time you eat at least 10 to 15 grams of protein, you trigger a burst of protein synthesis, which means your body is repairing and building muscle (it also means a greater calorie burn because of all this metabolic activity). And when you eat at least 30 grams, that period of synthesis lasts for about 3 hours—and that means even more muscle growth all day long.

Embrace a little fat. Years back, during the low-fat craze, we all tried to trim every ounce of fat from our diets. And what happened? We all got fatter. Now we understand that dietary fat plays a critical role in calorie control and fat metabolism. Oleic acid, an unsaturated fat found in olive oil, nuts, and avocados, helps quash hunger, according to a study

in the journal *Cell Metabolism*. During digestion, it's converted into a compound that indirectly triggers hunger-curbing signals to your brain. Omega-3 fatty acids found in naturally fatty foods like salmon and avocados also helps reduce body fat, lower triglycerides (a blood fat), and raise healthy HDL cholesterol. Just keep portions in check by eating fat in balance with the other elements of the Superfast Weight-Loss System. As long as pounds are peeling off, your fat intake should be fine.

Set limits on starch. Since 1980, the amount of food we eat has grown by up to 500 calories a day, nearly 80 percent of which can be attributed to carbohydrates; in that time, the prevalence of obesity has increased by 80 percent. Coincidence? I don't think so. The lesson: Cap your intake of the most carbohydrate-dense foods such as white breads, pasta, and rice, candy, baked goods, and potatoes. Think of starch as sugar in disguise. (One of my favorite descriptions of spaghetti: "Sugar on a string.") In fact, starch is nothing more than neatly packaged bundles of glucose, the basic building block of sugar stuck together by chemical bonds. These bonds start to dissolve the moment they make contact with the saliva in your mouth, immediately freeing the glucose to surge into your bloodstream. As a result, starch has an even greater impact on blood sugar than sucrose. It also encourages your body to store fat. When you do eat starch, try to choose whole grains or a small sweet potato, which at least contain some fiber to slow the down the blood-sugar surge. Or even better, try quinoa, a protein-packed grain with more fiber and fewer carbs than most. Limit yourself to two servings of starch a day.

Pile on the produce. These filling, good-for-you foods are your ticket to sticking with it. And they cannot be overdone. When researchers at the State University of New York Downstate Medical Center in New York City surveyed more than 2,000 low-carb dieters, they discovered that, on average, those who lost the most weight ate at least four servings of low-starch vegetables every day. That's likely because these foods are brimming with filling fiber (and water) that leaves you feeling full and satisfied on very few calories. And, of course, vegetables are loaded with essential vitamins and minerals that combat disease. Fruits have those nutrients, too, but keep your fruit intake a bit more in check. While low-cal-orie, high-nutrient fruits like berries and melons are encouraged in our superfast plan, bananas and other commonly consumed fruits like pineapples, oranges, grapes, and pears are not recommended because of their high fructose content.

Snack on nuts, seeds, and low-calorie fruits. Add nuts to your daily diet, but don't shovel fistfuls mindlessly—a serving of nuts should total 1 ounce, which is about 35 peanuts, 24 almonds, or 18 cashews. Limit yourself to two servings a day. A serving of low-calorie fruit is a ½ cup. You can also help yourself to a fruity protein shake when midafternoon hunger hits or after a workout.

Avoid liquid calories. Sugary soft drinks (including fruit juices) account for 1 in every 10 calories Americans consume. By making water and unsweetened tea your go-to beverages, you will take an enormous shortcut to weight loss and maintenance.

148

Average number of calories in 12 ounces of cola.

THE 15 BEST FAT-BURNING FOODS

These are foods that start winnowing your waistline the moment they enter your mouth by building muscle, promoting fat burning, or simply using energy (i.e., burn calories) just to digest them! Stock up today.

Almonds and other nuts (with skins)
Build muscle, reduce cravings

Dairy products (fat-free or low-fat milk, yogurt, cheese)
Build strong bones, fire up weight loss

Eggs
Build muscle, burn fat

Turkey and other lean meats
Build muscle, strengthen immune system

Berries
Improve satiety, prevent cravings

Enova oil (soy and canola oil)
Promotes fullness, not easily stored as fat

Continued on page 26

The Superfast Weight-Loss System

Peanut butter
Boosts testosterone, burns fat, builds muscle

Fatty fish (such as salmon, tuna, mackerel)
Trigger satiety, fire up fat burning

Grapefruit
Lowers insulin, regulates blood sugar and metabolism; be sure to eat the fleshy white membranes

Green tea
Fires up fat burning

Chili peppers
Spike metabolism

Spinach and leafy green vegetables
Fight free radicals and improve recovery for better muscle building

Whole grains (quinoa, brown rice, whole-grain cereal)
Small doses prevent body from storing fat

Beans and legumes
Build muscle, help burn fat, regulate digestion

Whey
Builds muscle, burns fat

Meal-by-Meal Guidelines

Remember, healthy eating needs to be easy and quick, otherwise you'll give up and run to the nearest drive-thru. So don't complicate it. Build your meals around protein and vegetables and you're good to go (and lose!). Here's a look at what 24 hours of Superfast Weight-Loss eating might look like.

MORNING: Crack those eggs. No matter how you scramble or serve them, they're a perfect part of the morning meal. Add some cheese, toss in sliced peppers and tomatoes, and add a serving of meat like lean sausage or Canadian bacon.

MIDMORNING: A handful of nuts, low-fat yogurt, a protein shake, or some string cheese and berries will keep you moving through any morning lull.

NOONISH: Lunch should be a big, meaty salad. Mix up greens and vegetables with tuna, chicken, or beef. For a change, you might have a burger with no bun, some egg salad or tuna wrapped in Romaine leaves, or simply the leftovers from last night's dinner.

MIDAFTERNOON: Pump up the protein to shake the sleepy 3 p.m. dip. A whey-protein smoothie or nut butter on celery will do the trick.

EVENING: Dinner is easy. Just pair your favorite meat with a heaping serving of recommended vegetables and you're on the program. Don't limit yourself to chicken and broccoli (though they're a stellar combination) every night or you'll get bored fast. Try roasting cauliflower and brussels sprouts in olive oil and garlic for a savory side dish. Grill asparagus and a skirt steak. Use your imagination and watch the pounds peel away.

For more ideas, check out the recipes in Chapter 11.

What to Drink

Fill your cup with beverages that have 5 calories or fewer per serving. Water is a no-brainer, but a bit boring. Stock up on herbal teas, pick up some Crystal Light, go ahead and enjoy your coffee (just skip the sugar). Diet soda is okay on rare occasions, but opt for healthier beverages whenever possible.

As for alcohol, cut it out entirely for the fastest weight-loss results. (Alcohol causes your body to store calories as fat.) Can't say adios to cerveza? Then close the bar after one or two beers (or cocktails or glasses of wine) per day. And avoid those mixers at all costs. Juices, sodas, and sugary blended drink mixes (like margarita mix) make the calories add up fast.

HIGH-QUALITY PROTEINS	LOW-STARCH VEGETABLES*		NATURAL FATS
Beef	Artichokes	Leafy greens	Avocados
Cheese	Asparagus	Mushrooms	Butter
Eggs	Bok choy	Onions	Coconut
Fish	Broccoli	Peppers	Cream
Pork	Brussels sprouts	Radishes	Nuts and seeds
Poultry	Carrots	Spinach	Olives, olive oil, and canola oil
Soy	Cauliflower	Tomatoes	
Whey and casein protein powder	Celery	Turnips	Full-fat salad dressings
	Cucumbers	Zucchini	

Any vegetables besides potatoes, peas, and corn are fair game.

How to Make It Work

If this way of eating is completely new, you might encounter a few bumps at first. Here's a troubleshooting guide for common glitches.

Gut troubles. Introduce the high-fiber veggies a bit at a time, so your body can make the enzymes it needs to digest them. If you suspect you're not getting enough fiber because you're eating fewer grains, try taking a fiber supplement.

Mood swings. When you change the way you eat, your body sometimes protests by making you grouchy or tired. This should only last a couple of days. If it lingers a week, be sure you're taking in enough fluids to stay hydrated. And by all means, eat enough fat. This diet is designed to make you a better fat burner, so you absolutely need to eat this important source of fuel.

Stuck scale. If the weight isn't coming off, do a quick calorie check. Maybe you're somehow consuming too many. Multiply your target body weight by 12. That's roughly how many calories you should aim for each day. Count them out for a few days so you know what that amount of food looks like. Many of us don't have a sense of proper portions.

AVOID THE SUGAR SPIKERS

Foods high in starch and sugars spike your blood sugar too quickly and cause a crash, slowing down your superfast route to a new body. Some common culprits to avoid (or in the case of fruit, simply limit):

Bananas

Biscuits

Candy

Chips

Cookies

Doughnuts

Grapes

Ice cream

Pasta (refined)

Rice (white)

Soda

Sweet tea

Fruit juices

White bread

Chapter 4:
15-Minute Total-Body Workouts

The Easiest Way to Build Calorie-Burning Muscle
and Lose Weight in Record Time.

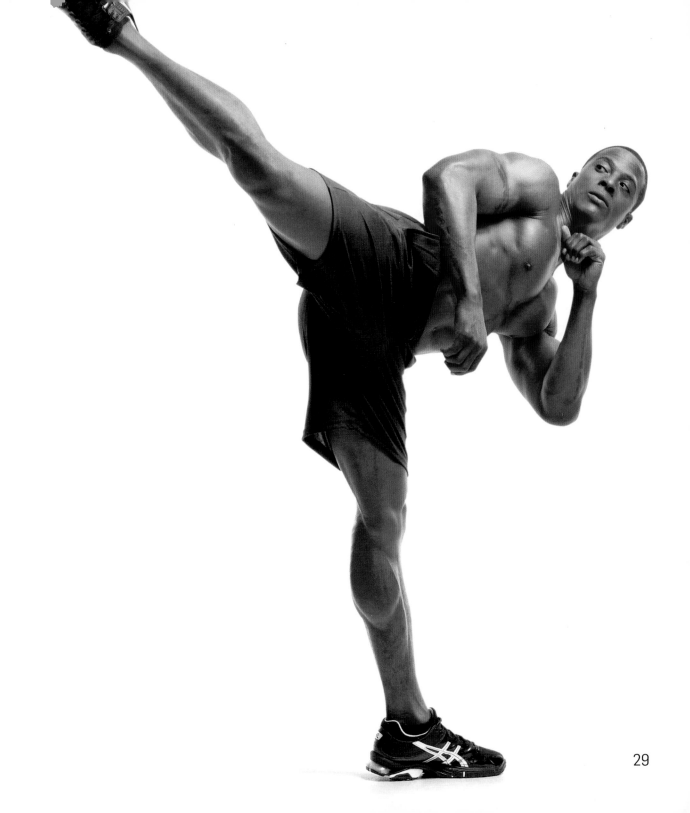

Superfast Total-Body Workouts

No more excuses. Anyone can carve out 15 minutes 4 days a week for something so important to their health and the way their body looks and feels. We're starting the meat of this book—the workouts—with a package of head-to-toe circuits that'll work for anyone—beginner to advanced. Each includes a mix of high-energy, challenging exercises that put your muscles to the test at every angle and velocity, guaranteeing that no muscle fiber is left untapped.

As a bonus (because we know that your body also includes your brain), we've also included mind-body workouts, like the 15-minute stress-busting workout, in here, too. It's a perfect complement to the resistance-training workouts and can be done anytime you want to blast stress and improve flexibility.

Begin with bodyweight . . .

If you're just getting back into training, we recommend you begin with our bodyweight-only workouts. Why? Well, they don't require any equipment so you can start immediately. And they are designed to stretch and strengthen key muscles throughout your body to bring them up to speed for the more advanced workouts later in this chapter and the more specialized ones found later in the book. That doesn't mean they are easy. These no-gym, no-equipment programs are some of the toughest, most effective workouts you can do, which is why they form the backbone of *Men's Health*'s popular *Belly Off! Diet* book and online programs. Work through these beginner, intermediate, and advanced calisthenics workouts and you'll have the strength and aerobic stamina to tackle the dumbbell and powerlifting workouts later on.

Find It Quick: Your 15-Minute Total-Body Circuit Plan

HOW TO DO A CIRCUIT

Circuits are fast and efficient workouts that combine the heart rate-elevating benefit of aerobics and the muscle building of resistance training. In a circuit, you do one set of each exercise, resting only briefly—10 to 30 seconds if at all—before moving to the next. Only after completing the list of exercises do you go back and repeat the exercises. Rest for 1 to 3 minutes between circuits.

Strength and Agility Workout/Beginner

Four moves. That's all it takes to fire up your fat burning and build lean, metabolism-charging muscle—that is, if it's done with enough intensity and perfect form. As mentioned in Chapter 1, you can lose 4 pounds of fat and add 2 pounds of muscle in just 8 weeks with a basic total-body routine. (Some guys will see even faster results!) This high-intensity interval routine, designed by Robert dos Remedios, CSCS, strength and conditioning coach at the College of the Canyons, in California, is a perfect get-back-in-shape workout for beginners.

START HERE: Perform each move for 30 seconds, take a quick rest break for up to 30 seconds, and then continue to the next exercise. Repeat the circuit as many times as you can until 15 minutes are up.

Judo Pushup

WORKS your chest, arms, back, and core.

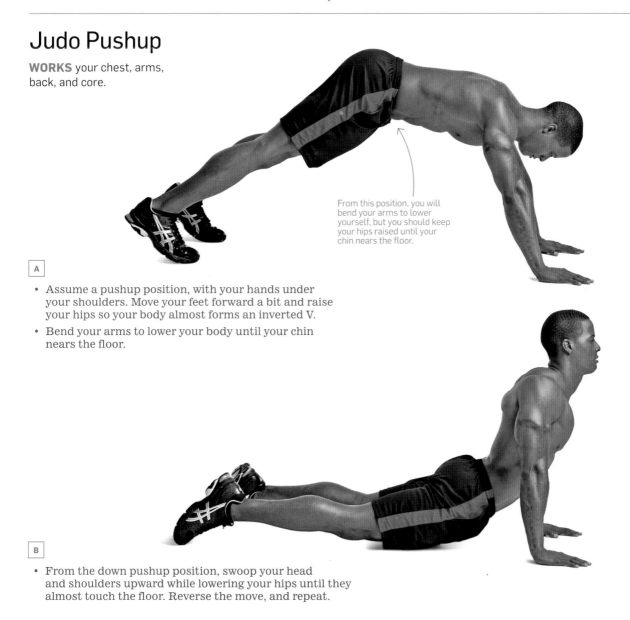

From this position, you will bend your arms to lower yourself, but you should keep your hips raised until your chin nears the floor.

A

- Assume a pushup position, with your hands under your shoulders. Move your feet forward a bit and raise your hips so your body almost forms an inverted V.
- Bend your arms to lower your body until your chin nears the floor.

B

- From the down pushup position, swoop your head and shoulders upward while lowering your hips until they almost touch the floor. Reverse the move, and repeat.

REPS: Do as many as you can in 30 seconds.

Strength and Agility Workout/Beginner

Seesaw Lunge

WORKS your quadriceps, glutes, hamstrings, and calves.

A

- Stand with your feet hip-width apart, hands on your hips.

B

- Step forward with your right leg into a lunge, and lower yourself until your left leg is bent 90 degrees and nearly touches the floor.

C

- In one motion, rock backward by straightening and lifting your right leg and stepping back with it into a reverse lunge.
- Now your left leg will be forward and your right leg will be bent 90 degrees and nearly touching the floor.
- Keep shifting between forward and back lunges with the same leg.
- Repeat the exercise, this time lunging forward and back with the left leg.

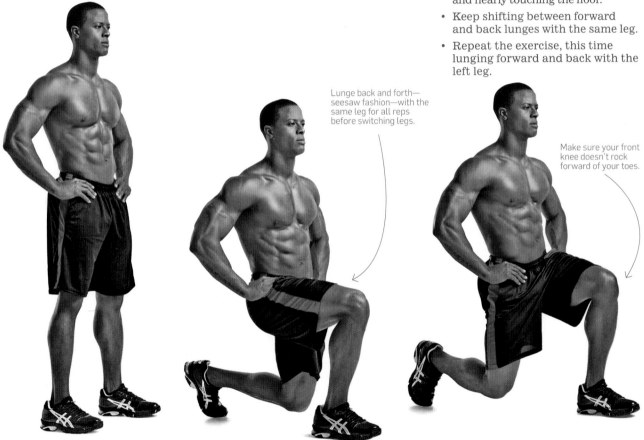

Lunge back and forth—seesaw fashion—with the same leg for all reps before switching legs.

Make sure your front knee doesn't rock forward of your toes.

REPS: Do as many as you can in 30 seconds with the right leg, then repeat with the left for 30 seconds.

Wall Slide

WORKS your lats, trapezius, and rear deltoids.

- Stand with your butt, upper back, and head against a wall. Raise your arms straight above your head, making sure your shoulders, elbows, and wrists also touch the wall.

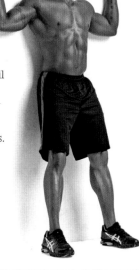

The halfway point; try to bend your arms until elbows are tucked at your sides.

B

- Maintaining these points of contact, bend your arms until your elbows are tucked in at your sides. You should feel a contraction in your shoulders and the muscles between your shoulder blades.
- Reverse the move.

REPS: Slowly, do as many as you can in 30 seconds.

Plank Reach

WORKS all of your abdominal muscles that support the spine.

TRAINER'S TIP: *This move can be difficult. Build up to it with staggered pushups: Place one hand a foot forward of the other.*

Try to straighten your arm completely.

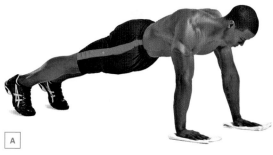

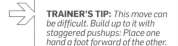

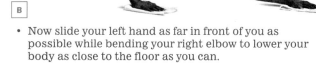

A

- Start in a pushup position on a smooth surface. Place your hands on small towels, Valslides, Core Sliders, or paper plates positioned on the floor directly under your shoulders.

REPS: Do as many as you can in 30 seconds, alternating arms.

B

- Now slide your left hand as far in front of you as possible while bending your right elbow to lower your body as close to the floor as you can.
- Slide your left hand back to the starting position as you push up with your right arm.
- Repeat, this time sliding your right hand forward and bending your left arm.

Your Body Is Your Barbell 1/Intermediate

Again, no gym or gear needed here. The next two workouts use athletic multi-muscle moves to raise your heart rate, so you incinerate fat while building muscle. As a bonus, they strengthen the core and hone your balance to resist injury wherever you play hard. Alternate workouts 1 and 2, leaving a day of rest in between.

START HERE:
Alternate between the Y Squat and the Spider-Man Pushup for three sets of each. Perform the remaining three exercises as a circuit (without rest). When finished with the Spider-Man Lunge, return to the Squat and Jump Combo and complete the three-exercise circuit twice more.

Y Squat

WORKS your quads, glutes, and hamstrings.

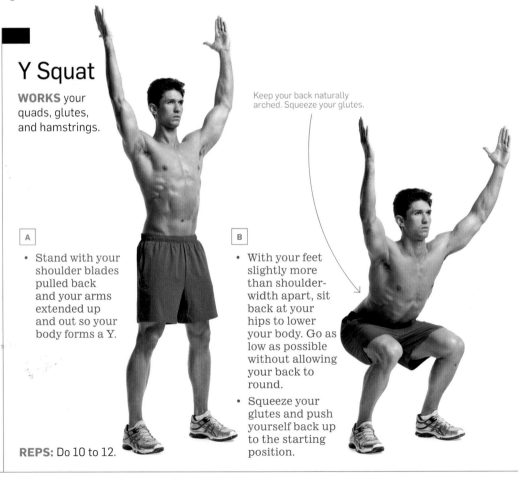

Keep your back naturally arched. Squeeze your glutes.

A
- Stand with your shoulder blades pulled back and your arms extended up and out so your body forms a Y.

B
- With your feet slightly more than shoulder-width apart, sit back at your hips to lower your body. Go as low as possible without allowing your back to round.
- Squeeze your glutes and push yourself back up to the starting position.

REPS: Do 10 to 12.

Spider-Man Pushup

WORKS your chest, arms, and core.

A

- Assume the classic pushup position with your legs straight and your abs tight.

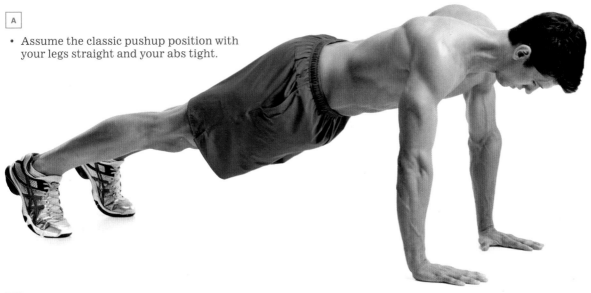

B

- As you lower your body, bend your right leg and rotate your right knee outward until it's outside your right elbow. Don't drag your foot, and try not to allow your torso to rotate.

- As you press yourself up, return the leg to the starting position and repeat, pulling your left knee to your left elbow. That's 1 rep.

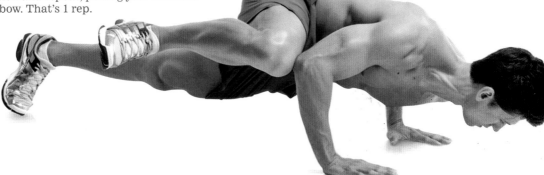

REPS: Do 5 to 6.

Your Body Is Your Barbell 1/Intermediate

Squat and Jump Combo

WORKS the fast-twitch muscle fibers in your legs.

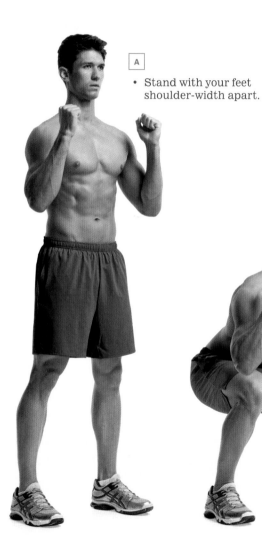

- Stand with your feet shoulder-width apart.

- Lower your body as far as you can by pushing your hips back and bending your knees.
- Pause, and then stand.

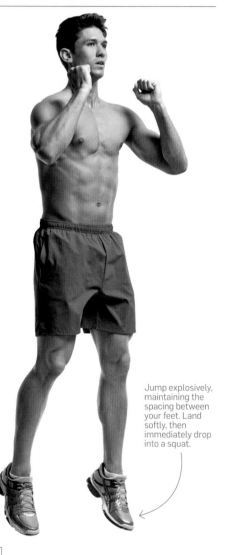

Jump explosively, maintaining the spacing between your feet. Land softly, then immediately drop into a squat.

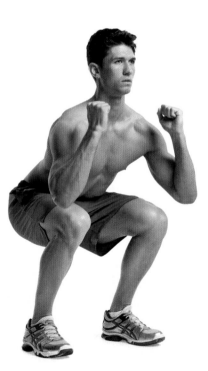

C

- Squat again, but after this one, jump as high as you can. That's 1 rep.
- Upon landing, perform a normal squat. Keep alternating between squats and jumps.

REPS: Do 8 to 10.

Single-Leg Romanian Deadlift

WORKS your lower back, core, and glutes.

A

- Stand on your left foot with your right foot raised behind you, arms hanging down in front of you.

B

- Keeping a natural arch in your spine, push your hips back and lower your hands and upper body toward the floor.
- Squeeze your glutes and press your heel into the floor to return to an upright position.
- Do all reps then repeat the exercise while standing on your right foot.

REPS: Do 8 to 10 per leg.

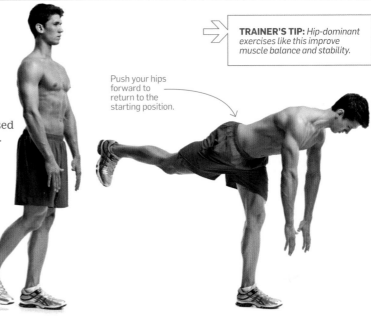

TRAINER'S TIP: *Hip-dominant exercises like this improve muscle balance and stability.*

Push your hips forward to return to the starting position.

Spider-Man Lunge

WORKS your chest, core, and legs.

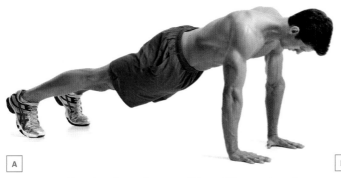

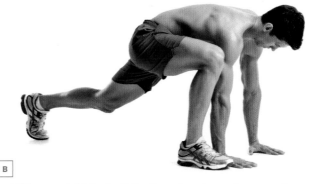

A

- Assume the classic pushup position with your hands directly beneath your shoulders, your legs straight, and your abs braced.

REPS: Do 8 to 10.

B

- Lift your right foot off the floor, bend your knee, and place the foot outside your right hand.
- Return to the starting position and lunge forward with your left leg toward your left hand. That's 1 rep.

39

Your Body Is Your Barbell 2/Intermediate

START HERE:
Alternate between the Bodyweight Squat and the Tucked-Elbow Push-up for three sets of each. Then perform the remaining three exercises consecutively as a circuit (again, without rest). Do three complete circuits of those three exercises.

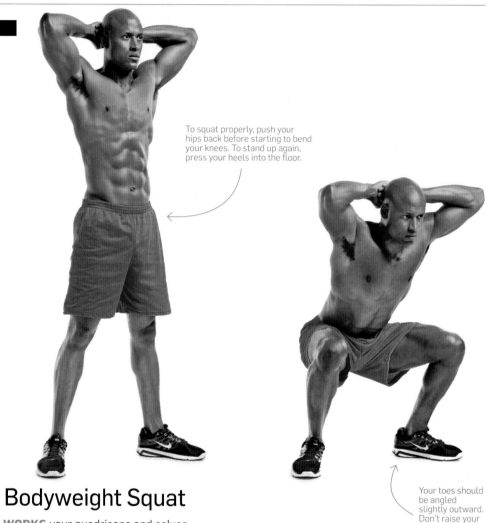

To squat properly, push your hips back before starting to bend your knees. To stand up again, press your heels into the floor.

Your toes should be angled slightly outward. Don't raise your heels as you drop into a squat.

Bodyweight Squat

WORKS your quadriceps and calves.

A

- Stand with your hands behind your head, chest out, and elbows back.

REPS: Do 10 to 12.

B

- Sit back at your hips and bend your knees to lower your body as far as you can without losing the natural arch of your spine.
- Squeeze your glutes and push yourself back to the starting position.

Tucked-Elbow Pushup

WORKS your biceps, triceps, and chest.

A

- Assume a standard pushup position, but instead of placing your hands shoulder-width apart, position them a bit closer together to make it easier to tuck your elbows in. Your arms should be straight.

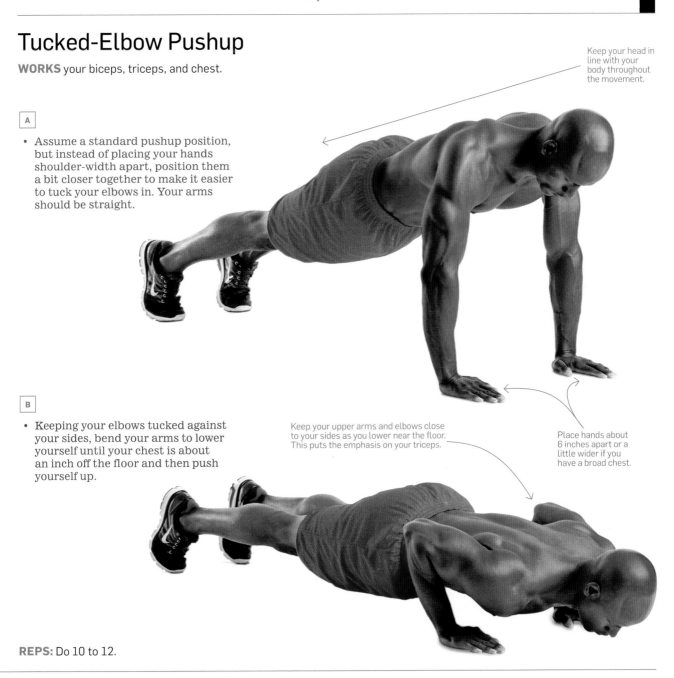

Keep your head in line with your body throughout the movement.

B

- Keeping your elbows tucked against your sides, bend your arms to lower yourself until your chest is about an inch off the floor and then push yourself up.

Keep your upper arms and elbows close to your sides as you lower near the floor. This puts the emphasis on your triceps.

Place hands about 6 inches apart or a little wider if you have a broad chest.

REPS: Do 10 to 12.

5-Second Forward Lunge

WORKS your quadriceps and calves.

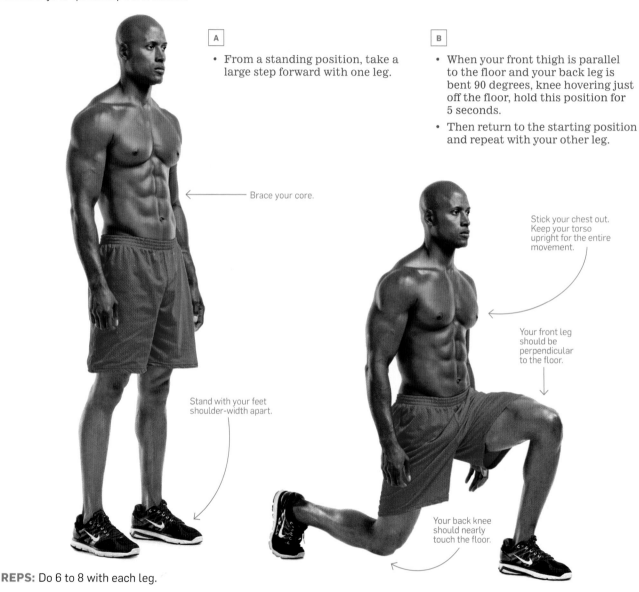

A

- From a standing position, take a large step forward with one leg.

B

- When your front thigh is parallel to the floor and your back leg is bent 90 degrees, knee hovering just off the floor, hold this position for 5 seconds.
- Then return to the starting position and repeat with your other leg.

Brace your core.

Stick your chest out. Keep your torso upright for the entire movement.

Your front leg should be perpendicular to the floor.

Stand with your feet shoulder-width apart.

Your back knee should nearly touch the floor.

REPS: Do 6 to 8 with each leg.

Stepup

WORKS your glutes and hamstrings.

> **TRAINER'S TIP:** *To make this move harder, hold your arms straight out in front of you, parallel to the floor, throughout the movement.*

Your entire foot should be on the bench, with your toes pointed forward.

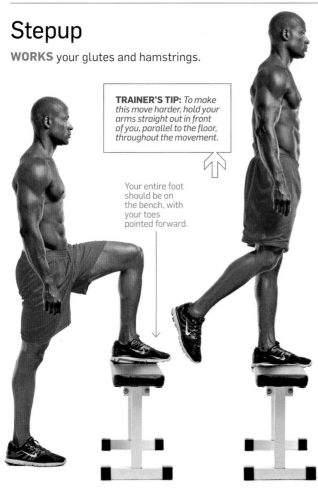

A
- Holding your arms at your sides, place one foot on a step that's about 2 feet off the floor.

B
- Push down through your heel to straighten your leg and lift your other leg.
- Return to the starting position. Complete all your reps with one leg before switching legs and repeating the movement.

REPS: Do 8 to 10 with each leg.

Jump

WORKS the fast-twitch muscles of your legs.

A
- Stand with your feet shoulder-width apart. Now dip down at your hips and knees.

B
- Explode up, jumping as high as you can. Land softly, and then lower yourself and repeat.

Drop your hips back to generate power.

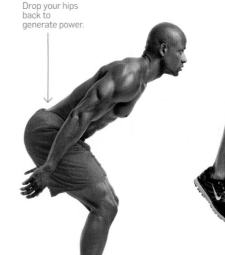

Land softly on your toes before sinking into your heels.

REPS: Do 10.

43

Belly Off! No-Gym Classic 1/Advanced

No-Gym Classic 1 and 2 are derived from our Belly Off! Diet Bodyweight 100 Workout. They combine resistance exercises and calisthenics for a highly effective full-body pump that you can do at home. Alternate between the two, resting a day in between. Later, team one or both with free-weight workouts to create your own program.

START HERE:
Alternate between the Shoulder Press Pushup and the Single-Leg Bench Getup for three sets of each. Then perform the remaining three exercises consecutively (again, without rest), doing the circuit three times.

Shoulder Press Pushup

WORKS your deltoids, chest, and triceps.

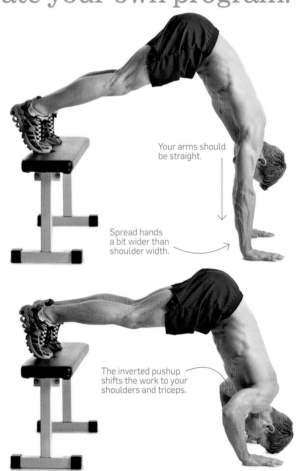

Your arms should be straight.

Spread hands a bit wider than shoulder width.

The inverted pushup shifts the work to your shoulders and triceps.

A

- Place your feet on a bench and hands on the floor a foot or two from the bench and slightly wider than shoulder-width apart.
- Pike your hips up in the air, so you are as vertical as possible.

B

- Slowly bend your arms to lower your head to the floor.
- Pause, and push with your shoulders and triceps back to the start position.

REPS: Do 10.

Single-Leg Bench Getup

WORKS your quadriceps and calves.

A

- Sit on a bench with your back upright and hold your arms straight out in front of your body at shoulder height, parallel to the floor.
- Raise your right foot off the floor.

B

- Without leaning forward, press through your heel to stand. (If this is too difficult, try sliding your foot slightly back toward your body in the starting position.)
- Sit down and repeat.

34

Percentage increase in your risk of death over a 14-year period if you spend 6 hours of leisure time a day seated.

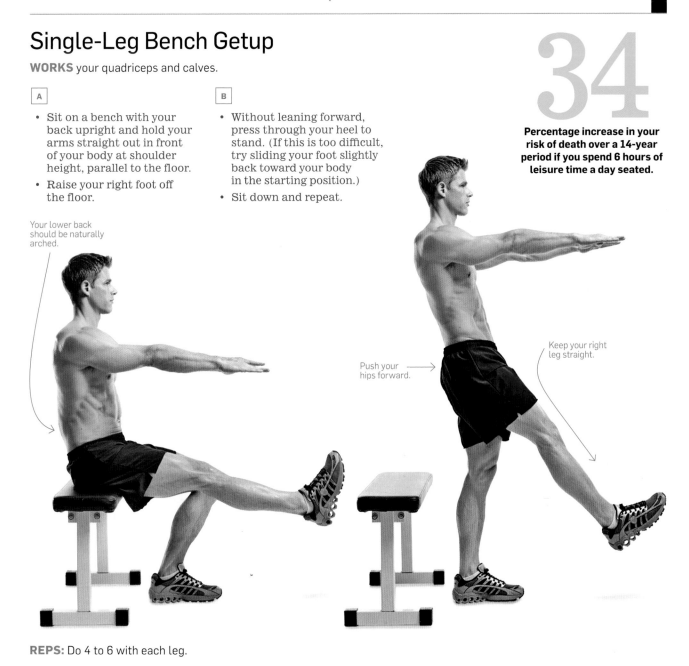

Your lower back should be naturally arched.

Push your hips forward.

Keep your right leg straight.

REPS: Do 4 to 6 with each leg.

Belly Off! No-Gym Classic 1/Advanced

Mountain Climber

WORKS your legs and lungs.

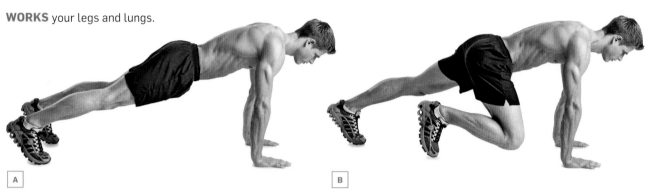

A

- Assume the classic pushup position with your hands on the floor directly under your shoulders and your legs straight behind you. This is the starting position.

REPS: Do 10 per leg.

B

- Lift one foot off the floor and bring your knee toward your chest.
- Straighten your leg back out, move your other knee to your chest, and return that leg to the starting position.
- Alternate right, left, right, left as fast as you can with good form.

Wide-Grip Pushup

WORKS your chest and arms.

 TRAINER'S TIP: *The greater the distance between your hands, the more stress on your chest and shoulders.*

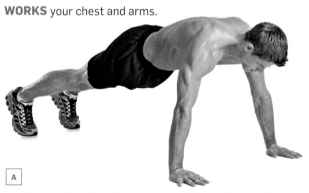

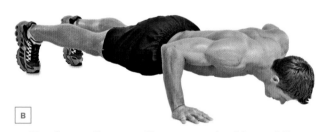

A

- Assume the classic pushup position with your legs straight and your abs tight.
- Instead of placing your hands directly under your shoulders, place them wider than shoulder-width apart.

REPS: Do 20.

B

- Bend your elbows and lower your chest toward the floor until your upper arms are parallel with the floor.
- Press back to the starting position.

Inverted Row

WORKS your trapezius, rear deltoids, and rhomboidei.

- Set a chinup bar or other bar at hip height.
- Lie underneath the bar with your heels on the floor and grab the bar, your hands 1 or 2 inches more than shoulder-width apart. Use an overhand grip.

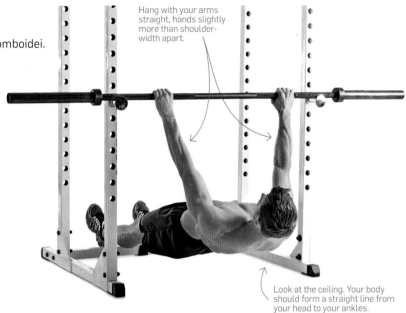

Hang with your arms straight, hands slightly more than shoulder-width apart.

Look at the ceiling. Your body should form a straight line from your head to your ankles.

- Keeping your body in a straight line, pull your chest up to the bar using your back muscles.
- Slowly lower yourself until your arms are straight.

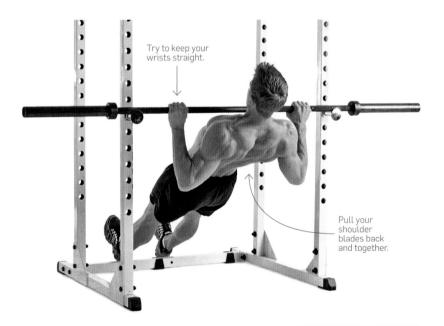

Try to keep your wrists straight.

Pull your shoulder blades back and together.

REPS: Do 12.

START HERE:
Alternate between the Front-Foot Elevated Split Squat and the Walking Offset Pushup for three sets of each. Then perform the remaining three exercises as a circuit (again, without rest between exercises). Do a total of three circuits, resting briefly after each one.

Front-Foot Elevated Split Squat

WORKS your quadriceps and calves.

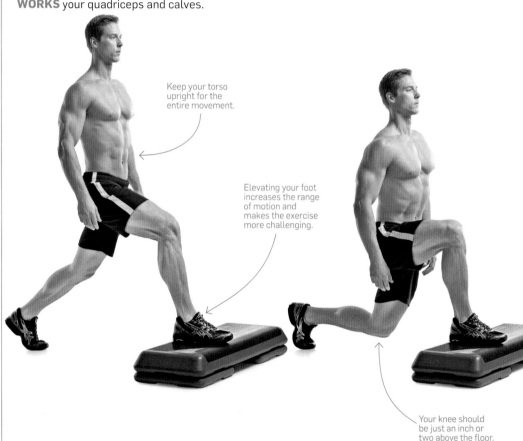

Keep your torso upright for the entire movement.

Elevating your foot increases the range of motion and makes the exercise more challenging.

Your knee should be just an inch or two above the floor.

A

- Stand with one foot 2 to 3 feet in front of the other, each in line with its corresponding buttock. Place the front foot on a 6-inch riser.

REPS: Do 12 per side.

B

- Keep your upper body erect as you descend until the top of your front thigh is parallel to the floor.
- Pause, then press back up to the starting position.

Walking Offset Pushup

WORKS your chest and core.

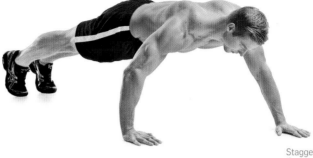

A

- Place your hands on the floor slightly wider than shoulder-width apart.
- Move one hand forward of your shoulder and the other a bit behind your shoulder.

Staggering your hands makes the pushup more challenging for your core and shoulders.

B

- Now, from this staggered hand stance, slowly lower yourself until your chest is 1 inch off the floor.
- Push through your chest, shoulders, and triceps to return to the start position.

C **D**

- After 2 reps, reverse the hand positions by walking your hands and feet forward one step.
- Repeat the exercise.

Alternate which hand is placed forward after every two reps.

Keep your body in a straight line at all times.

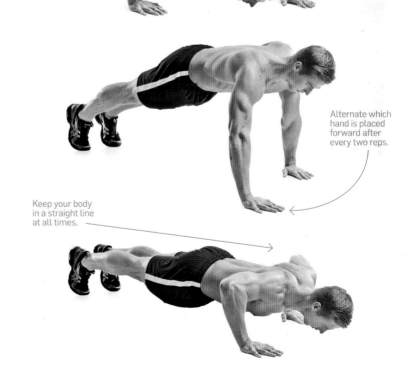

REPS: Do 8 per side.

Belly Off! No-Gym Classic 2/Advanced

Stability Ball Leg Curl

WORKS your glutes and hamstrings.

A

- Lie faceup on the floor with your calves on a stability ball and your arms at your sides, palms down.
- Squeeze your glutes and raise your hips off the floor so your body is in a straight line from your shoulders to your ankles.

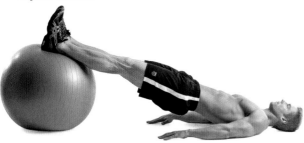

B

- Pause for a second, then bend your legs to roll the ball toward your butt.
- Straighten your legs to roll the ball back out away from you, then lower your body back to the starting position. That's 1 rep.

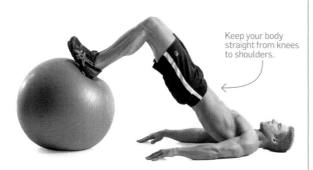

Keep your body straight from knees to shoulders.

REPS: Do 12.

Single-Leg Hip Raise

WORKS your glutes and hamstrings.

A

- Lie on your back, with your knees bent and feet flat on the floor.
- Brace your abs while you straighten your right leg to lift it off the floor so it is in line with your left thigh.

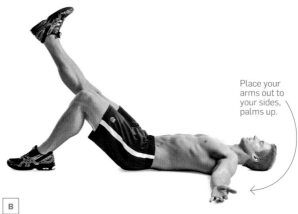

Place your arms out to your sides, palms up.

B

- Raise your hips so your body forms a straight line from your shoulders to your knees.
- Slowly lower your hips until they are an inch above the floor.
- Perform all reps for one leg and then switch sides.

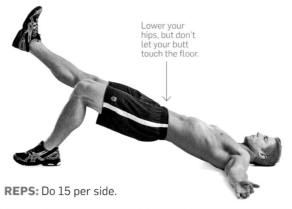

Lower your hips, but don't let your butt touch the floor.

REPS: Do 15 per side.

Chinup

WORKS your lats, biceps, and core.

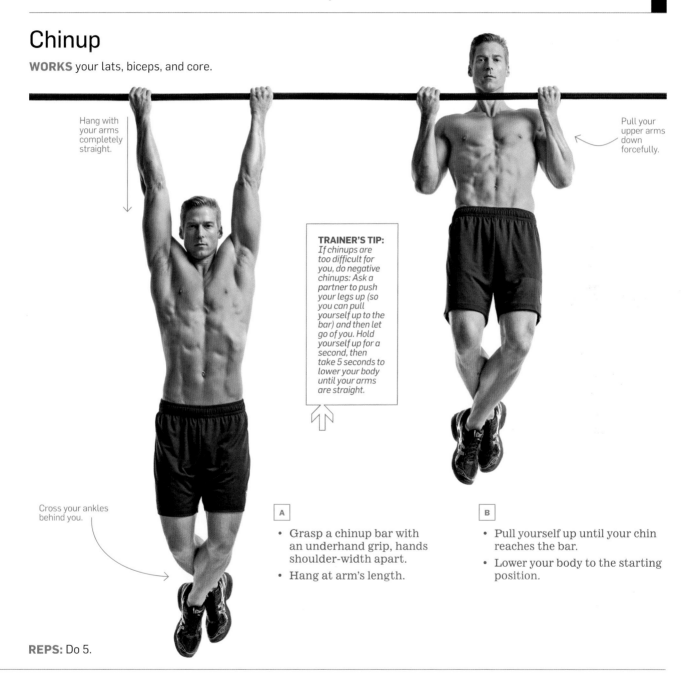

Hang with your arms completely straight.

Pull your upper arms down forcefully.

TRAINER'S TIP:
If chinups are too difficult for you, do negative chinups: Ask a partner to push your legs up (so you can pull yourself up to the bar) and then let go of you. Hold yourself up for a second, then take 5 seconds to lower your body until your arms are straight.

Cross your ankles behind you.

A

- Grasp a chinup bar with an underhand grip, hands shoulder-width apart.
- Hang at arm's length.

B

- Pull yourself up until your chin reaches the bar.
- Lower your body to the starting position.

REPS: Do 5.

Dumbbell Blast Workout 1: The Single

Dumbbells are pure genius. No other single piece of workout equipment is so simple yet so well designed and effective. Dumbbells are the ultimate free weights, allowing you to truly isolate your muscles. Because your dominant side (corresponding with right-handedness or left-handedness) tends to be stronger than the other, when you lift with a straight barbell, you can easily develop muscle imbalances that can lead to injury. Dumbbells eliminate that ability to compensate for weaker muscles. Each side of your body has to work equally hard, creating a balance of power and muscle symmetry. On the following pages, you'll find three excellent 15-minute total-body dumbbell workouts that build every single sinew of muscle. Mix them into your rotation.

START HERE:
This rapid-fire routine uses just one dumbbell. Do this workout as a circuit: Perform each exercise for 45 seconds before moving to the next. After completing one circuit, rest for 1 minute. Then do one or two more. Start with a 15-pound dumbbell. Increase the weight as the workout becomes easier.

Woodchopper

WORKS your arms, shoulders, and core.

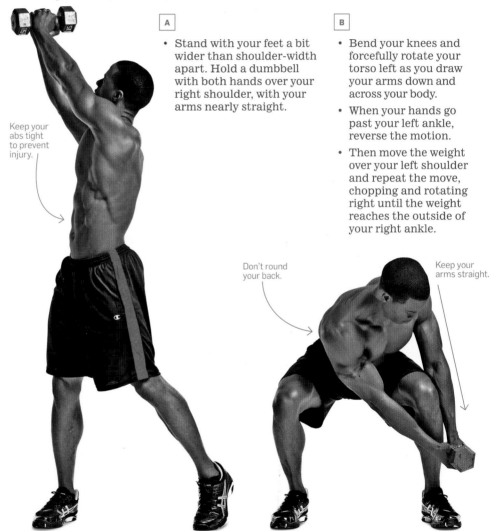

Keep your abs tight to prevent injury.

A

- Stand with your feet a bit wider than shoulder-width apart. Hold a dumbbell with both hands over your right shoulder, with your arms nearly straight.

B

- Bend your knees and forcefully rotate your torso left as you draw your arms down and across your body.
- When your hands go past your left ankle, reverse the motion.
- Then move the weight over your left shoulder and repeat the move, chopping and rotating right until the weight reaches the outside of your right ankle.

Don't round your back.

Keep your arms straight.

REPS: Do as many as you can quickly in 45 seconds, alternating sides.

Dumbbell Blast Workout 1: The Single

Arms-Out Squat

WORKS your quadriceps, hamstrings, shoulders, and back.

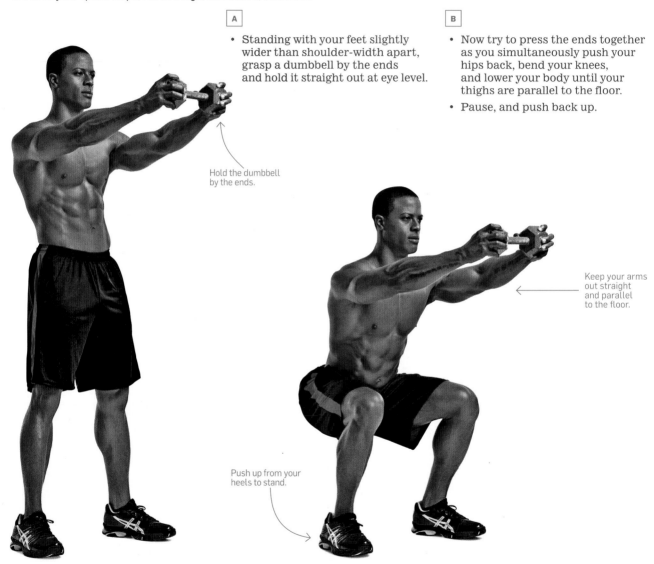

A

- Standing with your feet slightly wider than shoulder-width apart, grasp a dumbbell by the ends and hold it straight out at eye level.

Hold the dumbbell by the ends.

B

- Now try to press the ends together as you simultaneously push your hips back, bend your knees, and lower your body until your thighs are parallel to the floor.
- Pause, and push back up.

Keep your arms out straight and parallel to the floor.

Push up from your heels to stand.

REPS: Do as many as you can in 45 seconds.

Standing Pressout

WORKS your shoulders and back.

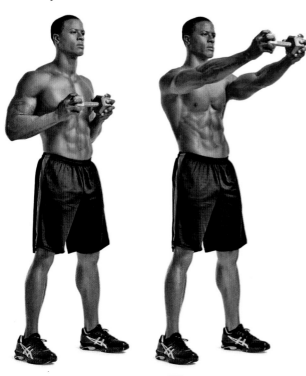

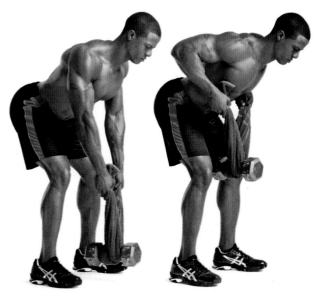

Towel Row

WORKS your middle and upper back, and shoulders.

TRAINER'S TIP: *Grasping a towel increases the demand on your forearm muscles as you work your back.*

A
- With your feet shoulder-width apart, hold a dumbbell by its ends against your chest.

B
- Try to press the ends together as you simultaneously push the dumbbell away from your body and slightly up (to eye level) until your arms are straight.
- Pause, and pull the dumbbell back as you squeeze your shoulder blades together.

REPS: Do as many as you can in 45 seconds.

A
- Secure a towel around a dumbbell's handle. Grab an end of the towel with each hand and stand with your feet shoulder-width apart, knees slightly bent.
- Bend at your hips, keep your lower back flat, and lower your torso until it's almost parallel to the floor.

B
- Pull the towel ends to either side of your abdomen.
- Pause and lower the towel ends and repeat without standing back upright.

REPS: Do as many as you can in 45 seconds.

Dumbbell Blast Workout 2: The Buildup

Perform three circuits, lifting a slightly heavier weight (if possible) each round. Start with 12 reps for the first circuit, then reduce reps by 2 for each subsequent circuit. Rest only between circuits. Beginners should lift 20 to 30 pounds and rest 60 to 90 seconds; intermediates, 30 to 40 pounds, 45 to 60 seconds; advanced lifters, 40 to 50 pounds, and 30 to 45 seconds.

Straight-Leg Deadlift

WORKS your glutes and hamstrings.

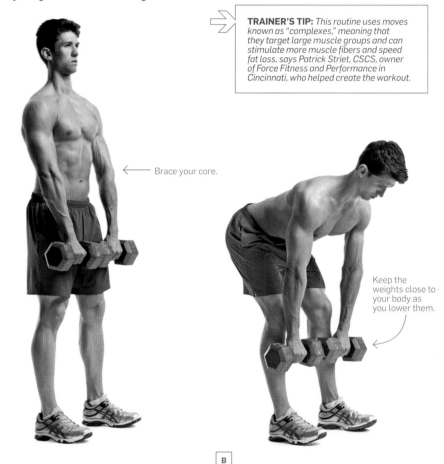

Brace your core.

Keep the weights close to your body as you lower them.

TRAINER'S TIP: *This routine uses moves known as "complexes," meaning that they target large muscle groups and can stimulate more muscle fibers and speed fat loss, says Patrick Striet, CSCS, owner of Force Fitness and Performance in Cincinnati, who helped create the workout.*

A
- Using an overhand grip, hold the dumbbells in front of your thighs.
- Stand with your feet hip-width apart and knees slightly bent.

B
- Bend at your hips to lower your torso until it's almost parallel to the floor.
- Pause, and raise back up.

REPS: Do 12, 10, and 8, respectively, for the three circuits.

Thrusters

WORKS your total body, especially the quads and shoulders.

A

- Stand with your feet shoulder-width apart, holding a pair of dumbbells next to your shoulders.

B

- Sit back with your hips into a squat until your thighs are parallel to the floor.

C

- As you stand up, press the dumbbells over your head.
- Then lower them back down to your shoulders. That's 1 rep.

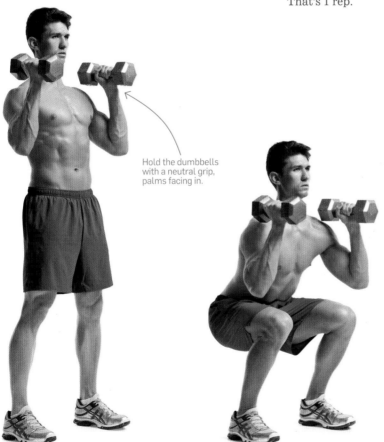

Hold the dumbbells with a neutral grip, palms facing in.

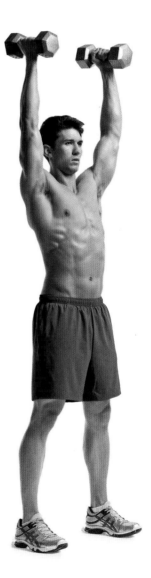

REPS: Do 12, 10, and 8, respectively, for the three circuits.

Dumbbell Blast Workout 2: The Buildup

Bent-Over Row

WORKS your upper back.

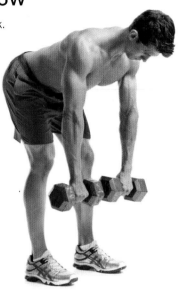

A

- Stand with your feet hip-width apart while holding a pair of dumbbells in front of your thighs. Bend at your hips and knees and lower your torso until it's almost parallel to the floor, allowing your arms to hang straight down toward the floor, palms facing you.

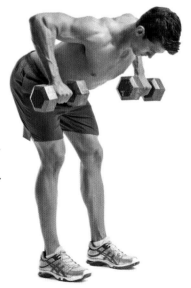

B

- Bend your elbows and pull the dumbbells to the sides of your torso.
- Pause, and then slowly lower them.

REPS: Do 12, 10, and 8, respectively, for the three circuits.

Squat Thrust

WORKS your total body, especially the quads, calves, and chest.

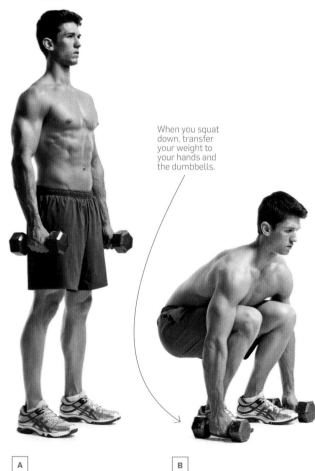

When you squat down, transfer your weight to your hands and the dumbbells.

A

- Stand holding a pair of dumbbells at your sides.

B

- Squat down and place the dumbbells on the floor to the outside of your feet. Keep your arms straight.

REPS: Do 12, 10, and 8, respectively, for the three circuits.

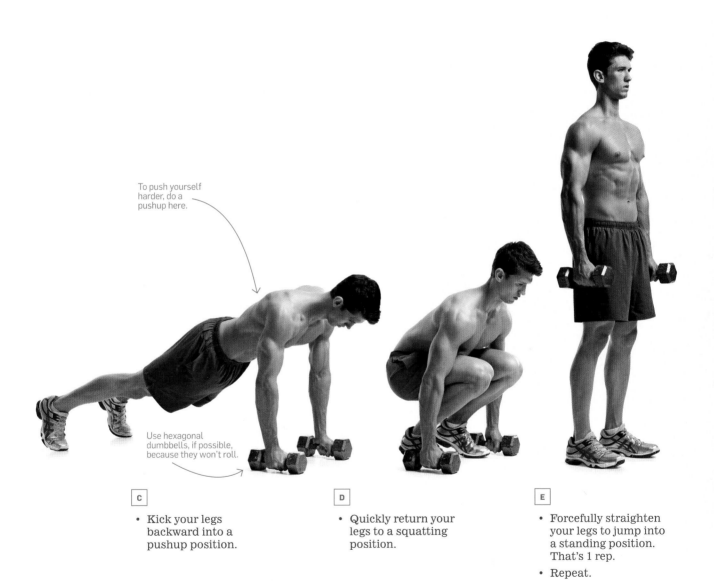

To push yourself harder, do a pushup here.

Use hexagonal dumbbells, if possible, because they won't roll.

C

- Kick your legs backward into a pushup position.

D

- Quickly return your legs to a squatting position.

E

- Forcefully straighten your legs to jump into a standing position. That's 1 rep.
- Repeat.

Dumbbell Blast Workout 3: Fast and Furious

START HERE:

This old-school dumbbell routine builds muscle and melts unwanted flab the old-fashioned way—hard work, no rest. Do this four-exercise circuit with no break between exercises. After completing a circuit, rest for 90 seconds before doing it again. Do three complete circuits.

Incline Bench Press

WORKS your upper chest, deltoids, and triceps.

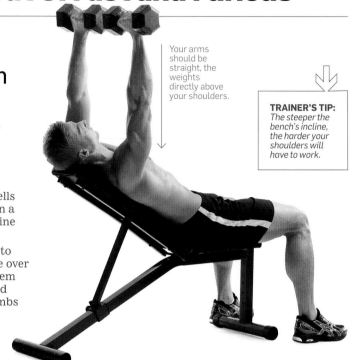

Your arms should be straight, the weights directly above your shoulders.

> **TRAINER'S TIP:**
> The steeper the bench's incline, the harder your shoulders will have to work.

A

- Grab a pair of dumbbells and lie on your back on a bench set to a low incline (15 to 30 degrees).
- Lift the dumbbells up to arm's length so they're over your chin, and hold them with your palms turned toward your feet (thumbs facing each other).

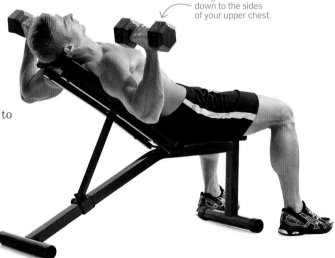

Bring the dumbbells down to the sides of your upper chest.

B

- Slowly lower the weights to your upper chest, pause, then push them back up over your chin.

REPS: Do 10 to 12.

One-Arm Snatch

WORKS your total body, especially the legs, hips, back, and shoulders.

> **TRAINER'S TIP:** *If you're using a heavy dumbbell, bring it down to your shoulders with both hands, then lower it to the floor.*

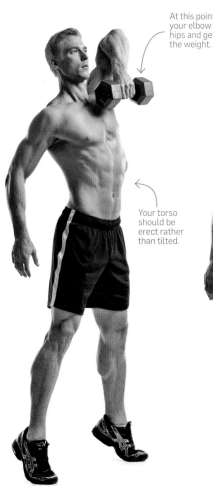

At this point, drop your elbow and hips and get under the weight.

Your torso should be erect rather than tilted.

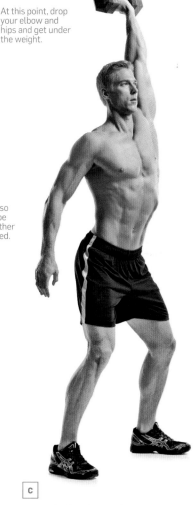

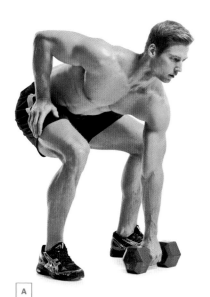

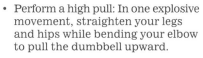

A

- Hold a dumbbell in your left hand with an overhand grip.
- Set your feet shoulder-width apart, bend your knees and place the dumbbell on the floor.

REPS: Do 10 with each arm.

B

- Perform a high pull: In one explosive movement, straighten your legs and hips while bending your elbow to pull the dumbbell upward.
- At the dumbbell's highest point, slide into the catching phase, drop your hips, and drive under the weight by rotating your wrist under the dumbbell.

C

- Quickly straighten your arm so the dumbbell is now over the top of your shoulder. Return and repeat.
- After completing all reps, repeat the exercise with the dumbbell in your right hand.

Dumbbell Blast Workout 3: Fast and Furious

Seated Calf Raise

WORKS your calves.

A

- Place a step in front of a bench, grab a pair of dumbbells, and sit down.
- Set the balls of both feet on the step, and hold a dumbbell vertically on each knee.
- Lower both heels as far as you can without touching the floor.

B

- Push off the balls of your feet and lift your heels as high as you can.
- Pause, then repeat.

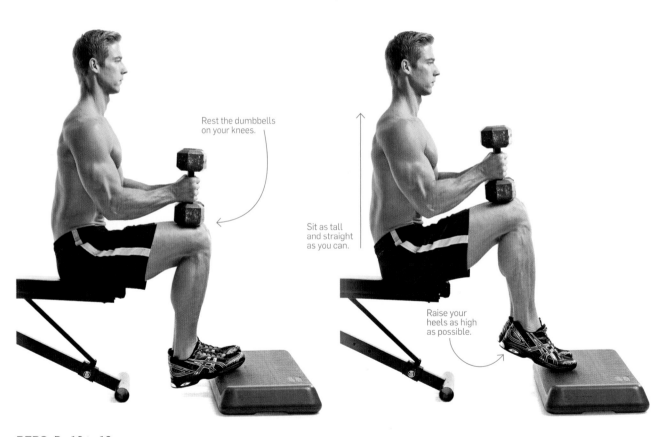

Rest the dumbbells on your knees.

Sit as tall and straight as you can.

Raise your heels as high as possible.

REPS: Do 10 to 12.

Chest-Supported Row

WORKS your upper back and shoulders.

A

- Grab a pair of dumbbells and lie chest down on an adjustable bench set to a low incline.
- Let the dumbbells hang at arm's length from your shoulders, your palms facing each other.

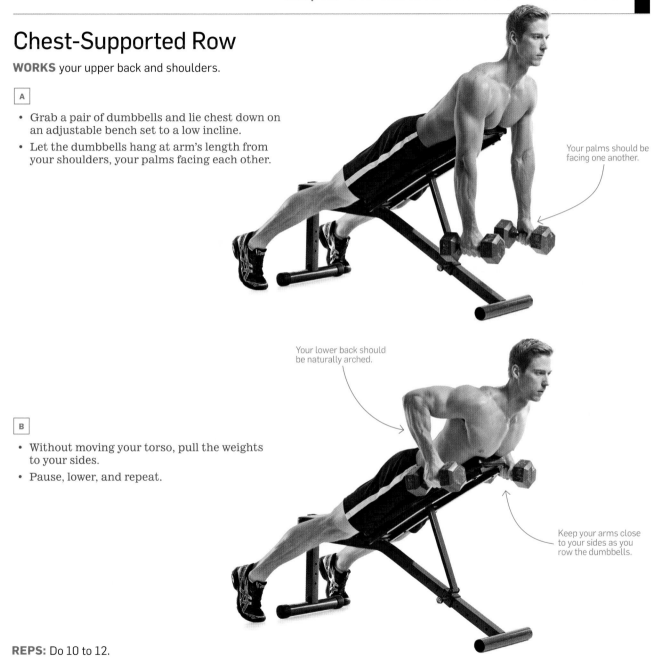

Your palms should be facing one another.

Your lower back should be naturally arched.

B

- Without moving your torso, pull the weights to your sides.
- Pause, lower, and repeat.

Keep your arms close to your sides as you row the dumbbells.

REPS: Do 10 to 12.

The Muscle Definer Workout 1

If you want to build well-defined muscles that really pop, the best strategy calls for lifting with high intensity and heavy weights. The power exercises in the following two workouts do just that, targeting your fast-twitch muscle fibers, which have great potential for growth in both size and strength.

START HERE:
Do this circuit three times, adding a little more weight each time. Try to perform each move quickly while maintaining control of the weight. Rest 60 seconds between circuits.

Dumbbell Standing Press

WORKS your shoulders.

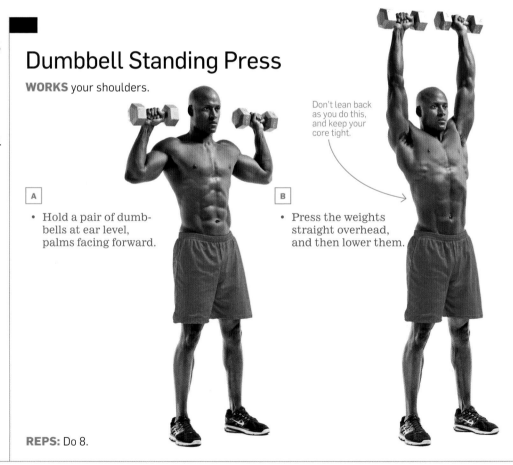

A
- Hold a pair of dumbbells at ear level, palms facing forward.

Don't lean back as you do this, and keep your core tight.

B
- Press the weights straight overhead, and then lower them.

REPS: Do 8.

Romanian Deadlift, Row, Shrug

WORKS your back, shoulders, triceps, and legs.

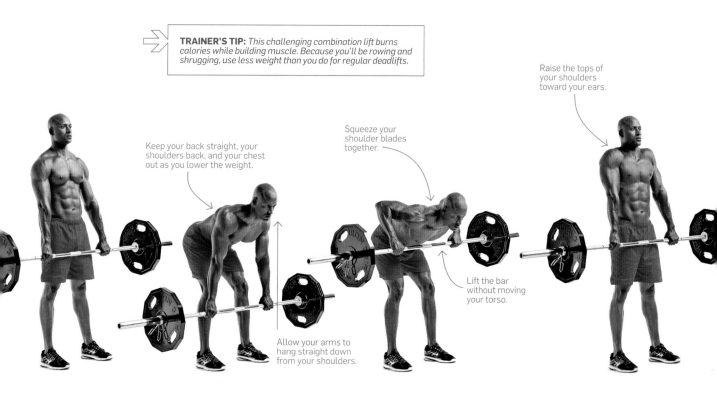

TRAINER'S TIP: *This challenging combination lift burns calories while building muscle. Because you'll be rowing and shrugging, use less weight than you do for regular deadlifts.*

Keep your back straight, your shoulders back, and your chest out as you lower the weight.

Squeeze your shoulder blades together.

Raise the tops of your shoulders toward your ears.

Lift the bar without moving your torso.

Allow your arms to hang straight down from your shoulders.

A

- Stand with your feet shoulder-width apart.
- Using an overhand grip (hands about shoulder-width apart), hold a barbell in front of your thighs.

REPS: Do 5.

B

- Push your hips backward and lower the bar below your knees.
- Bend at the hips.

C

- When your back is flat and parallel to the floor, pull the bar up to your sternum and lower it.

D

- Stand up, keeping the bar as close to your body as possible.
- Shrug your shoulders toward your ears. That's 1 rep.

The Muscle Definer Workout 1

Dumbbell Lunge

WORKS your quadriceps and calves.

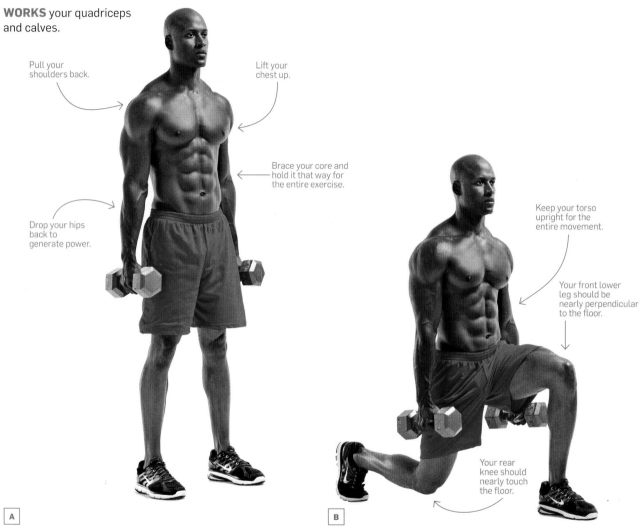

Pull your shoulders back.

Lift your chest up.

Brace your core and hold it that way for the entire exercise.

Drop your hips back to generate power.

Keep your torso upright for the entire movement.

Your front lower leg should be nearly perpendicular to the floor.

Your rear knee should nearly touch the floor.

A

- Stand holding dumbbells at your sides, palms facing inward.

REPS: Do 10.

B

- Step forward with your left foot and lower your body until your front and back knees are bent 90 degrees and your back knee is about an inch off the floor.
- Push back up and repeat with the other leg.
- That's 1 rep.

Dumbbell Rotation

WORKS your core.

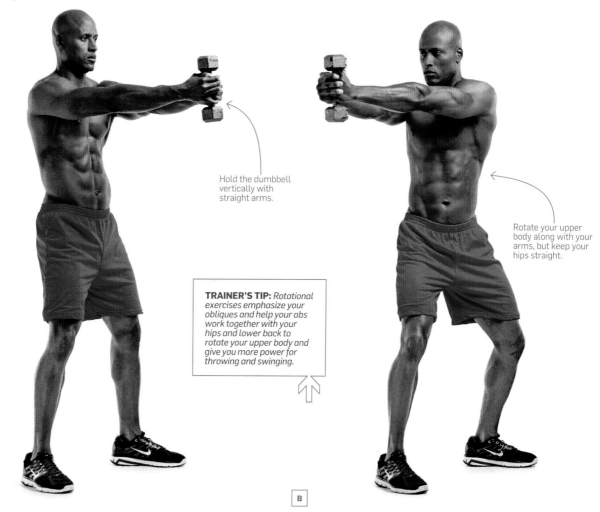

Hold the dumbbell vertically with straight arms.

Rotate your upper body along with your arms, but keep your hips straight.

TRAINER'S TIP: *Rotational exercises emphasize your obliques and help your abs work together with your hips and lower back to rotate your upper body and give you more power for throwing and swinging.*

A

- Hold a dumbbell vertically with both hands.
- Raise it until your arms are parallel with the floor.

REPS: Do 15 reps per side.

B

- Rotate the dumbbell to just past one shoulder (without moving your lower body). Return to the starting position and repeat.

The Muscle Definer Workout 2

Do this circuit three times, adding a little more weight after every circuit. Rest 60 seconds between circuits.

Diagonal Lift and Press

WORKS your quads, shoulders and core.

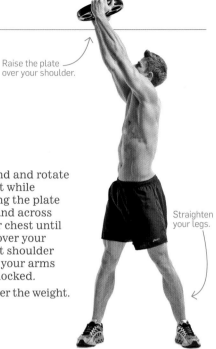

Raise the plate over your shoulder.

Straighten your legs.

A

- Hold a weight plate in front of your thighs.
- With your feet shoulder-width apart, squat and rotate your torso (and the plate) to the left.

REPS: Do 10, 5 to each side.

B

- Stand and rotate right while lifting the plate up and across your chest until it's over your right shoulder and your arms are locked.
- Lower the weight.

Goblet Squat

WORKS your quads and calves.

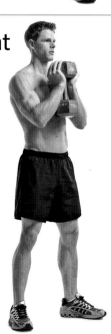

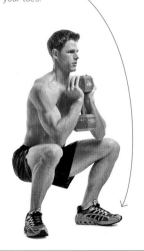

Press up through your heels. Don't put pressure on your toes.

A

- Stand with your feet slightly wider than shoulder-width apart.
- Grasp a dumbbell vertically with both hands cupping the top weight. Hold it against your chest.

REPS: Do 8 to 10.

B

- Keeping your back naturally arched, push your hips back, bend your knees, and lower your body until the tops of your thighs are at least parallel to the floor.
- Pause, then push yourself back up to the start. If that's too hard, do a bodyweight squat instead.

Dumbbell Push Press

WORKS your quads and shoulders.

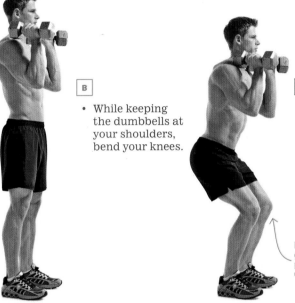

A

- Stand holding a pair of dumbbells just outside of your shoulders, with your arms bent and palms facing each other.
- Set your feet shoulder-width apart, your knees slightly bent.

B

- While keeping the dumbbells at your shoulders, bend your knees.

C

- Explosively push up with your legs as you press the weights straight over your shoulders.
- Lower the dumbbells back to the starting position and repeat.

Bend your knees to generate more power to press the dumbbells overhead.

REPS: Do 8 to 10.

Dumbbell Deadlift

WORKS your glutes, hamstrings, and core.

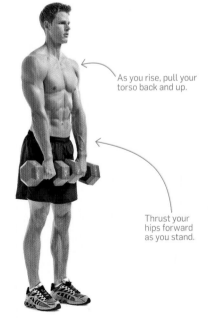

A

- Set heavy dumbbells on the floor and stand between them with your feet shoulder-width apart.
- Bend at your hips and knees, and grab the dumbbells with an overhand grip.

Your arms should be straight, and your lower back slightly arched.

Keep your chest up.

B

- Without allowing your lower back to round, stand up with the dumbbells.
- Lower the dumbbells to the floor.

As you rise, pull your torso back and up.

Thrust your hips forward as you stand.

REPS: Do 8 to 10.

The Classic Powerlifter Workout

You don't need 15 exercises to build great power, just three. Powerlifters focus on these training classics—the barbell squat, bench press, and deadlift—because, when done right, they train every major muscle and move thousands of pounds in a single workout. The key is using a heavy weight and pushing yourself on each lift.

START HERE: Do two light sets of barbell squats, resting for 90 seconds in between. Next, load the bar with a weight you can lift only six times with good form. Perform 5 flawless reps, then rest for 2 minutes before moving on. Do the same for the other two exercises.

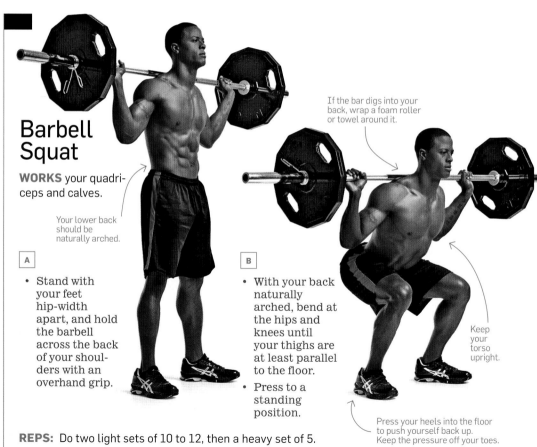

Barbell Squat

WORKS your quadriceps and calves.

Your lower back should be naturally arched.

If the bar digs into your back, wrap a foam roller or towel around it.

Keep your torso upright.

A

- Stand with your feet hip-width apart, and hold the barbell across the back of your shoulders with an overhand grip.

B

- With your back naturally arched, bend at the hips and knees until your thighs are at least parallel to the floor.
- Press to a standing position.

Press your heels into the floor to push yourself back up. Keep the pressure off your toes.

REPS: Do two light sets of 10 to 12, then a heavy set of 5.

Barbell Bench Press

WORKS your chest, front deltoids, and triceps.

Keep your wrists straight.

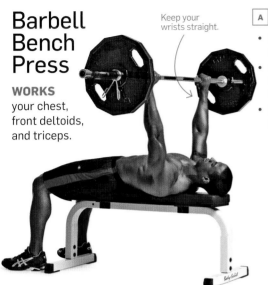

A

- Lie on a bench with your feet flat on the floor.
- Grab the bar with your hands more than shoulder-width apart, and hold it over your chest.
- Squeeze your shoulder blades down and together.

B

- As you lower the weight to your chest, pull your elbows toward your sides.
- Pause, then push the weight back up while by driving your head and upper body into the bench.

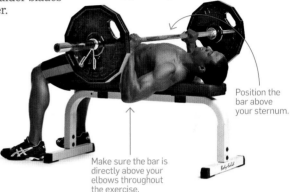

Position the bar above your sternum.

Make sure the bar is directly above your elbows throughout the exercise.

REPS: Do two light sets of 10 to 12, then a heavy set of 5.

Barbell Deadlift

WORKS your glutes, hamstrings, core, shoulders, hips, and back.

A

- Stand with a bar on the floor in front of you so it just touches your shins.
- Push your hips back and grasp the bar with an overhand grip, your hands just outside your calves.

B

- Keeping your back straight and your chest up, drive your heels into the floor and move your hips forward to stand up and raise the weight.
- Lower the bar back to the floor.

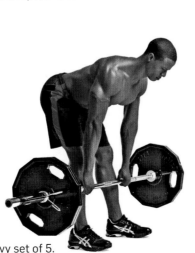

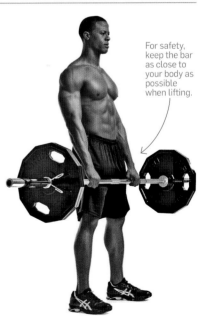

For safety, keep the bar as close to your body as possible when lifting.

REPS: Do two light sets of 10 to 12, then a heavy set of 5.

Total-Body Stress-Buster Workout

Send stress packing with this explosive ultimate-fighter-inspired workout. Its high-energy athletic maneuvers will shoot your fat-burning furnace into the red and chisel every muscle from your head to your fast-moving feet.

START HERE:
Perform as many reps as you can in 60 seconds, then move to the next exercise and so on. After completing all seven moves back to back, rest for 60 seconds, then repeat the circuit.

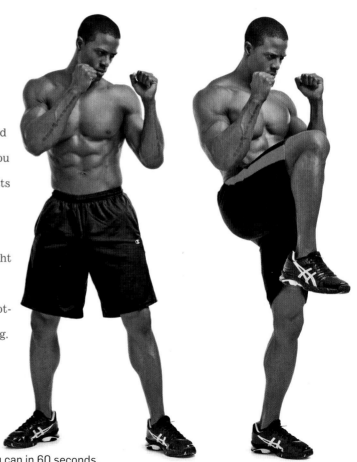

Knee Thrust

A

- Assume a left-foot-lead boxing-style stance (or right-foot lead if you are a southpaw), knees slightly bent, fists in front of your chin, palms facing in.

B

- Quickly raise your right knee toward your chest, drive it back down, and, without changing your left-foot-lead stance, do the same with your left leg.
- That's 1 rep.

REPS: Do as many as you can in 60 seconds.

Squat Thrust with Knee Thrust

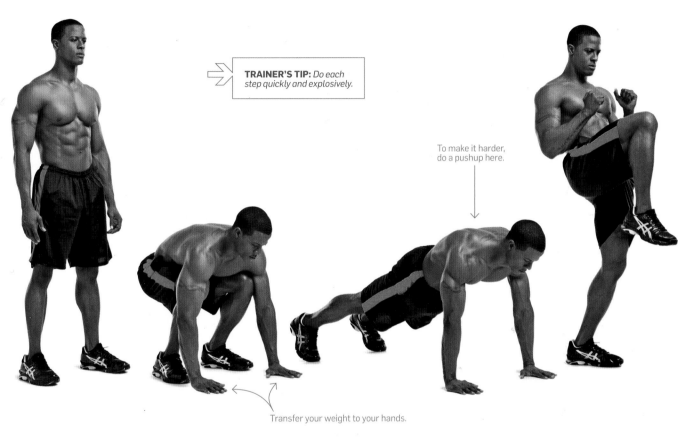

TRAINER'S TIP: *Do each step quickly and explosively.*

To make it harder, do a pushup here.

Transfer your weight to your hands.

A
- Stand with your feet hip-width apart, arms at your sides.

B
- Bend your knees and lower your hands to the floor.

C
- Jump both feet back so you're in a pushup position.
- Keep your back straight and your core braced.

D
- Jump your feet back up to your hands, quickly stand, then pull your right knee toward your chest.
- Return to start and repeat the sequence with the left leg.
- That's 1 rep.

REPS: Do as many as you can in 60 seconds.

Total-Body Stress-Buster Workout

Speed Jump Rope

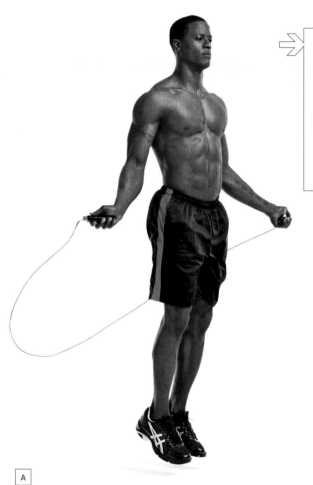

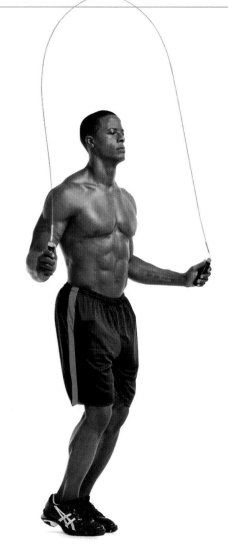

TRAINER'S TIP:
To make it harder, add a double under, in which you pass the rope under your feet twice in a single jump. But don't just jump higher; keep your hands by your waist and quickly rotate your wrists to create the right rope speed.

A

- Stand with your feet hip-width apart and your knees slightly bent, holding the ends of a jump rope.
- Push off the floor with the balls of your feet and point your toes downward, while making small circles with your wrists.

REPS: Do as many as you can in 60 seconds.

B

- Land softly on your toes, immediately pushing off again.
- Focus on jumping over the rope as quickly as possible.

Front Kick

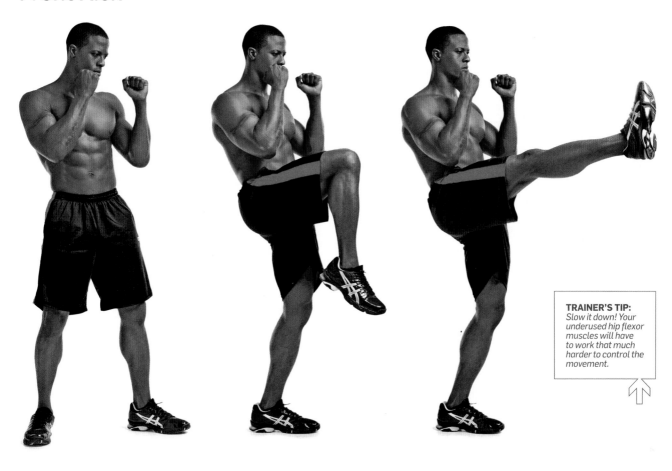

TRAINER'S TIP:
Slow it down! Your underused hip flexor muscles will have to work that much harder to control the movement.

A

• Assume a left-foot lead boxing stance, fists at chin height.

B

• Raise your right knee toward your chest.

C

• Kick straight out as if you're slamming a door closed with your heel.

• Quickly bring your leg back, placing it staggered behind your left.

• Repeat with your left leg (that's 1 rep), and continue alternating.

REPS: Do as many as you can in 60 seconds.

Total-Body Stress-Buster Workout

Situp with Punch

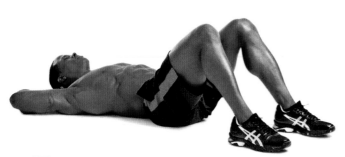

A

- Lie on your back with your knees bent, your feet flat on the floor, and hands behind your head.

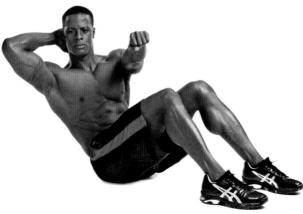

B

- Brace your abs, sit up, and punch across your body six times with your left arm.
- Return to the starting position, sit up, and punch across your body six times with your right arm.
- That's 1 rep.

REPS: Do as many as you can in 60 seconds.

Straight Punch

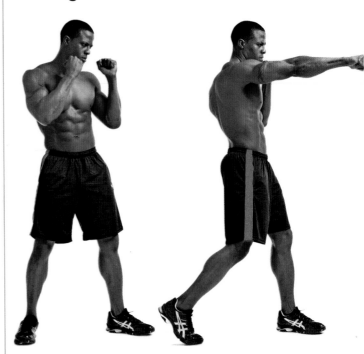

A

- Assume a left-foot-lead boxing stance with your fists up, palms facing each other.

TRAINER'S TIP: *Pace your breathing with your punches and exhale with each punch, even if it makes your breath quick and shallow.*

B

- Rotate your hips to the left and extend your right arm, twisting your forearm so your fingernails face the floor and your arm is in line with your shoulder.
- Return to the starting position, then repeat on the opposite side with your right foot forward and extending your left arm.
- That's 1 rep.

REPS: Do as many as you can in 60 seconds, alternating sides.

Side Kick

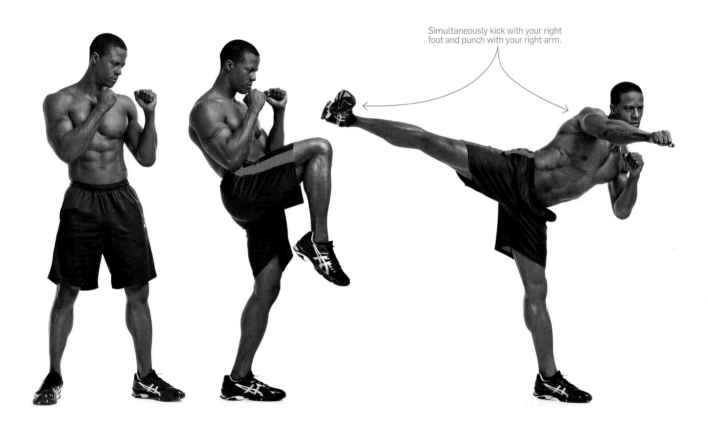

Simultaneously kick with your right foot and punch with your right arm.

A

- Assume a left-foot-lead boxing stance, fists up.

B

- Raise your right knee toward your chest.

C

- Rotate your hips and left foot and kick your right leg to the side, pushing through the heel, while punching with your right arm.
- Quickly bring your right leg down, placing it staggered in front of your left. Bring your right arm back in.
- Repeat with your left leg and arm.
- That's 1 rep.

REPS: Do as many as you can in 60 seconds, alternating sides.

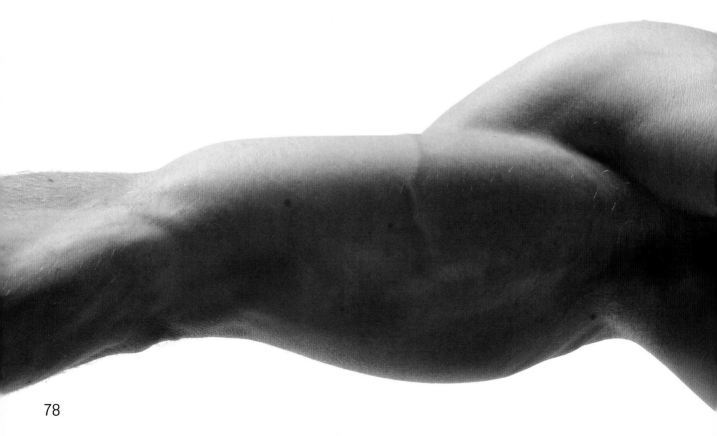

Chapter 5:
15-Minute Fat-Burning Workouts

Jack Up Your Metabolism with These Fast-Paced Cardio Programs, and Melt Away Pounds. Are You Ready for This?

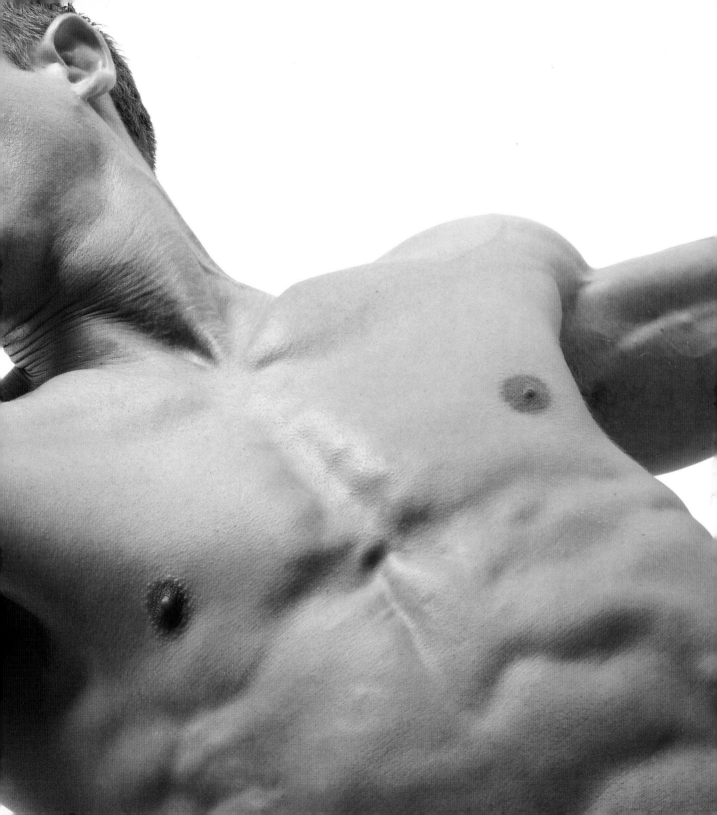

Superfast Metabolic Workouts

This chapter of workouts is designed for anyone with a stubborn layer of extra insulation that just won't budge. These high-energy strength-training routines incinerate tough-to-lose weight by jacking up your heart rate during exercise and keeping your metabolic rate—the rate at which your body burns calories during rest—elevated for up to 48 hours after you've banged out your final move. Take note: These workouts are intense; you should finish the final rep of each move wishing you could breathe out of your ears as well as your nose. You'll find five flab-melting metabolic workouts on the following pages. While they're designed to boost calorie burn, these programs are also terrific for boosting stamina and strength.

For best results...

To get the most from these metabolic workouts, choose the ones that most closely suit your goals. Or add one of these workouts to others of your choice in the book. For these metabolic workouts, it's important to do the prescribed number of sets and reps for each exercise, using a weight heavy enough that you can barely squeeze out the last rep of your final set with perfect form. You'll start seeing results in 2 weeks. But you'll start feeling it working immediately.

Find It Quick: Your 15-Minute Fat-Burning Program

p.82
You're Melting: Workout A
Barbell Rollout
Crossover Dumbbell Stepup
Elevated-Feet Inverted Row
Barbell Front Squat
Pushup

p.88
You're Melting: Workout B
Cable Core Press
Offset Reverse Dumbbell Lunge
Chinup
Zercher Good Morning
Dumbbell Alternating Shoulder
  Press and Twist

p.92
Strength, Stamina, Speed, and Sweat
In-Place Heidens
Dumbbell Goblet Squat with Pulse
Spider-Man Pushup
Bodysaw

p.96
The Superhero Workout
Spider-Man Pullup
Hulk Super Leap
Superman Back Extension
Thor's Hammer

p.100
The Supersweat Supersets
Plyometric Pushup
Dumbbell Bench Press
Explosive Stepup
Alternating Dumbbell Stepup
V-Up
Weighted Stability Ball Situp

2-MINUTE BELLY TORCHERS

7 a.m.
Wake up and do 2 minutes of jumping jacks, high-knee skips, and pushups.

Noon
Drink 16 ounces of water midday and you could burn calories 24 percent faster for an hour.

3 p.m.
Walk briskly around the office. A recent Mayo Clinic study found that lean people walk an average of 3.5 miles a day more than overweight people do. Plus, you'll look busy!

You're Melting: Workouts A and B

The following two full-body fat fryers are ideal for whittling those last couple of inches off your middle. The workouts, designed by Craig Rasmussen, CSCS, of Results Fitness in Santa Clarita, California, feature simple exercises choreographed into challenging routines that rev up metabolism. Alternate between workout A and workout B, allowing a day of rest after each session. (You can pick another 15-minute workout for your third workout of the week.)

Check Your Work

It's easy to slack off during workouts. Finding your target heart rate (HTR) ranges and checking your exertion level manually or with a heart rate monitor can help you make sure you're working hard enough. Use the formula below. Try to stay between your minimum and maximum target heart rate during workouts and push yourself near your maximum during the toughest HIIT segments.

Step 1. Calculate your maximum heart rate (MHR).	220 − _____ (your age) = _____ (MHR)
Step 2. Calculate your resting heart rate (RHR).	_____ (beats in 10 sec.) x 6 = _____ (RHR)
Step 3. Calculate your heart-rate reserve (HRR).	_____ (MHR) − _____ (RHR) = _____ (HRR)
Step 4. Determine your minimum target rate during exercise (minimum target heart rate).	(_____ [HRR] x 0.65) + _____ (RHR) = _____ (MIN THR)
Step 5. Determine your maximum target rate during exercise (maximum target heart rate).	(_____ [HRR] x 0.85) + _____ (RHR) = _____ (MAX THR)

START HERE:
For exercise 1, do two sets of 10 reps, resting for 60 seconds after each set. Then perform exercises 2a and 2b as a pair, resting for 60 seconds after each set. Do two sets of the pair. Follow the same sequence of reps, sets, and rest periods for exercises 3a and 3b.

■

EXERCISE 1
Barbell Rollout

TRAINER'S TIP:
Maintain proper alignment by keeping your neck in line with your spine at all times.

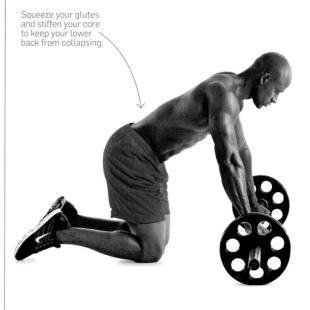

Squeeze your glutes and stiffen your core to keep your lower back from collapsing.

A

- Load a barbell with 10-pound plates and affix collars.
- Kneel on the floor and grab the bar with an overhand, shoulder-width grip.
- Position your shoulders directly over the barbell and keep your lower back naturally arched.

B

- Slowly roll the bar forward, extending your body as far as you can without letting your hips sag.
- Pause for 2 seconds, and reverse the move to return to the starting position.

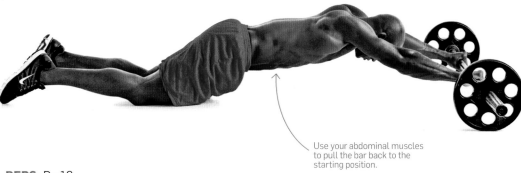

Use your abdominal muscles to pull the bar back to the starting position.

REPS: Do 10.

You're Melting: Workout A

Crossover Dumbbell Stepup

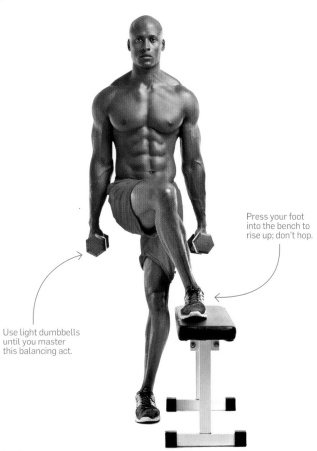

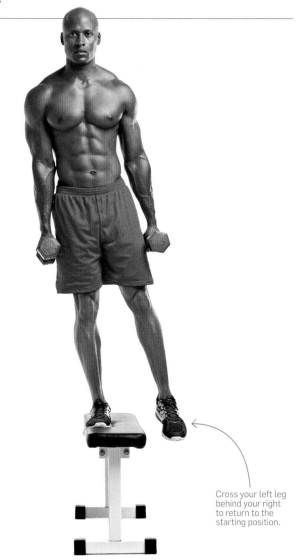

Press your foot into the bench to rise up; don't hop.

Use light dumbbells until you master this balancing act.

Cross your left leg behind your right to return to the starting position.

A

- Grab a pair of dumbbells and stand along the right side of a bench.
- Place your right foot on the bench by crossing it in front of your left leg.

REPS: Do 12 with each leg.

B

- Press your right foot into the bench and push your body up until both legs are straight. (Your left leg will naturally move across the bench.)
- Lower yourself by crossing your left leg behind your right and bending your right leg. Do all the reps, then repeat the exercise starting with your left leg.

EXERCISE 2b
Elevated-Feet Inverted Row

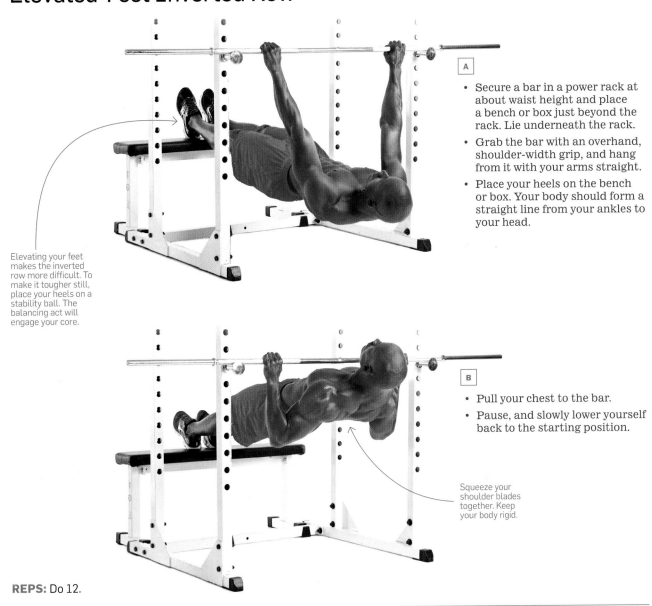

A

- Secure a bar in a power rack at about waist height and place a bench or box just beyond the rack. Lie underneath the rack.
- Grab the bar with an overhand, shoulder-width grip, and hang from it with your arms straight.
- Place your heels on the bench or box. Your body should form a straight line from your ankles to your head.

Elevating your feet makes the inverted row more difficult. To make it tougher still, place your heels on a stability ball. The balancing act will engage your core.

B

- Pull your chest to the bar.
- Pause, and slowly lower yourself back to the starting position.

Squeeze your shoulder blades together. Keep your body rigid.

REPS: Do 12.

You're Melting: Workout A

Barbell Front Squat

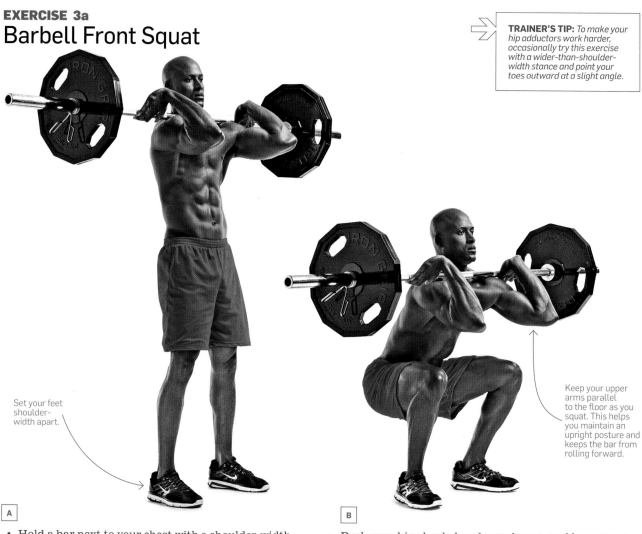

TRAINER'S TIP: *To make your hip adductors work harder, occasionally try this exercise with a wider-than-shoulder-width stance and point your toes outward at a slight angle.*

Set your feet shoulder-width apart.

Keep your upper arms parallel to the floor as you squat. This helps you maintain an upright posture and keeps the bar from rolling forward.

A

- Hold a bar next to your chest with a shoulder-width, overhand grip.
- Raise your upper arms until they're parallel to the floor, letting the bar roll back so that it's resting on the front of your shoulders.
- Engage your core and keep your back naturally arched.

REPS: Do 12.

B

- Push your hips back, bend your knees, and lower your body until the tops of your thighs are at least parallel to the floor.
- Pause, then drive your heels into the floor to push yourself back up to the starting position.

EXERCISE 3b
Pushup

Throughout the exercise, brace your abs as if you're expecting to be punched in the belly. This helps keep your hips from sagging and your body rigid.

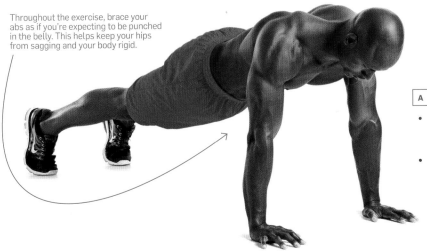

A

- Assume a pushup position with your arms straight and your hands slightly beyond shoulder width.
- Your body should form a straight line from your head to your ankles.

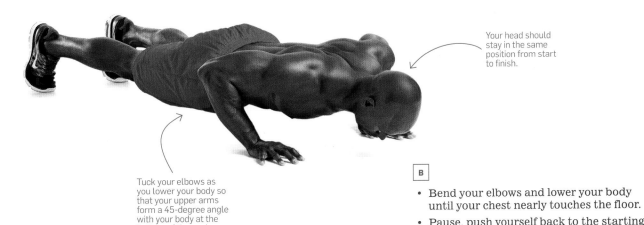

Your head should stay in the same position from start to finish.

Tuck your elbows as you lower your body so that your upper arms form a 45-degree angle with your body at the bottom of the pushup.

B

- Bend your elbows and lower your body until your chest nearly touches the floor.
- Pause, push yourself back to the starting position, and repeat.

REPS: Do 12.

You're Melting: Workout B

START HERE:
Perform two sets of exercise 1, resting for 60 seconds after each set. Then do exercises 2a and 2b as a pair, resting for 60 seconds after each set. Do two sets of exercises 2a and 2b. Follow the same sequence with exercises 3a and 3b.

EXERCISE 1

Cable Core Press

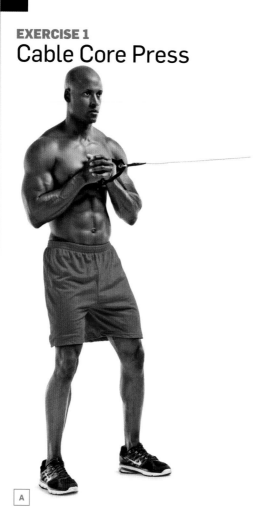

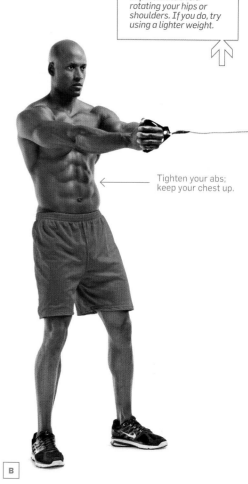

TRAINER'S TIP: *It's important to avoid rotating your hips or shoulders. If you do, try using a lighter weight.*

Tighten your abs; keep your chest up.

A

- Attach a stirrup handle to the middle pulley of a cable station.
- Stand with your left side facing the weight stack.
- Step back so the cable is taut. Hold the handle against your chest.

REPS: Do 10 on each side.

B

- Slowly press your arms forward until they're completely straight.
- Pause for 5 seconds, and reverse the movement.
- Do all your reps slowly and then turn around and work your other side.

EXERCISE 2a
Offset Reverse Dumbbell Lunge

EXERCISE 2b
Chinup

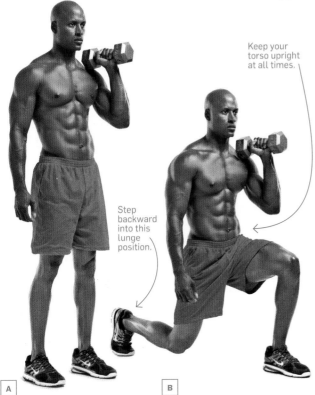

Keep your torso upright at all times.

Step backward into this lunge position.

A

B

- Stand holding a dumb-bell in your left hand next to your shoulder.
- Keep your torso straight; don't lean.

- Step backward with your right foot into a reverse lunge and lower your body until your back knee almost touches the floor.
- Push yourself back to the starting position and repeat.
- Do all your reps, and then move the weight to your right hand and lunge backward with your left leg.

REPS: Do 12 with each leg.

A

B

- Grab a chinup bar with a shoulder-width, underhand grip and hang at arm's length.

- Squeeze your shoulder blades down and back, bend your elbows, and pull the top of your chest to the bar.
- Pause, slowly lower your body back to the starting position, and repeat.

REPS: Do as many as you can but not more than 12.

You're Melting: Workout B

Zercher Good Morning

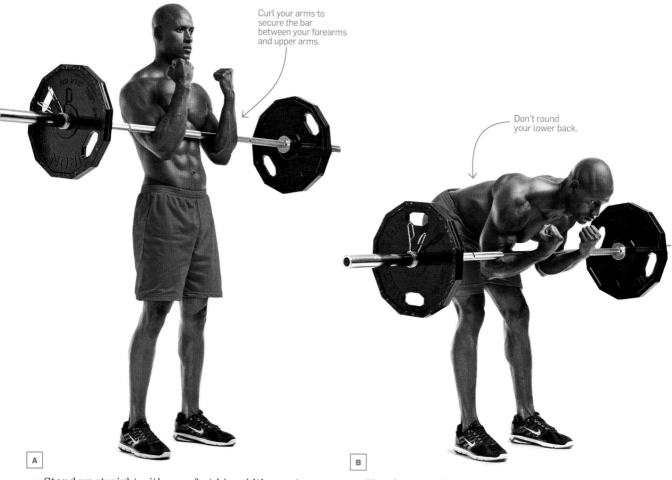

Curl your arms to secure the bar between your forearms and upper arms.

Don't round your lower back.

A

- Stand up straight with your feet hip-width apart and hold a barbell in the crooks of your bent arms. (You can use a bar pad or towel wrapped around the bar for cushioning.)

B

- Keeping your lower back naturally arched, bend forward at your hips as far as you comfortably can.
- Pause, then raise your torso back to the starting position.

REPS: Do 12.

EXERCISE 3b
Dumbbell Alternating Shoulder Press and Twist

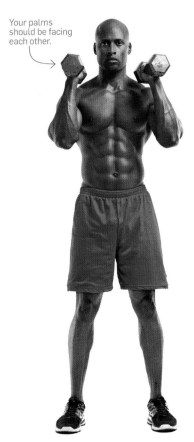

Your palms should be facing each other.

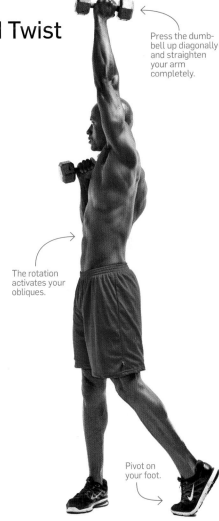

Press the dumbbell up diagonally and straighten your arm completely.

The rotation activates your obliques.

Pivot on your foot.

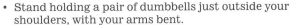

A

- Stand holding a pair of dumbbells just outside your shoulders, with your arms bent.
- Your feet should be shoulder-width apart and your knees slightly bent.

REPS: Do 12.

B

- Press the dumbbell in your left hand up at a slight diagonal to the right above your shoulder as you simultaneously rotate your torso to the right, pivoting on the ball of your left foot.
- Reverse the movement to the starting position, then rotate to your left and press the dumbbell in your right hand up. That's 1 rep.

Strength, Stamina, Speed, and Sweat

Like the average American, you're probably parked on your ass most of the workday. So why sit when you go to the gym to work out. Take a stand and fry fat instead. Stay away from benches and workout machines with seats. Instead, use this workout to keep moving, train your muscles in multiple directions, and accelerate fat loss.

START HERE: Perform the following four exercises as a circuit. Rest just 60 to 90 seconds between circuits. And keep doing as many circuits as you can in 15 minutes.

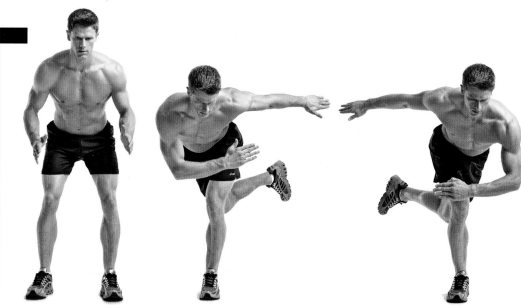

In-Place Heidens

- Assume an athletic stance with your hips pushed back and your knees slightly bent.

REPS: Do as many as you can in 30 seconds.

- Explosively hop off your right leg, swinging your arms and moving left.
- Stick the landing on your left foot, pause.

C
- Now push off your left foot and swing right, landing on your right foot without touching the floor with your left foot. Keep bounding back and forth.

Dumbbell Goblet Squat with Pulse

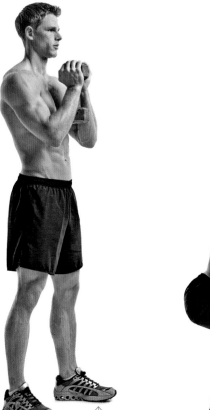

Angle your feet out slightly.

5

Percentage of U.S. adults who complete a challenging workout on any given day.

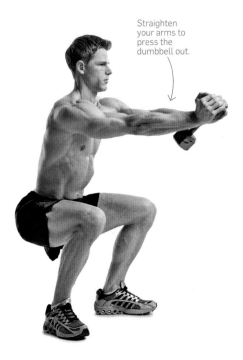

Straighten your arms to press the dumbbell out.

A

- Hold a dumbbell vertically at chest level, using both hands to cup one end. Your feet should be shoulder-width apart.

REPS: Do 8 to 10.

B

- Brace your abs and lower your body by pushing your hips back and bending your knees until your thighs are parallel with the floor.

C

- Pause, and press the weight in front of you until your arms are fully extended and parallel with the floor.

- Bring the weight back to your chest and stand. That's 1 rep.

93

Strength, Stamina, Speed, and Sweat

Spider-Man Pushup

A

- Assume a standard pushup position, with your body aligned from ankles to head.

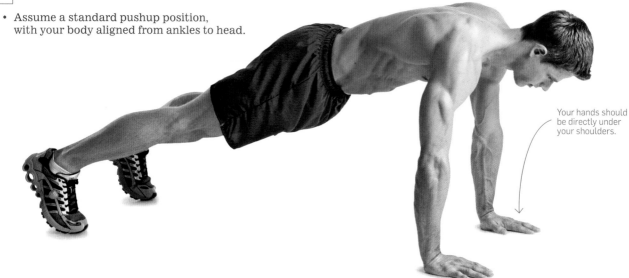

Your hands should be directly under your shoulders.

B

- As you lower your body toward the floor, lift your right foot, swing your right leg out sideways, and try to touch your elbow with your knee. Return to the starting position, and repeat with your left leg.

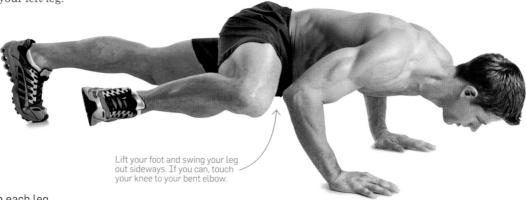

Lift your foot and swing your leg out sideways. If you can, touch your knee to your bent elbow.

REPS: Do 5 to 6 with each leg.

Bodysaw

- Place a towel on the floor and position your toes on it as you assume a plank position, with your forearms on the floor and your elbows directly underneath your shoulders.

TRAINER'S TIP: *If your hips sag, you've pushed out too far.*

B

- Brace your abs and squeeze your glutes, then "push" yourself back with your arms to slide the towel and your feet backward.

- You'll feel your core engage. Now, return to the starting position by pulling yourself forward. That's 1 rep.

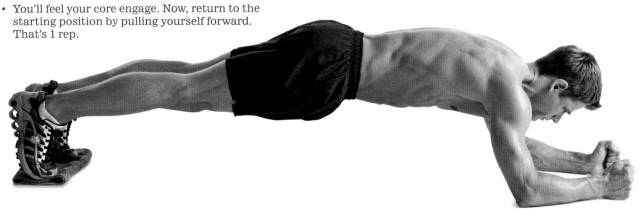

REPS: Do 8 to 10.

The Superhero Workout

You may never be able to leap tall buildings in a single bound, but you can look a lot more buff than George Reeves did as Superman in the 1950s TV show. Build Man-of-Steel muscles with these superhero-inspired exercises. They'll leave you in a pool of sweat, so take care to remove your cape before you get going.

START HERE: Perform two to three back-to-back sets of each exercise in this routine. Rest for 30 to 60 seconds between sets.

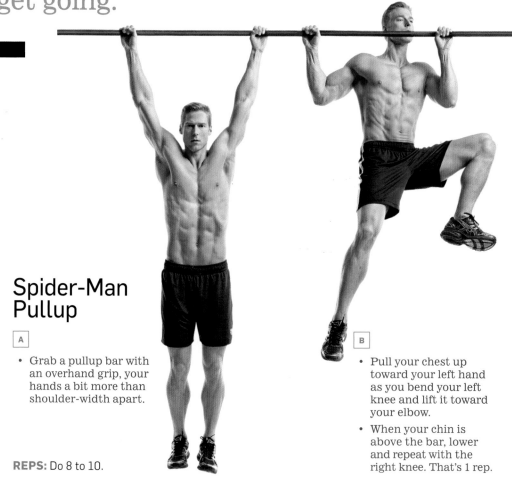

Spider-Man Pullup

A

- Grab a pullup bar with an overhand grip, your hands a bit more than shoulder-width apart.

REPS: Do 8 to 10.

B

- Pull your chest up toward your left hand as you bend your left knee and lift it toward your elbow.
- When your chin is above the bar, lower and repeat with the right knee. That's 1 rep.

Hulk Super Leap

 A

- Stand on a thick exercise mat with your feet spread wider than your shoulders.
- Bend at the hips and knees to quickly lower your body about halfway into a squat position.

 B

- Swing your arms overhead as you explode upward, jumping as high as you can.
- Land as softly as possible and then immediately drop down to the half-squat position and repeat.

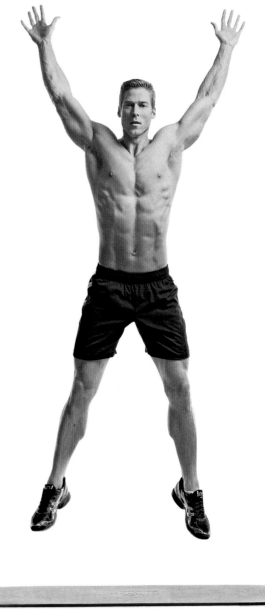

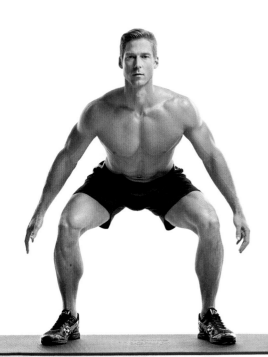

REPS: Do 8 to 10.

The Superhero Workout

Superman Back Extension

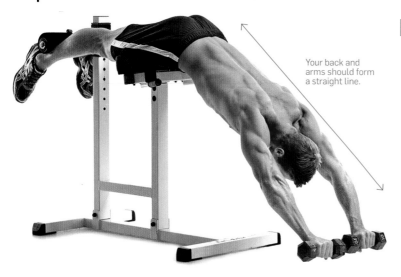

Your back and arms should form a straight line.

A

- Lie facedown at the back-extension station with your feet anchored.
- Hold a pair of dumbbells with your arms hanging down.
- Bend at the waist to allow your head to lower toward the floor.

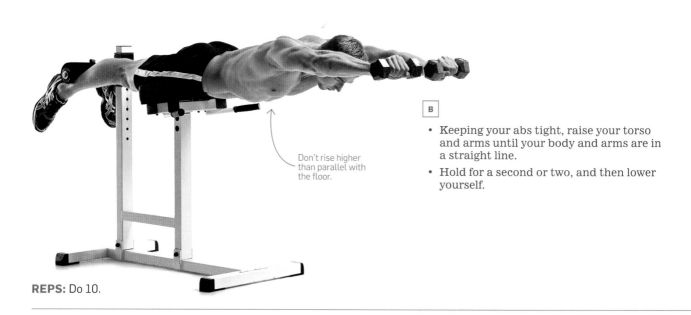

Don't rise higher than parallel with the floor.

B

- Keeping your abs tight, raise your torso and arms until your body and arms are in a straight line.
- Hold for a second or two, and then lower yourself.

REPS: Do 10.

Thor's Hammer

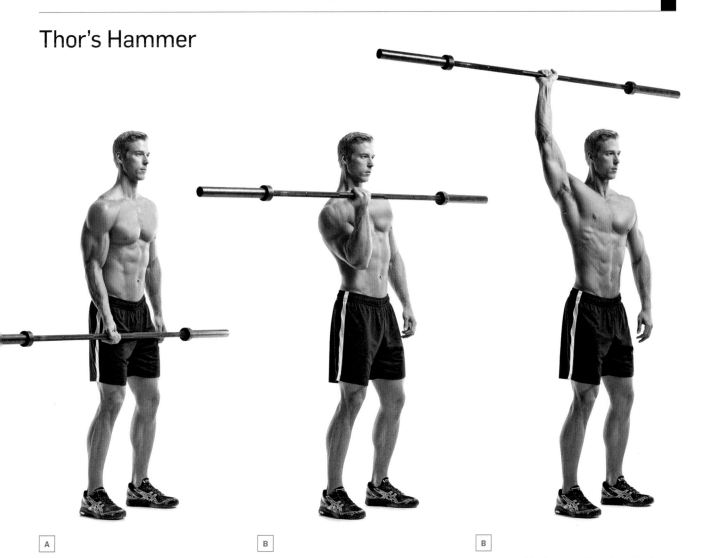

A
- Grab the center of a barbell with your right hand, palm facing up; hold it in front of your thighs.

REPS: Do 6 to 10 on each side.

B
- Curl the bar toward your shoulder.

B
- Press the bar overhead and rotate your palm so it faces forward at the top.
- Stretch and push the weight as high as you can.
- Lower the bar, switch arms, and repeat.

The Supersweat Supersets

A "superset" is when you do two exercises in a row with no rest in between. Often a superset pairs exercises that work opposing muscle groups so one body part rests while the other works. But in this three-superset series, we pair moves that hit the same muscles in very different ways to create a rigorous workout for extreme calorie burning.

START HERE:
Do 6 repetitions of each of the two exercises in each superset without resting between moves. After completing a superset, rest for 2 minutes before moving on to the next one.

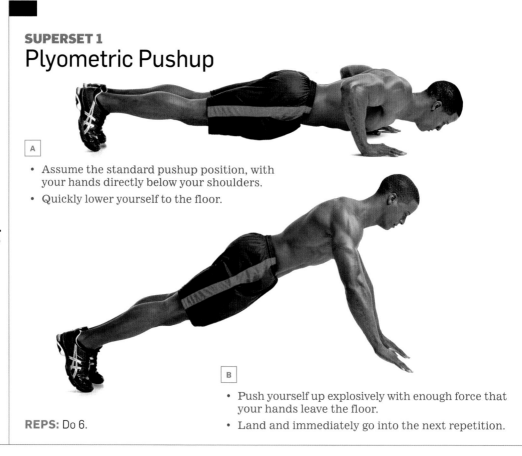

SUPERSET 1
Plyometric Pushup

A
- Assume the standard pushup position, with your hands directly below your shoulders.
- Quickly lower yourself to the floor.

B
- Push yourself up explosively with enough force that your hands leave the floor.
- Land and immediately go into the next repetition.

REPS: Do 6.

Dumbbell Bench Press

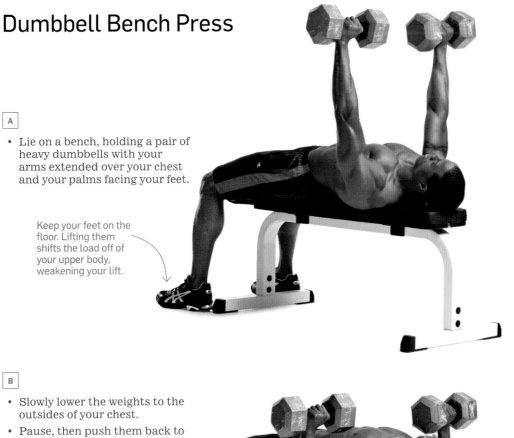

A

- Lie on a bench, holding a pair of heavy dumbbells with your arms extended over your chest and your palms facing your feet.

Keep your feet on the floor. Lifting them shifts the load off of your upper body, weakening your lift.

BENCH BETTER

During the lowering part of bench pressing with either a barbell or dumbbells, squeeze your shoulder blades together. This will help you build upper-body energy so that you can press the bar up with more force, says Craig Rasmussen, CSCS, a fitness coach at Results Fitness in Santa Clarita, California. "As you pull the weight down, lift your chest to meet the barbell," he says. "This will aid your efforts to create a springlike effect when you start to push the bar back up."

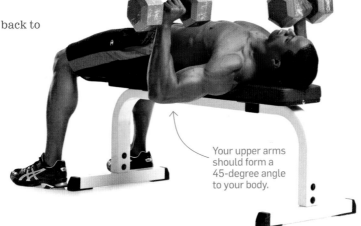

B

- Slowly lower the weights to the outsides of your chest.
- Pause, then push them back to the starting position.

Your upper arms should form a 45-degree angle to your body.

REPS: Do 6.

101

The Supersweat Supersets

Explosive Stepup

Alternating Dumbbell Stepup

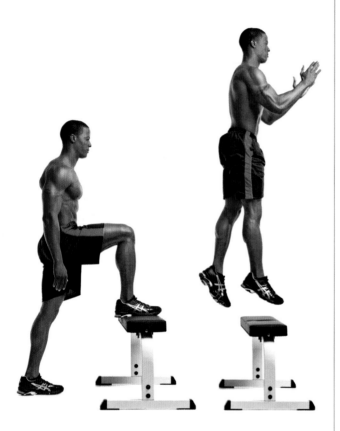

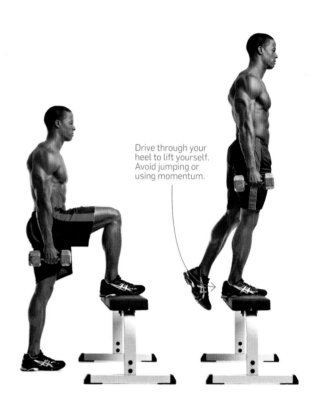

Drive through your heel to lift yourself. Avoid jumping or using momentum.

A

- Stand with your right foot on a sturdy step or bench and your left foot flat on the floor.

REPS: Do 6, alternating feet.

B

- Keeping your torso upright, push hard off the bench to thrust yourself into the air.
- Cycle your legs so your left foot lands softly on the bench and your right foot lands on the floor.

A

- Holding dumbbells at your sides, palms facing in, stand with a bench in front of you.
- Place your right foot on the bench.

REPS: Do 6.

B

- Step up, with your left foot hanging off the bench, then back down.
- Repeat, this time stepping up with the left foot. That's 1 rep.

SUPERSET 3

V-Up

 A

- Lie on the floor with your legs straight and your arms extended behind your head.

B

- Contract your abs to lift your torso and arms off the floor as you bring your legs toward you.

- Touch your toes with your hands at the top of the movement if you can, then return to the starting position.

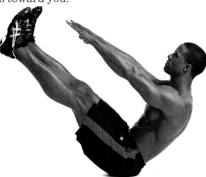

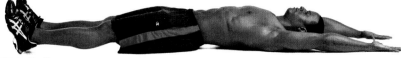

REPS: Do 6.

Weighted Stability Ball Situp

A

- Lie back on a stability ball, holding a dumbbell with both hands against your chest.

You should be supported by the ball from your hips to your shoulder blades.

B

- Curl up, stopping just short of upright. Slowly lower yourself to the starting position.

Engage your abs to lift yourself. Avoid using momentum.

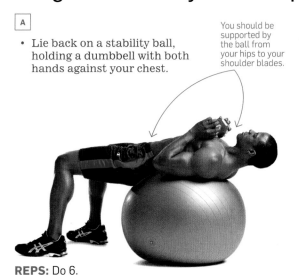

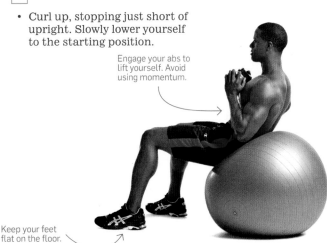

Keep your feet flat on the floor.

REPS: Do 6.

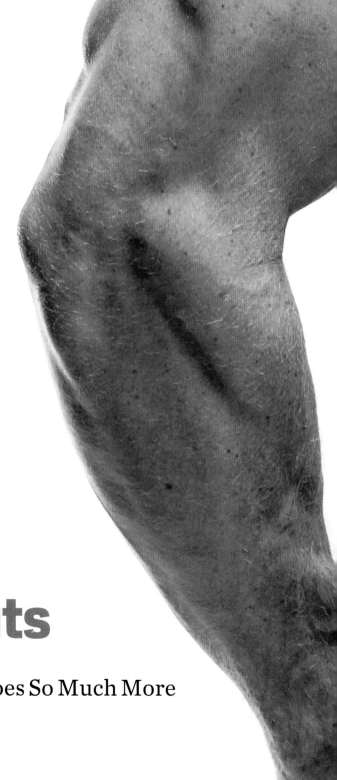

Chapter 6:
15-Minute Abs & Core Workouts

Flatten, Shape, and Strengthen
the Critical Muscle Group That Does So Much More
Than Look Good Shirtless.

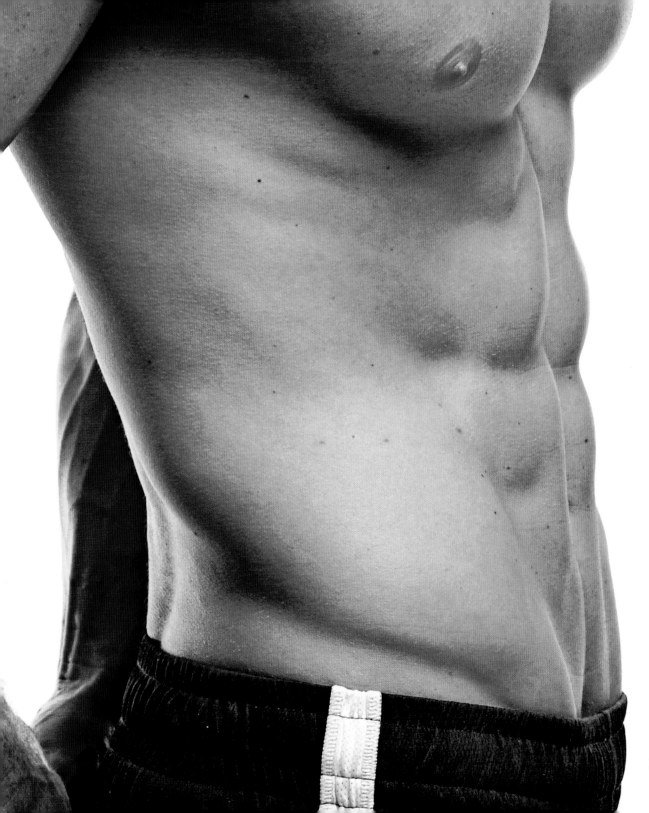

105

Superfast Exercises for Your Abs

Everybody wants a flat belly, one that doesn't jiggle and ooze out over the belt line. A lean, hard waist is a badge that says you pay attention to what you eat and you keep fit. You're disciplined, responsible, and healthy, three things women tend to look for in a guy. But beyond vanity and attraction, there are many other reasons to shore up your core. Like a hub on a bicycle wheel, your core is critical to the strength and stability of your entire body. If your core is weak, you are weak.

Renowned fitness coach Mark Verstegen, author of *Core Performance*, says strengthening your abs and all the back and oblique muscles that support your spine is like giving yourself a full-body makeover. It will make you feel younger, stronger, even smarter:

• The stronger your core, the taller and leaner you will look because this muscular scaffolding holds in your belly and lengthens your skeleton.

• Working the deep abdominal muscles and supporting muscles running up and down the spine creates a corset-like brace that prevents back injuries.

• A well-tuned core improves reaction speed and even mental function. Since your spine is the messenger between body and brain, having a stable and aligned spine allows your brain to receive messages more efficiently, says Verstegen.

For these reasons and many more, this may be the most important chapter in this book. Your core deserves your focused effort. The best news is that it requires only 15 minutes of your time.

Find It Quick: Your 15-Minute Abs and Core Circuits

ABS ANATOMY LESSON

Your core, the girdle of muscles that stabilize the spine, is made up of more than 2 dozen muscles. Get to know the key players:

Rectus abdomins: The six-pack muscles in front of your belly that are activated when you do crunches

Transverse abdominis: Deep muscles under the six-pack that pull your abdominal wall inward

Obliques: The abs muscles on the sides of your torso that help you bend to the side and resist rotation

Hip flexors: The muscles that allow you to flex your hips and lift your upper legs to walk and run are essential for core strength

Lower back: The many muscles here play a critical role in core mechanics by keeping your spine stable when you bend backward

The No-Crunch Core Workout

Some gluttons for punishment love crunches. Most normal people don't, and that's okay because you don't need them to build great abs. Crunches work only a small part of the abs. This workout, however, engages your entire core, plus your back and butt because slouchy shoulders and weak glutes contribute to a bulging belly.

START HERE:
Do these moves back-to-back with no rest between them. When you finish the first circuit, catch your breath, then do another.

Reverse Wood Chop

- Hold a medicine ball in both hands next to your left hip and bend your knees slightly.

B

- Keeping your arms straight, raise the ball up and across your body until you're standing straight and the ball is above your right shoulder. Lower back to the starting position. That's 1 rep.

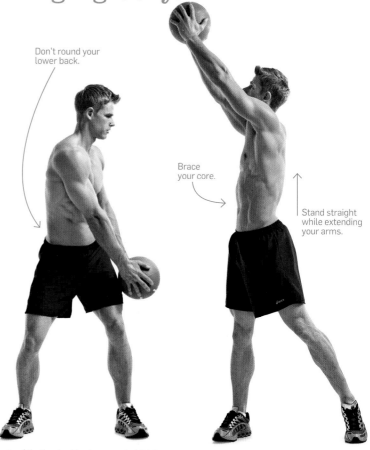

Don't round your lower back.

Brace your core.

Stand straight while extending your arms.

REPS: Do 10, then repeat with the ball at your right hip.

Single-Arm Lunge

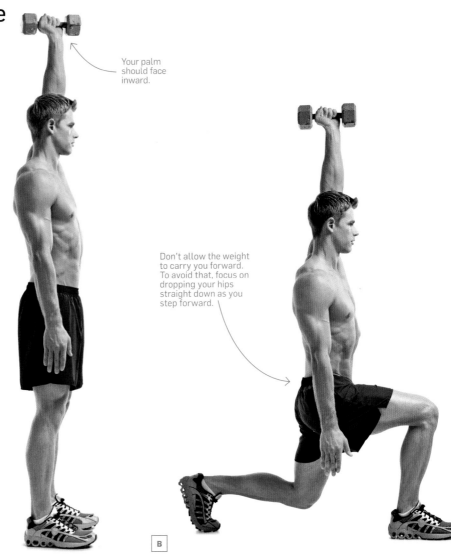

Your palm should face inward.

Don't allow the weight to carry you forward. To avoid that, focus on dropping your hips straight down as you step forward.

A

- Hold a dumbbell in your left hand and raise your left arm above your head. Keep your elbow close to your ear throughout the movement.

B

- Step forward with your right foot, lowering until the top of your thigh is parallel to the floor. Push off your left foot to stand. That's 1 rep.

REPS: Do 8 to 10, then hold the dumbbell in your right hand and lunge with your left leg.

The No-Crunch Core Workout

Reverse Plank with Leg Raise

A

- Sit on the floor with your legs
  outstretched and your hands behind
  your butt, fingers forward. Press
  onto your hands and raise your hips
  so your body forms a straight line
  from your heels to your head. This is
  a reverse plank.

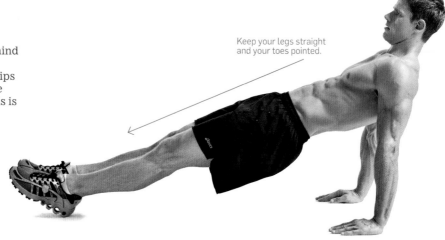

Keep your legs straight
and your toes pointed.

B

- Without lowering your hips, lift your
  right leg to at least 45 degrees.
  Hold for 3 seconds, then lower your
  leg and repeat.

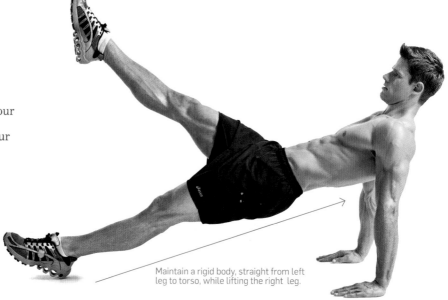

Maintain a rigid body, straight from left
leg to torso, while lifting the right leg.

REPS: Do 10 with each leg.

Single-Arm Bent-Over Row

Bend your knees slightly.

Don't rotate your torso as you row the weight.

A

- Hold a dumbbell in your right hand, bend your knees, and lean forward from your hips. Let the dumbbell hang naturally. Use a neutral grip, palm facing in. Lay your left hand on your lower back, palm up.

B

- Brace your abs and pull the weight up to chest height without rotating your torso. Return to the starting position. That's 1 rep.

REPS: Do 10 to 12, then repeat with the dumbbell in your left hand.

Half-Seated Leg Circle

A

- Sit on the floor with your legs fully extended and raise your feet a few inches off the ground.
- Lean back on your elbows, with your fingers near the sides of your hips.

B

- Keeping your lower back pressed into the floor, engage your core and lift your legs to about 45 degrees. Point your toes, press your thighs together, and trace large clockwise circles with your legs. Then trace circles counterclockwise.

Draw circles with your legs turning clockwise, then counterclockwise.

REPS: Do 12 in each direction.

The No-Crunch Core Workout

Rock 'n' Roll Core

A

- Assume a plank position with your straight body elevated between your toes and your forearms flat on the floor.

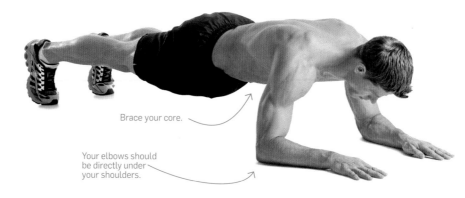

Brace your core.

Your elbows should be directly under your shoulders.

B

- Keeping your hands in place and using your feet as the pivot point, twist your body to the left as far as possible without losing your balance.

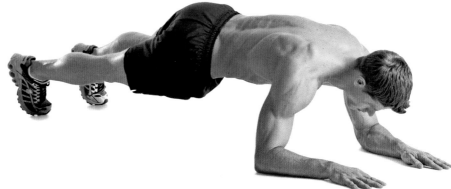

Don't change your lower-back posture as you twist your body.

C

- Twist your body to the right. Twisting in both directions equals 1 rep.

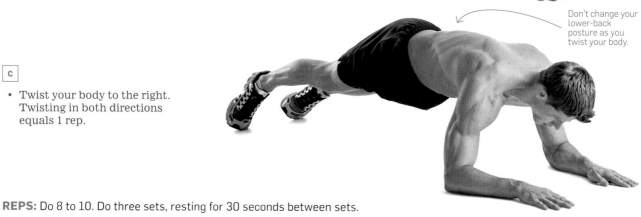

REPS: Do 8 to 10. Do three sets, resting for 30 seconds between sets.

Hammer Toss

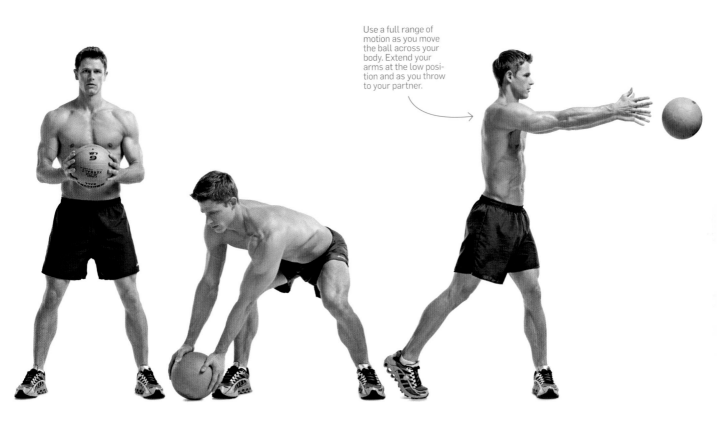

Use a full range of motion as you move the ball across your body. Extend your arms at the low position and as you throw to your partner.

A

- Grab a 5-pound medicine ball and stand with your feet shoulder-width apart, knees slightly bent.
- Hold the ball with both hands in front of your chest.

B

- Lower your hips and touch the ball to the floor outside your right foot.

C

- Stand up quickly, bringing the ball across the front of your body, and toss it to a partner, releasing to the left at about shoulder height.
- Have the partner toss it back. That's 1 rep.

REPS: Do 10, then repeat to the other side.

Six-Pack Abs Workout 1

The exercises here will appeal to those masochists who like the feeling of abs on fire. These two six-pack workouts are packed with all-star trunk flexion moves that target the rectus abdominis as well as the inner and outer obliques. This pair is for people who want washboards fast and are willing to put up with pain to get there. Enjoy!

START HERE:
Do the following six exercises as a circuit with no rest between moves. After completing the circuit, rest for 1 minute, then do another round.

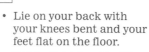

Long-Arm Weighted Crunch

- Lie on your back with your knees bent and your feet flat on the floor.
- Hold a light dumbbell in each hand and extend your arms straight back beyond your head.

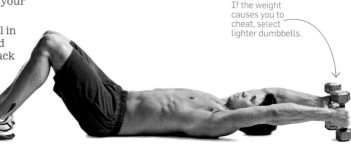

If the weight causes you to cheat, select lighter dumbbells.

B

- Now crunch your rib cage toward your pelvis, keeping your shoulders still and your arms straight.
- Don't generate momentum with your arms.

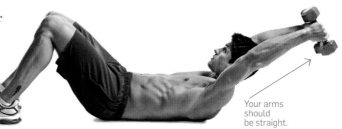

Your arms should be straight.

REPS: Do 12 to 15.

Seated Abs Crunch

A

- Sit on the edge of a bench. Grip the edge of the pad and lean back slightly, extending your legs down and away and keeping your heels off the floor.

B

- Bend your knees and slowly raise your legs toward your chest. At the same time, lean forward with your upper body, allowing your chest to approach your thighs.
- Return to the starting position.

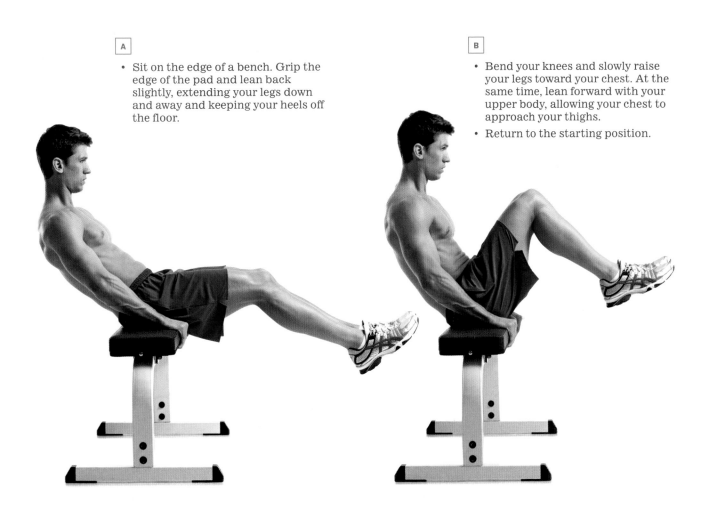

REPS: Do 12 to 15.

Six-Pack Abs Workout 1

Medicine-Ball Leg Drops

A

- Lie faceup on the floor and squeeze a light medicine ball between your ankles.
- Keep your legs nearly straight and hold them directly above your hips.

You can use a basketball instead if the medicine ball is too heavy.

Keep the same bend in your knees from start to finish.

Brace your core.

B

- Allow your legs to drop straight down as far as possible without touching the floor.
- In the same motion, return your legs to the starting position as fast as possible. That's 1 rep.

At this position, it should feel as if you're "throwing on the brakes."

REPS: Do 10 to 12.

Weighted One-Sided Crunch

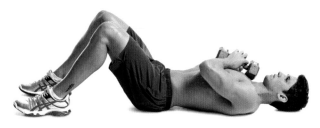

A

- Lie on your back with your knees bent and your feet flat on the floor, and hold a dumbbell with both hands by your right shoulder.

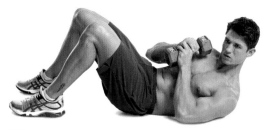

B

- Curl your torso up and rotate to the left.
- Lower yourself, finish the set on that side, then switch directions and repeat, holding the dumbbell next to your left shoulder.

REPS: Do 8 to 10 on each side.

Kneeling Cable Crunch

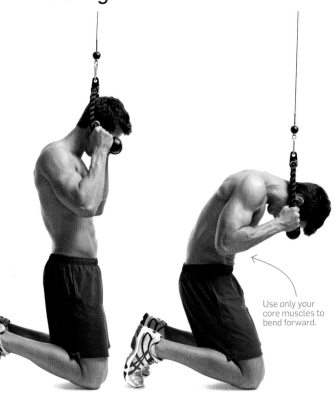

Use only your core muscles to bend forward.

A

- Kneel facing the pulley of a cable machine that has a rope attached to the high cable. Hold the ends of the rope along the sides of your face.

B

- Crunch forward, aiming your chest at your pelvis.
- Return to the starting position, then repeat the movement, this time aiming your chest toward your left knee.
- Return, then repeat to your right. That's 1 rep.

REPS: Do 8 to 10.

Crunch/Side-Bend Combo

A

- Lie on your back with your knees bent, feet on the floor, and hands behind your ears.
- Curl up so your shoulder blades are off the floor.

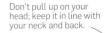

Don't pull up on your head; keep it in line with your neck and back.

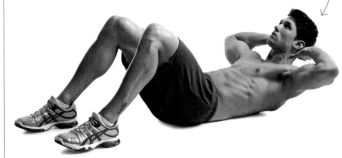

B

- Bend at the waist to your left, aiming your left armpit toward your left hip.
- Straighten, then bend to your right. That's 1 rep.
- Lower yourself to the starting position and repeat.

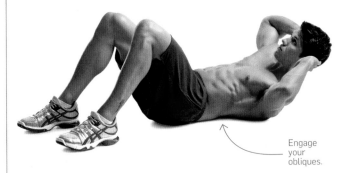

Engage your obliques.

REPS: Do 8 to 10.

117

Six-Pack Abs Workout 2

START HERE:
Do the following five exercises as a circuit with no rest between moves. After completing the circuit, rest for 1 minute, then do another round.

Stability Ball Pike

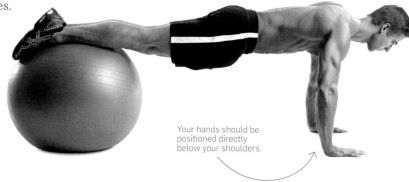

A

- Assume a pushup position with your arms completely straight underneath your shoulders.
- Rest your shins on a stability ball, so that your body forms a straight line from your head to your ankles.

Your hands should be positioned directly below your shoulders.

 B

- Without bending your knees, roll the stability ball toward your body by raising your hips as high as you can.
- Pause, then return the ball to the starting position by lowering your hips and rolling the ball backward.

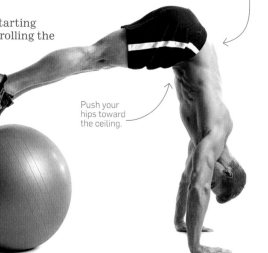

Don't round your lower back.

Push your hips toward the ceiling.

REPS: Do 8 to 10.

Reverse Crunch

A

- Lie faceup on an incline situp bench.
- Hold a foam roller between your calves and hamstrings to help keep your legs in proper position.
- Grasp the bench behind your head for leverage.

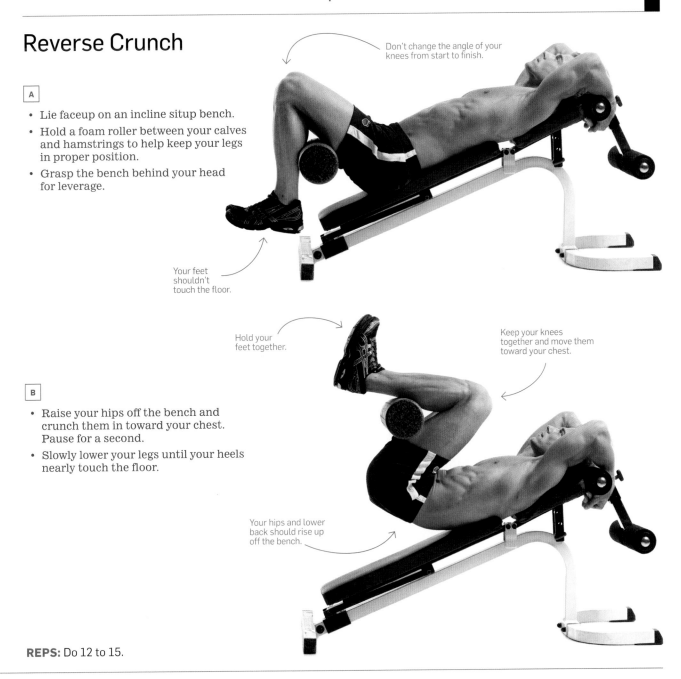

Don't change the angle of your knees from start to finish.

Your feet shouldn't touch the floor.

Hold your feet together.

Keep your knees together and move them toward your chest.

B

- Raise your hips off the bench and crunch them in toward your chest. Pause for a second.
- Slowly lower your legs until your heels nearly touch the floor.

Your hips and lower back should rise up off the bench.

REPS: Do 12 to 15.

119

Six-Pack Abs Workout 2

Stability Ball Leg Curl

A

- Lie on your back on the floor with your calves resting on a stability ball and your arms at your sides.
- Squeeze your glutes to raise your hips off the floor so your body is in a straight line from your shoulders to your ankles.

B

- Pause for a second, and then bend your legs and roll the ball toward your butt.
- Straighten your legs to roll the ball back out away from you, and then lower your body to the floor. That's 1 rep.

REPS: Do 10 to 12.

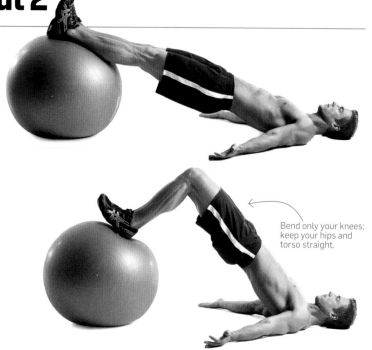

Bend only your knees; keep your hips and torso straight.

Prone Cobra

A

- Lie facedown on the floor with your legs straight and your arms next to your sides, palms down.
- Contract your glutes and the muscles of your lower back, and raise your head, chest, arms, and legs off the floor.
- Simultaneously rotate your arms so that your thumbs point toward the ceiling.
- At this time, your hips should be the only parts of your body touching the floor.

REPS: Do 1 for 60 seconds.

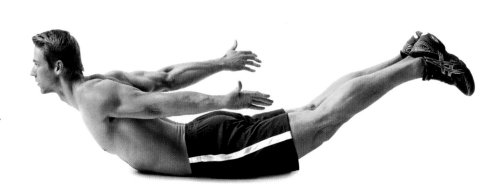

Hanging Leg Raise

Don't lean back as you raise your legs. Use your abs and hip flexors to squeeze your knees to your chest.

A

- Grab a chinup bar with an overhand, shoulder-width grip (or use elbow supports, if available), and hang from the bar with your knees slightly bent and your feet together.

B

- Simultaneously bend your knees, raise your hips, and curl your lower back underneath you as you lift your thighs toward your chest.

- Pause when the fronts of your thighs reach your chest, and then slowly lower your legs back to the starting position.

REPS: Do 8 to 10.

The Obliques Obliterator Workout

Despite their kind of cutesy name, love handles are doughy side overhangs that can wreck the trim-looking lines of guys who otherwise have admirably flat guts. This routine is designed to tone and strengthen your obliques—the muscles on the sides of your torso that help you bend and rotate—for a tight midsection all the way around.

START HERE:
Perform these moves as a circuit with no breaks between exercises. After finishing the circuit, rest for 1 minute, then do one more.

Oblique V-Up

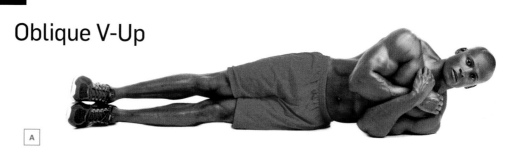

A

- Lie on your side with your body in a straight line.
- Fold your arms across your chest.

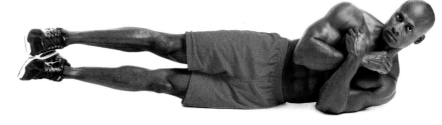

B

- Keeping your legs together, lift them off the floor as you raise your top elbow toward your hip.
- The range of motion is short, but you should feel an intense contraction in your obliques.

REPS: Do 10 on each side of your body.

Saxon Side Bend

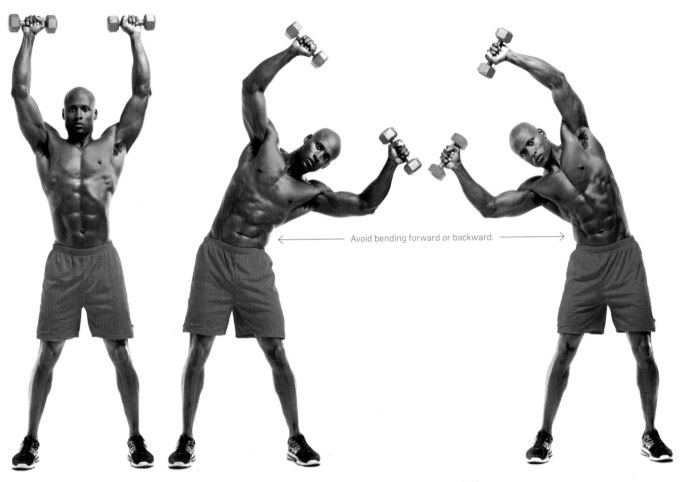

Avoid bending forward or backward.

A
- Hold a pair of lightweight dumbbells over your head, in line with your shoulders, with your elbows slightly bent.

REPS: Do 10 per side.

B
- Keep your back straight, and slowly bend directly to your left side as far as possible without twisting your upper body.

C
- Pause, return to an upright position, then bend to your right side as far as possible.

The Obliques Obliterator Workout

Speed Rotation

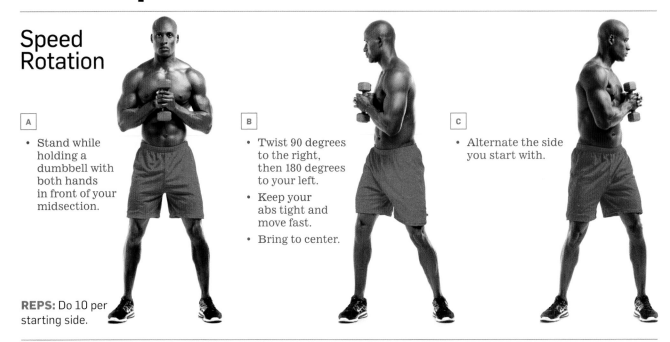

A
- Stand while holding a dumbbell with both hands in front of your midsection.

B
- Twist 90 degrees to the right, then 180 degrees to your left.
- Keep your abs tight and move fast.
- Bring to center.

C
- Alternate the side you start with.

REPS: Do 10 per starting side.

Medicine Ball Torso Rotation

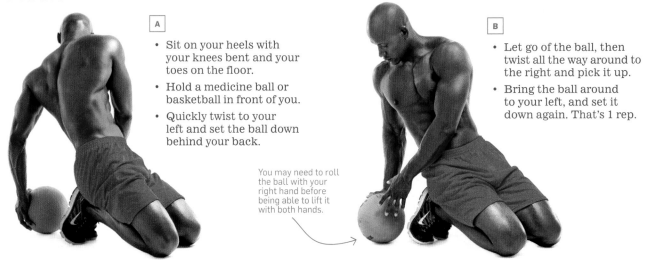

A
- Sit on your heels with your knees bent and your toes on the floor.
- Hold a medicine ball or basketball in front of you.
- Quickly twist to your left and set the ball down behind your back.

You may need to roll the ball with your right hand before being able to lift it with both hands.

B
- Let go of the ball, then twist all the way around to the right and pick it up.
- Bring the ball around to your left, and set it down again. That's 1 rep.

REPS: Do 10 to each side.

Two-Handed Wood Chop

- Grab a dumbbell and hold it with both hands above your right shoulder.
- Rotate your torso to your right. You can pivot on your left foot if you wish.

B

- Flex your abs and swing the dumbbell down and to the outside of your left thigh, bending at your hips.
- Reverse the movement to return to the start, finish the set, and repeat on the other side.

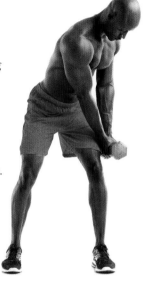

REPS: Do 10 on each side.

Side Jackknife

- Lie on your left side on the floor and stack your feet. Place your right hand on the back of your head.
- Raise your torso by propping yourself up on your left elbow and forearm beneath your shoulder.

B

- Lift your legs toward your torso while keeping your torso stationary.
- Pause to feel the contraction on the right side of your waist.
- Then slowly lower your legs and repeat.

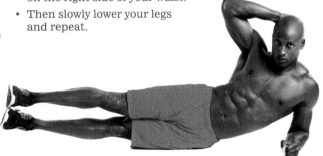

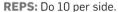

REPS: Do 10 per side.

Build Your Own 15-Minute Core Workout

We know how it is. Sometimes you want a no-brainer workout—just follow the directions and get on with your day. But other times you want to call the shots and do your own thing. That's why we provided this DIY workout. Below, you'll find 19 more belly-blasting, core-building moves. Mix and match to create your own core circuit.

START HERE: ▄▄
Choose any five core exercises on the following pages. Do them circuit style, moving from one exercise to the next with no rest. Recover for 1 minute, then repeat the circuit twice more.

Side Bridge

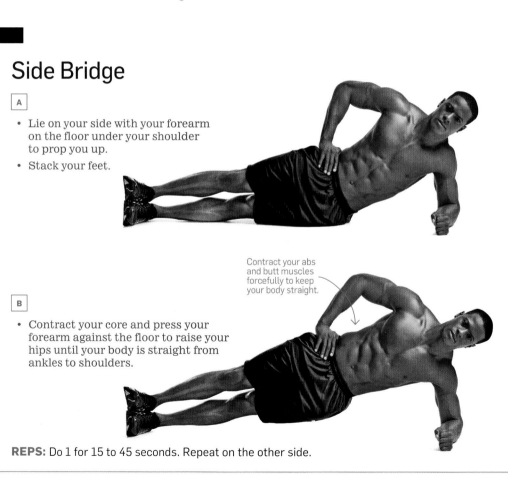

A
- Lie on your side with your forearm on the floor under your shoulder to prop you up.
- Stack your feet.

Contract your abs and butt muscles forcefully to keep your body straight.

B
- Contract your core and press your forearm against the floor to raise your hips until your body is straight from ankles to shoulders.

REPS: Do 1 for 15 to 45 seconds. Repeat on the other side.

Plank with Diagonal Arm Lift

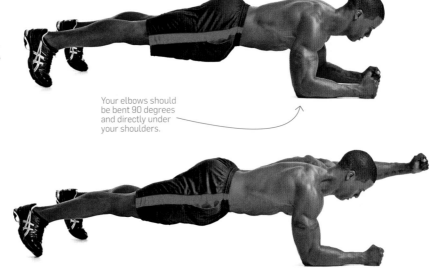

A

- Assume a modified pushup position with your feet shoulder-width apart, forearms on the floor.

B

- Keeping your torso steady, raise your right arm and point to the right, to 2 o'clock.
- Hold for 2 seconds, then lower and repeat with your left arm, raising it and pointing to 10 o'clock. That's 1 rep.

Your elbows should be bent 90 degrees and directly under your shoulders.

REPS: Do 6 to 8.

Single-Leg Lowering Drill

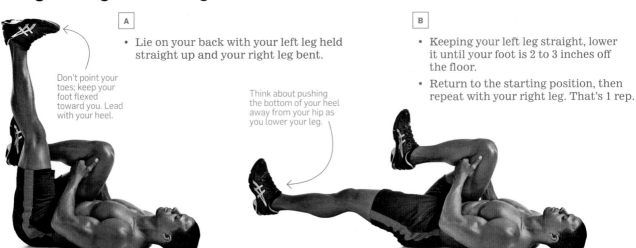

A

- Lie on your back with your left leg held straight up and your right leg bent.

Don't point your toes; keep your foot flexed toward you. Lead with your heel.

Think about pushing the bottom of your heel away from your hip as you lower your leg.

B

- Keeping your left leg straight, lower it until your foot is 2 to 3 inches off the floor.
- Return to the starting position, then repeat with your right leg. That's 1 rep.

REPS: Do 8 to 12.

Build Your Own 15-Minute Core Workout

Stability Ball Knee Tuck

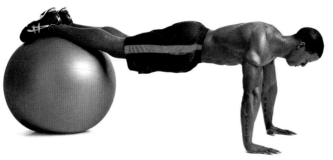

A

- Assume the pushup position with your shins resting on a stability ball, hands slightly more than shoulder-width apart.

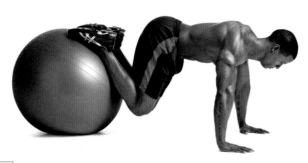

B

- Keeping your abs tight, draw your knees toward your chest until your toes are on top of the ball.
- Slowly straighten your legs so the ball rolls back to the starting position.

REPS: Do 8 to 12.

Glute Bridge March

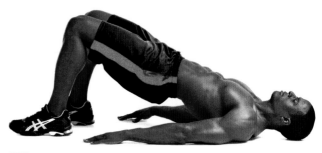

A

- Lie with your knees bent and your arms and heels on the floor.
- Push down through your heels and squeeze your glutes to raise your body into a straight line from your knees to your shoulders.

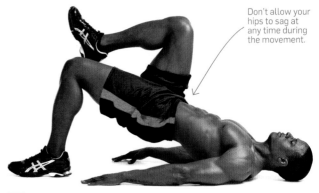

Don't allow your hips to sag at any time during the movement.

B

- Next, bring your right knee toward your chest.
- Reverse the move, then repeat with your left leg. That's 1 rep.

REPS: Do 8 to 10.

Prone Oblique Roll

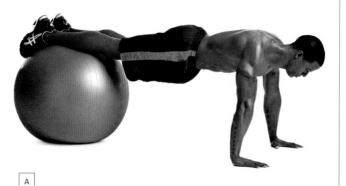

A

- Get in a plank position with your shins about hip-width apart on a stability ball and your hands shoulder-width apart on the floor.

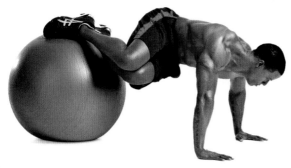

B

- Keeping your feet on the ball, draw your right knee toward your right shoulder (the left just comes along for the ride).
- Return to center, then draw your left knee toward your left shoulder. That's 1 rep.

REPS: Do 12 to 15.

Walk the Plank and Rotate

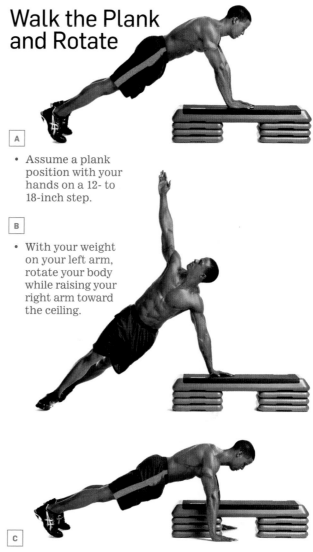

A

- Assume a plank position with your hands on a 12- to 18-inch step.

B

- With your weight on your left arm, rotate your body while raising your right arm toward the ceiling.

C

- Return to the plank position and step your right arm down to the right of the bench, then your left arm down to the left of the bench.
- Step back up, leading with your left arm. That's 1 rep.

REPS: Do 8 to 10 on each side.

Build Your Own 15-Minute Core Workout

Canoe

TRAINER'S TIP: *Grasp the handle of the dumbbell with one hand over the other. "Paddle" slowly, as if against the resistance of water, to gain the full benefit.*

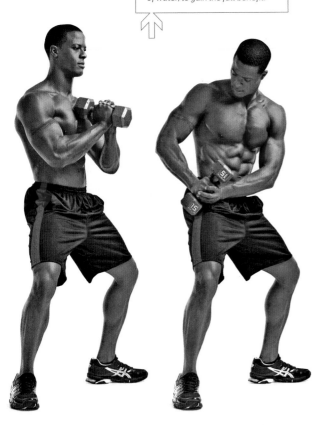

A

- Stand with your feet 3 feet apart, and with your knees slightly bent.
- Hold a dumbbell in front of your chest.

B

- Keeping your hips still, bring the dumbbell down to your right hip, stroking it backward like a canoe paddle.
- Return to the starting position and "paddle" to the left hip. That's 1 rep.

REPS: Do 10.

Alternating Dumbbell Row

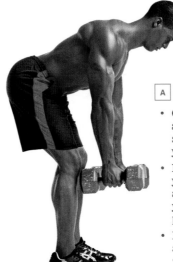

A

- Grab a pair of dumbbells and stand with your feet shoulder-width apart and your knees slightly bent.
- Bend at your hips, keeping your lower back naturally arched, and lower your torso until it's almost parallel to the floor.
- Let the dumbbells hang at arm's length from your shoulders.

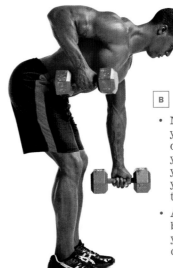

B

- Now pull the dumbbell in your right hand to the side of your torso by raising your upper arm, bending your elbow, and squeezing your shoulder blade toward your spine.
- As you lower that dumbbell, row the dumbbell in your left hand to the side of your torso. That's 1 rep.

REPS: Do 8 to 10.

130

Side Plank with Reach-Under Rotation

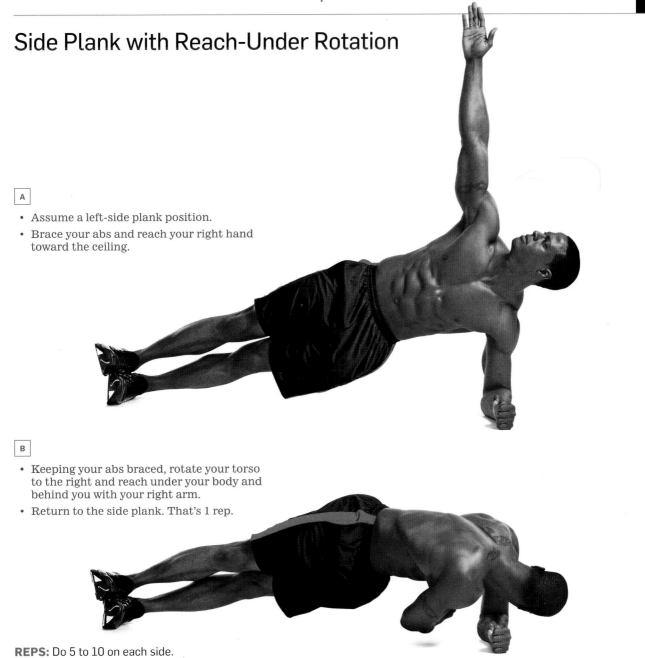

A

- Assume a left-side plank position.
- Brace your abs and reach your right hand toward the ceiling.

B

- Keeping your abs braced, rotate your torso to the right and reach under your body and behind you with your right arm.
- Return to the side plank. That's 1 rep.

REPS: Do 5 to 10 on each side.

Build Your Own 15-Minute Core Workout

Abs Chopper

A

- Lie on your back with your hands clasped beyond your head.

B

- Contract your abs and crunch up, bringing your hands over to the outside of your right thigh.
- Lower to the starting position and repeat to the left, alternating sides.

TRAINER'S TIP: *As you get stronger, grab a 3- to 5-pound dumbbell with both hands and do 12 reps per weighted set.*

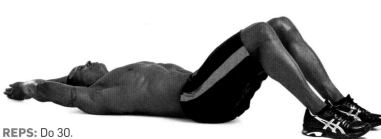

REPS: Do 30.

The Matrix

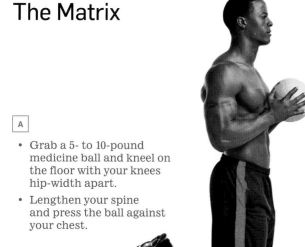

A

- Grab a 5- to 10-pound medicine ball and kneel on the floor with your knees hip-width apart.
- Lengthen your spine and press the ball against your chest.

B

- Slowly lean back as far as possible, keeping your knees planted.
- Hold the reclined position for 3 seconds, then use your core to slowly come up to the starting position.

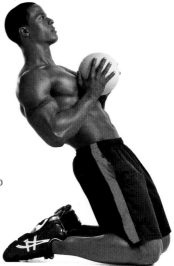

REPS: Do 12 to 15.

T-Stabilizer

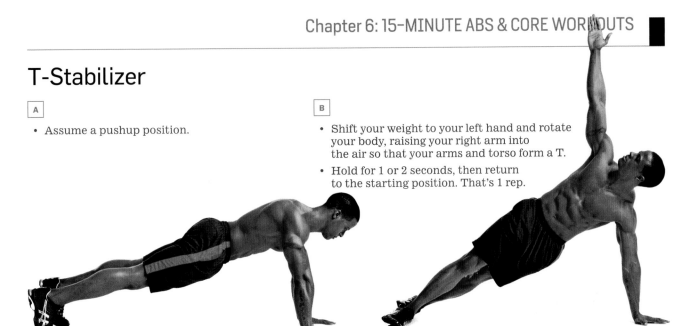

A

- Assume a pushup position.

B

- Shift your weight to your left hand and rotate your body, raising your right arm into the air so that your arms and torso form a T.
- Hold for 1 or 2 seconds, then return to the starting position. That's 1 rep.

REPS: Do 8 to 10.

Double-Leg Stretch

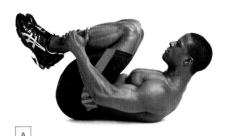

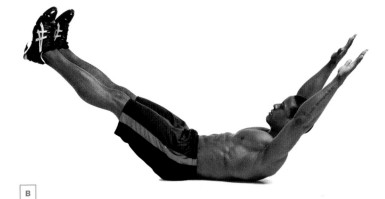

A

- Lie on the floor, bend your knees, hold onto your shins, and curl your shoulders up off the floor.

REPS: Do 5 to 10.

B

- Keeping your hips down and your lower back pressed into the floor, extend your legs up and out at a 45-degree angle to the floor as you reach your arms up (biceps near ears) to form a wide U shape with your body.
- Hold this position, pressing your ribs down toward the floor.
- Use your abs to bring your legs and arms back to the starting position.

Build Your Own 15-Minute Core Workout

Back Extension Leg Raise

A

- Rest your hips and belly on a stability ball.
- Straighten your legs and position your toes hip-width apart on the floor.
- Extend your arms in line with your shoulders.

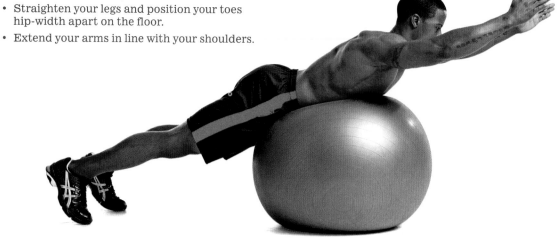

B

- Lift your right leg about 6 inches off the floor while reaching your arms as far out as possible. That's 1 rep.

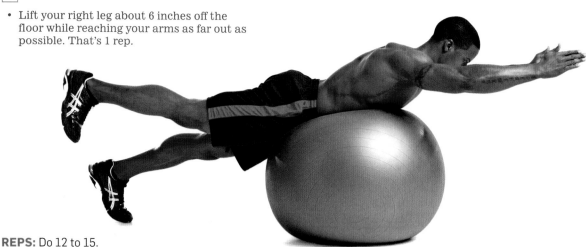

REPS: Do 12 to 15.

Stability Ball Plank Rocker

A

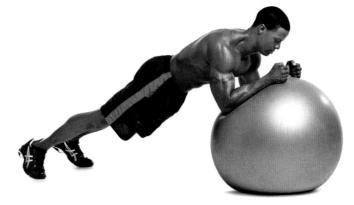

- Assume a plank position by leaning your forearms on a stability ball.
- Your body should form a straight line from your head to your ankles.

B

- Brace your core and push your arms forward, rolling the ball under your forearms. Pull your arms back in and repeat for 5 reps.

 TRAINER'S TIP: *A variation of this core exercise is Stirring the Pot. Instead of moving your arms forward, backward, and diagonally, you move your arms in a circular motion as if stirring a cauldron with both hands. Do five clockwise circles and five counterclockwise circles.*

C

- Now push and pull your arms first diagonally right, then left, rolling the ball underneath your forearms. That's 1 rep; repeat for 5 reps.

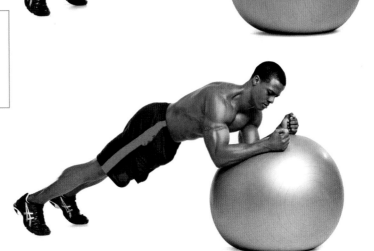

REPS: Do 5 in each direction.

Build Your Own 15-Minute Core Workout

Stability Ball Knee-Up

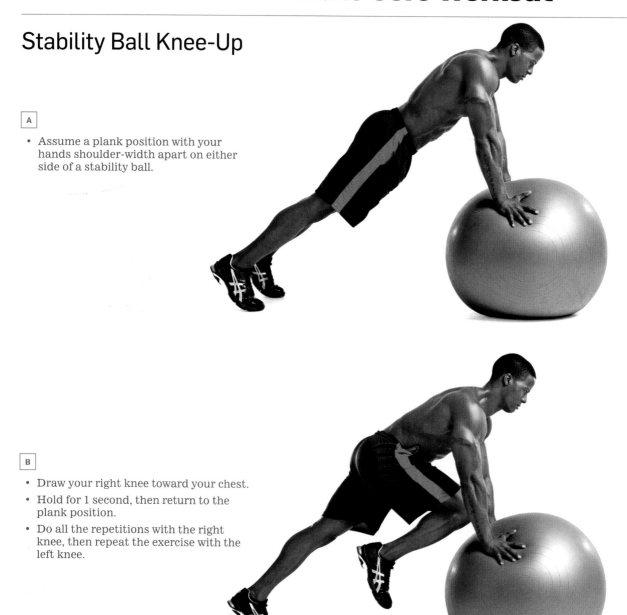

A

- Assume a plank position with your hands shoulder-width apart on either side of a stability ball.

B

- Draw your right knee toward your chest.
- Hold for 1 second, then return to the plank position.
- Do all the repetitions with the right knee, then repeat the exercise with the left knee.

REPS: Do 12 to 15 with each leg.

Arm Pull Over Straight-Leg Crunch

A

- Grab a pair of 10- to 12-pound dumbbells and lie on your back with your arms beyond your head.
- Raise your legs to a 45-degree angle.

B

- Bring your arms up over your chest and lift your shoulders off the mat while raising your legs until they're perpendicular to the floor.
- Return to the starting position (don't let your legs touch the floor).

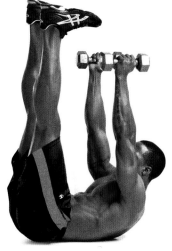

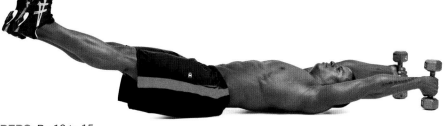

REPS: Do 12 to 15.

The Sprinter

A

- Lie on your back with your hands at your sides, legs straight, and heels hovering 6 to 12 inches off the floor.

B

- Start sitting up while elevating your right arm with the elbow bent so it resembles a sprinter's pumping motion.
- At the peak of the situp, bring your left knee to your chest.
- Return to the starting position, keeping your legs raised, and repeat with the opposite arm and leg.
- That's 1 rep.

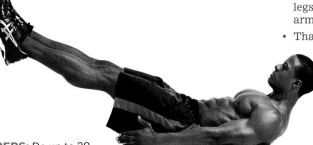

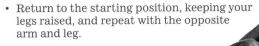

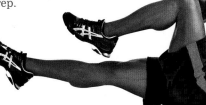

REPS: Do up to 20.

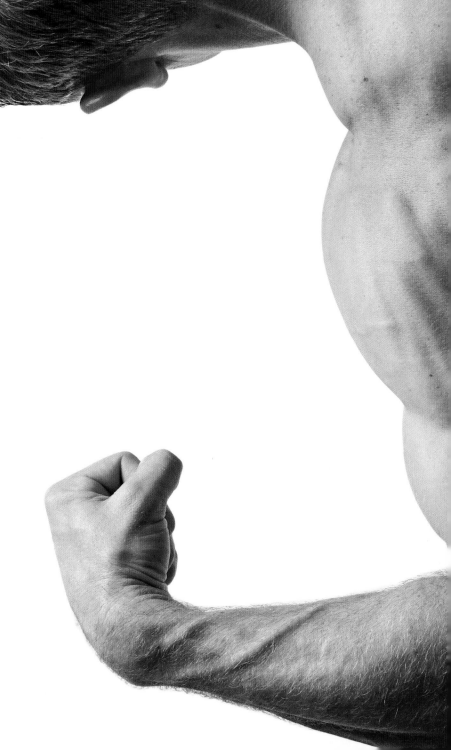

Chapter 7:
15-Minute Shoulders & Arms Workouts

Guns, Pythons, Pipes: Whatever You Call 'Em, These Programs will Build Their Mass Fast.

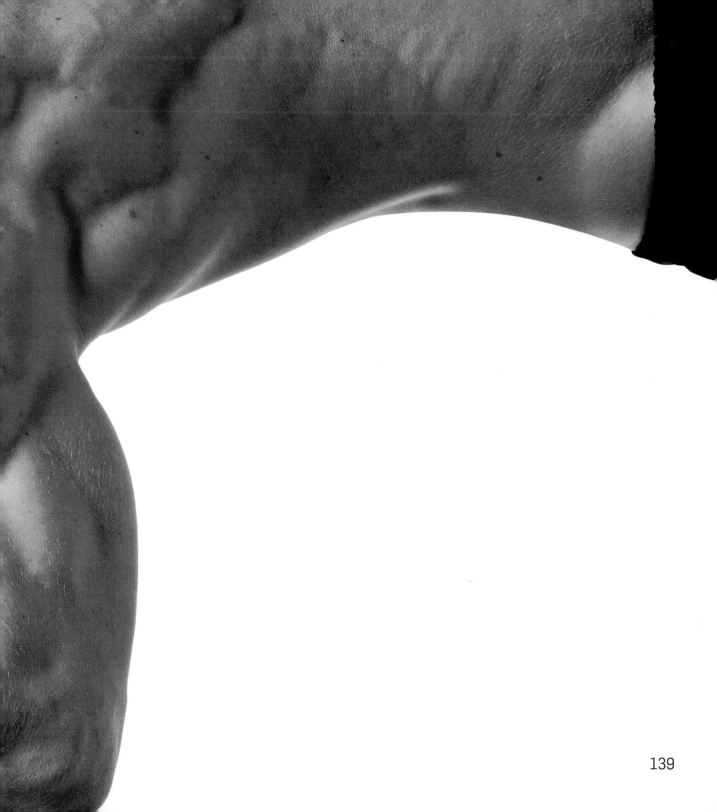

139

Build Arms & Shoulders Superfast

Your arms and shoulders make a big first impression. A well-defined upper body doesn't just look good on the beach or underneath a crisp white oxford. It also broadcasts strength and confidence anywhere, and may even make you a little bit taller. You see, the muscles of your upper back help pull your shoulders down and back so you stand up tall, instead of being slumped over like Quasimodo. As an added benefit, when your shoulders are naturally pulled back, your pecs become more pronounced. So you look and feel great whether you're buttoned down in an Armani three-piece or chilling in your favorite T-shirt.

The basics...

In this chapter you'll find workouts that tackle your triceps, biceps, shoulders, upper back and chest. For the best results, do one (or more) of the upper-body workouts, honing in on the areas you need the most help with, two days a week. You can do more, just be sure to leave a day of rest between workouts for recovery. (You can always piggyback any of these routines onto another 15-minute workout for when you have more time for a total-body workout.) Do the prescribed number of sets and reps for each exercise, opting for a weight at which you can barely squeeze out the last rep of your final set with perfect form.

Find It Quick: Your 15-Minute Arms and Shoulders Programs

DUMBBELLS OR DRUGS?

Building more muscle on your frame can help your body regulate blood sugar more efficiently. In a study, UCLA scientists found that people with low muscle mass were 67 percent more likely to be insulin resistant than their more muscular counterparts. Insulin resistance is a warning sign for type 2 diabetes.

Dumbbell Total Arms Workout

Dumbbells are made for arms and shoulders workouts because they allow you to do moves through a big range of motion. Every man should own at least two pairs of these versatile tools—a light pair for wrist and rotator cuff work and heavy for curls and presses. Hexagonal-head dumbbells are our favorite style because they don't roll on the floor (and they double as sledgehammers in a pinch).

The back-to-basics routine found on these pages hits your arms from hands to shoulders at every angle for deep definition. You'll get the best pump from these moves if you concentrate on perfect form.

START HERE: Do the exercises in this workout as a circuit, completing all reps of one move before jumping to the next exercise. Avoid resting between exercises if you can. After finishing the last exercise, recover for no more than 60 seconds, then repeat the circuit once more.

Concentration Curl

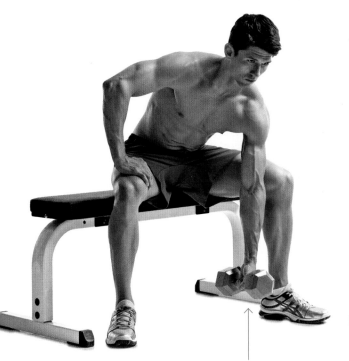

Let your arm hang completely straight. Keep your upper body motionless as you begin to curl.

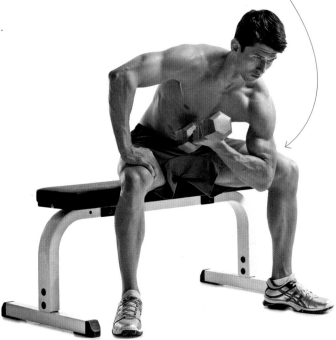

Keep your upper arm braced against your thigh as you slowly curl the weight to your shoulder.

A

- Sit on an exercise bench or a chair with your knees wider than shoulder-width apart and your feet flat on the floor.
- Grasp a dumbbell with your left hand, palm facing inward. Bend over slightly and rest the back of your upper left arm against your inner left thigh.
- Place your right hand on your right thigh or knee for support.

B

- Curl the dumbbell up toward your shoulder, keeping your upper left arm and elbow tucked against your inner thigh at all times.
- Lower the weight and repeat.

REPS: Do 8 to 12, then switch to the opposite side and curl with your right arm.

Dumbbell Total Arms Workout

Seated Triceps Extension

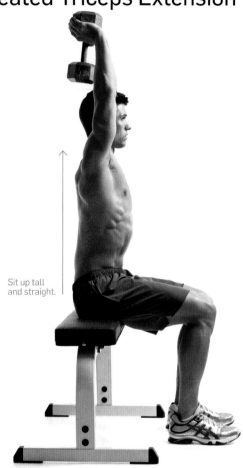

A

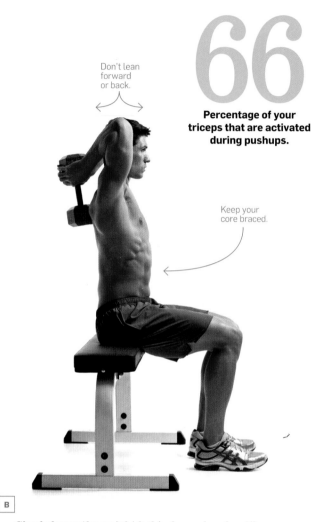

Don't lean
forward
or back.

66

**Percentage of your
triceps that are activated
during pushups.**

Keep your
core braced.

Sit up tall
and straight.

B

- Sitting on a chair or an exercise bench with your back straight, place your feet firmly on the floor and grasp a single dumbbell with both hands.
- Raise the weight above your head, rotating it so it is vertical and the top plate rests comfortably on the palms of your hands, thumbs around the handle. This is the starting position.

REPS: Do 8 to 12.

- Slowly lower the weight behind your head until your forearms touch your biceps and press it back up to the starting position. Repeat.
- Keep your upper arms stationary as you lower the weight and press it back up.

Wrist Curl

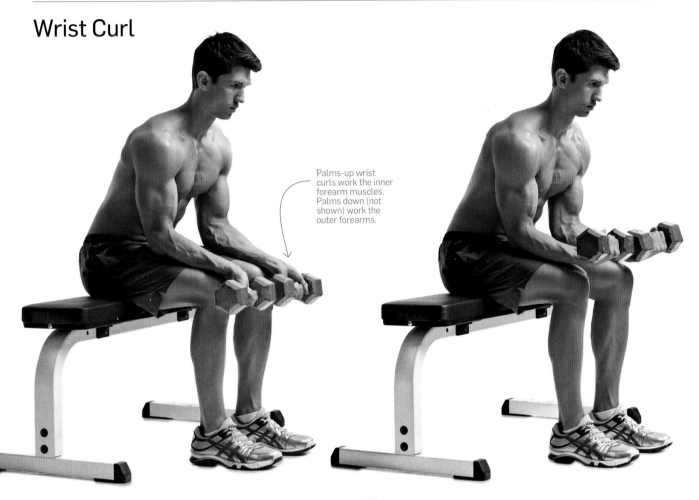

Palms-up wrist curls work the inner forearm muscles. Palms down (not shown) work the outer forearms.

A

- Sit on an exercise bench or a chair with your knees about 2 feet apart and your feet flat on the floor.
- With a dumbbell in each hand, palms up, lean forward and place your forearms on your upper thighs so your wrists are hanging over your knees.
- Slowly bend both wrists down as far as you can.

REPS: Do 12 to 15 each way, palms up and palms held down.

B

- Using only your wrists, curl the weights up as high as possible. Lower and do all your reps.
- Now rotate your wrists to the palms-down position to do reverse wrist curls.
- Bend your wrists up to raise the dumbbells as high as you can. Lower them slowly and repeat.

Dumbbell Total Arms Workout

Alternating Grip Hammer Curl

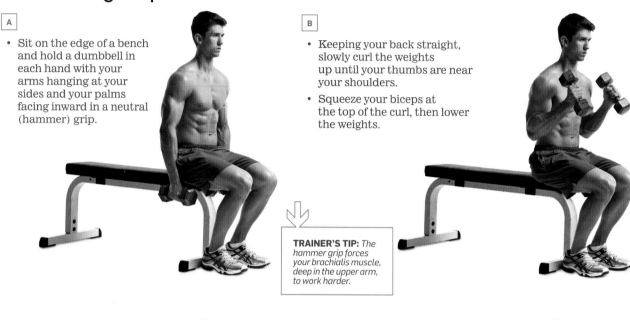

A

- Sit on the edge of a bench and hold a dumbbell in each hand with your arms hanging at your sides and your palms facing inward in a neutral (hammer) grip.

B

- Keeping your back straight, slowly curl the weights up until your thumbs are near your shoulders.
- Squeeze your biceps at the top of the curl, then lower the weights.

TRAINER'S TIP: *The hammer grip forces your brachialis muscle, deep in the upper arm, to work harder.*

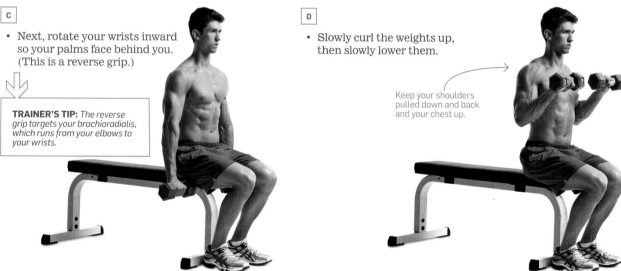

C

- Next, rotate your wrists inward so your palms face behind you. (This is a reverse grip.)

TRAINER'S TIP: *The reverse grip targets your brachioradialis, which runs from your elbows to your wrists.*

D

- Slowly curl the weights up, then slowly lower them.

Keep your shoulders pulled down and back and your chest up.

REPS: Do 8 to 12, alternating grips with each curl.

Cross-Shoulder Extension

A

- Lie on an incline bench and hold a light dumbbell overhead in your right hand, with your palm facing left.
- Place your left hand on your right triceps for support.

B

- Slowly bend your right arm to lower the weight to your left shoulder, keeping your wrist straight throughout the exercise. (You may need to tilt your head to the right to keep it out of the way.)
- Raise the weight back overhead and repeat.

REPS: Do 12, then switch arms for the next set.

Standing Scaption

The weights should point to 10 o'clock and 2 o'clock at the top of the move.

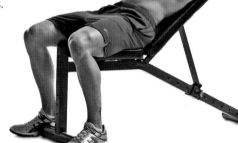

A

- Stand holding a light pair of dumbbells in front of your thighs with a neutral grip (your palms facing each other).

REPS: Do 8 to 12.

B

- Keeping your arms straight, slowly raise them in front of you at about 45-degree angles to the sides.
- Raise them to eye level.
- Slowly lower your arms and repeat.

Arms and Dangerous

Big arms make you look like you mean business. But like police officers, they also serve and protect. Biceps help you tote anything—from groceries to quarter kegs—with ease. Triceps work as shock absorbers to protect your elbow joints when they are called upon to brace your upper body or break your fall.

START HERE: Do the exercises as a circuit, moving from one to the next without resting. After completing one circuit, rest for 60 seconds, then do one more circuit.

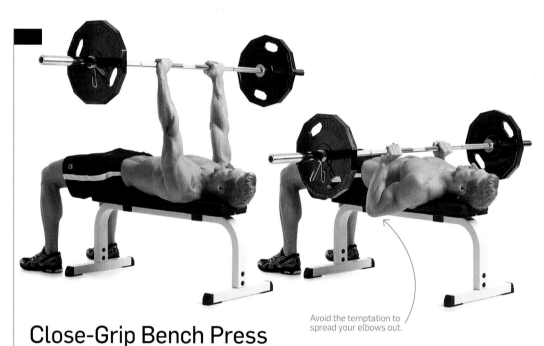

Avoid the temptation to spread your elbows out.

Close-Grip Bench Press

A
- Lie faceup on a bench with your feet flat on the floor. Grab the bar with an overhand grip, your hands just shy of shoulder-width apart.

REPS: Do 8 to 12.

B
- Lower the bar to your chest, bringing your elbows close to the sides of your chest.
- Press the weight back up and repeat.

Barbell Curl

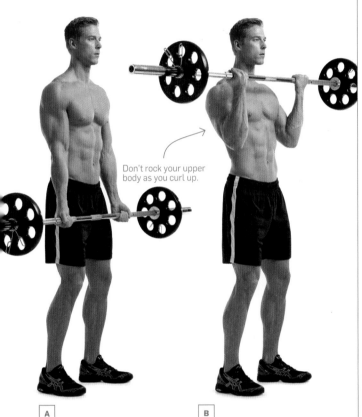

Don't rock your upper body as you curl up.

A

- Stand holding a barbell in front of your thighs with an underhand grip, your hands shoulder-width apart.

B

- Keeping your back straight and your elbows at your sides, slowly curl the bar up in a semicircular motion until your forearms touch your biceps.
- Pause, then slowly lower the bar to about an inch in front of your thighs before repeating the move.

REPS: Do 8 to 12.

Cable Incline-Bench Triceps Extension

A

- Attach a rope to a low-pulley cable and place an incline bench a couple of feet in front of the pulley.
- Grab the rope and lie faceup on the bench with your arms straight above your shoulders and near your ears.

B

- Without moving your upper arms, bend your elbows to 90 degrees. Pause, then straighten your arms.

REPS: Do 8 to 12.

Arms and Dangerous

Cable Single-Arm Curl

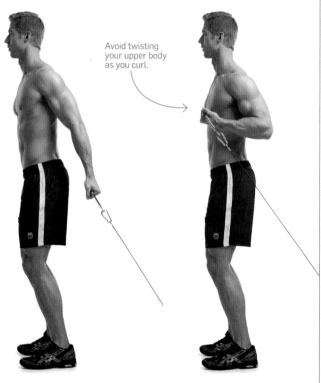

Avoid twisting your upper body as you curl.

A

- Stand with your back to the weight stack of a cable station and grab the low-pulley handle with your left hand.
- Step forward so your left hand is a few inches behind you and your arm is straight.

B

- Keeping your elbow in place, curl the handle up until it reaches the side of your chest. Pause, then slowly lower your arm.

REPS: Do 8 to 12.

Twisting Rope Pulldown

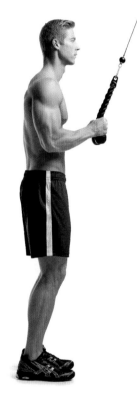
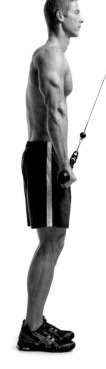

A

- Attach a rope handle to a high-pulley cable and grab an end with each hand. Spread your hands about 6 to 8 inches apart.
- Keeping your upper arms tucked at your sides, pull the rope down until your forearms are parallel to the floor. This is the starting position.

B

- Slowly pull the rope down until your fists reach your thighs, then rotate your wrists so your palms face out, away from your body.
- Squeeze your triceps for a second, then reverse the move to return to the starting position.

REPS: Do 8 to 12.

Pause Reverse Curl

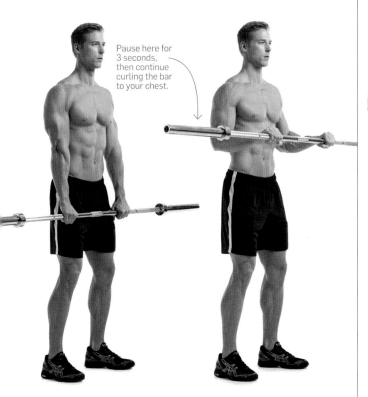

Pause here for 3 seconds, then continue curling the bar to your chest.

A

- Stand holding a light barbell with an overhand grip (palms down) in front of your thighs.
- Press your elbows to your sides throughout the movement.

B

- Slowly curl the bar up until your forearms are parallel to the floor. Pause for 3 seconds, then continue to curl the bar until it reaches your chest.
- Slowly lower the bar until your forearms are again parallel to the floor. Pause for another 3 seconds, then lower the bar to the starting position.

REPS: Do 8 to 12.

Overhead Cable Triceps Extension

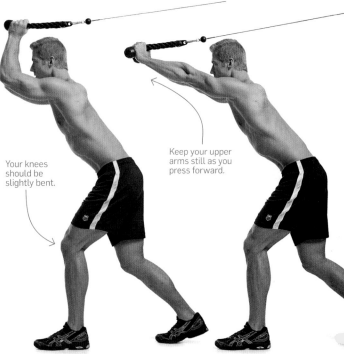

Your knees should be slightly bent.

Keep your upper arms still as you press forward.

A

- Attach a rope handle to a high-pulley cable and grab an end with each hand.
- Stand with your back to the weight stack, lean forward with one foot ahead of the other, and hold the rope just over your head with your arms bent.

B

- Without moving your upper arms, straighten your arms in front of you to work your triceps.
- Pause, then slowly allow the resistance to pull your hands back over your head.

REPS: Do 8 to 12.

The Deltoid Definer Workout

Shoulders are one of the most often neglected parts of a lifter's body because they're not typically thought of as the "show" muscles. How wrong that thinking is. Broad, sculpted, cannonball shoulders top off the perfect total body. Bigger shoulders will make your arms look bigger, your waist look slimmer, and your back appear broader for that classic V shape. The key to fully developing your shoulders is exercising the heads of each of the three muscles that make up this group known as the deltoids: the anterior (front) deltoid, the lateral (middle) deltoid, and the posterior (rear) deltoid. Here's a workout that will make yours pop.

3

Increase (in inches) in shoulder range of motion after just 5 weeks of weight lifting, according to a study at the University of North Dakota.

START HERE:
The shoulder is the most unstable joint in your body. Protect it with a 60-second warmup of arm circles before you do this workout. Just hold your arms out to form a T and make tight and wide circles in each direction. The workout: Do two sets of each exercise, resting 30 seconds between sets. Finish both sets before moving to the next lift.

Negative Shoulder Press

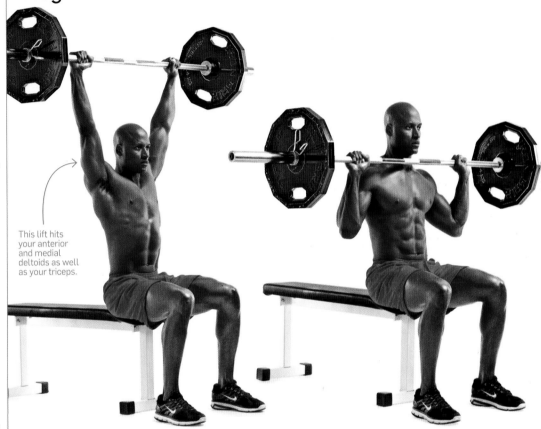

This lift hits your anterior and medial deltoids as well as your triceps.

A

- Place a bench in front of a squat rack. Use half the weight you can lift 8 to 10 times with perfect form.
- Grab the bar with your hands slightly wider than shoulder width and sit on the bench. Raise the weight overhead.

REPS: Do 8 to 12.

B

- Take 6 seconds to lower the barbell to the front of your chest.
- Then press the bar overhead for a count of three.

153

The Deltoid Definer Workout

Barbell Front Raise

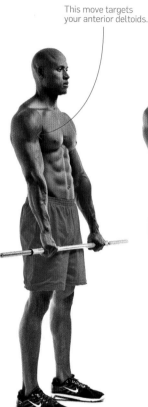

This move targets your anterior deltoids.

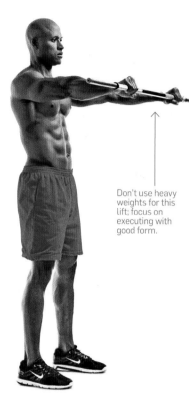

Don't use heavy weights for this lift; focus on executing with good form.

A

- Stand with your feet hip-width apart and hold a light barbell with your hands shoulder-width apart. Your arms should hang straight down, palms facing the fronts of your thighs.

B

- Keeping your arms straight, slowly lift the bar up and out in front of you until your arms are parallel to the floor.
- Pause, then slowly lower the bar until your hands barely touch your thighs.

REPS: Do 8 to 12.

Seated Lateral Raise

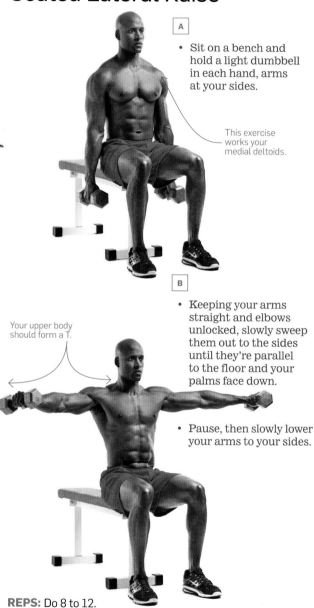

A

- Sit on a bench and hold a light dumbbell in each hand, arms at your sides.

This exercise works your medial deltoids.

B

Your upper body should form a T.

- Keeping your arms straight and elbows unlocked, slowly sweep them out to the sides until they're parallel to the floor and your palms face down.

- Pause, then slowly lower your arms to your sides.

REPS: Do 8 to 12.

Bent-Over Cable Raise

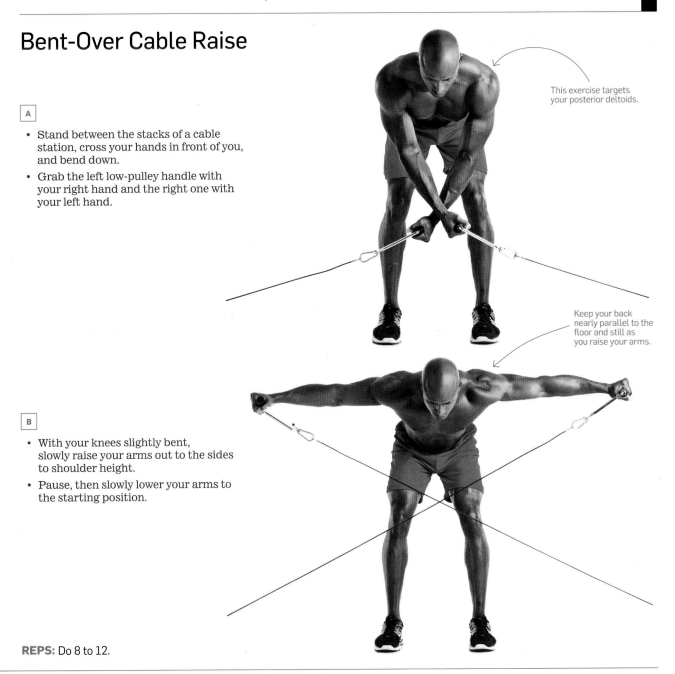

This exercise targets your posterior deltoids.

A

- Stand between the stacks of a cable station, cross your hands in front of you, and bend down.
- Grab the left low-pulley handle with your right hand and the right one with your left hand.

Keep your back nearly parallel to the floor and still as you raise your arms.

B

- With your knees slightly bent, slowly raise your arms out to the sides to shoulder height.
- Pause, then slowly lower your arms to the starting position.

REPS: Do 8 to 12.

Shoulders and Arms Combo Workout 1

Powerful arms and shoulders are a key foundation for developing the large muscles in your back and chest, since you're only as strong as your weakest links. The rest of this chapter contains three different workouts using combination lifts that will keep the whole chain stable and strong.

START HERE:
Do three sets of each exercise, resting for 60 seconds after each set. Complete all sets before moving on to the next lift.

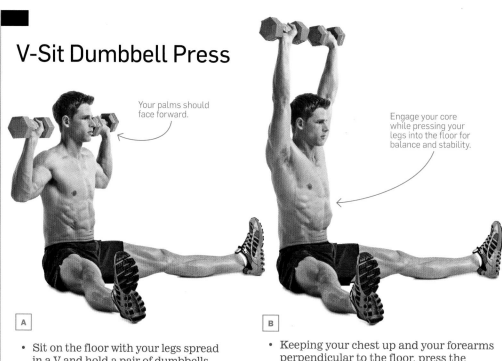

V-Sit Dumbbell Press

Your palms should face forward.

Engage your core while pressing your legs into the floor for balance and stability.

A

- Sit on the floor with your legs spread in a V and hold a pair of dumbbells at your shoulders.
- Squeeze your glutes and press your hamstrings and calves against the floor.

REPS: Do 12.

B

- Keeping your chest up and your forearms perpendicular to the floor, press the weights up until your arms are extended. Pause, then slowly lower your arms.

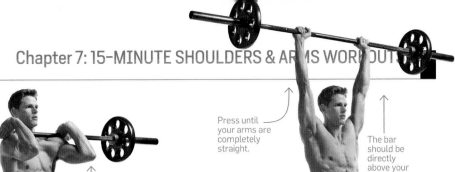

Olympic Military Press

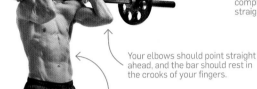

Press until your arms are completely straight.

The bar should be directly above your shoulders.

Your elbows should point straight ahead, and the bar should rest in the crooks of your fingers.

Brace your core to support your spine throughout the movement.

A

- Stand holding a barbell just in front of your shoulders with your hands slightly more than shoulder-width apart.

B

- Press the weight above you and slightly back so that, at the top of the motion, your arms are even with your ears or just behind them.
- Contract your arms for a second, then slowly lower the weight to the starting position.

REPS: Do 12.

Single-Leg Lateral Raise

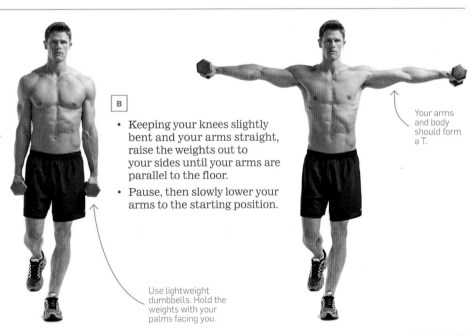

A

- Stand on one leg and hold a pair of light dumbbells at your sides, palms toward you.

B

- Keeping your knees slightly bent and your arms straight, raise the weights out to your sides until your arms are parallel to the floor.
- Pause, then slowly lower your arms to the starting position.

Your arms and body should form a T.

TRAINER'S TIP: *To maintain your single-leg balance, pick an object in the distance to focus on.*

REPS: Do 6 on each leg.

Use lightweight dumbbells. Hold the weights with your palms facing you.

Shoulders and Arms Combo Workout 2

START HERE:
Perform two sets of each move before switching to the next exercise. Rest for 60 seconds between sets.

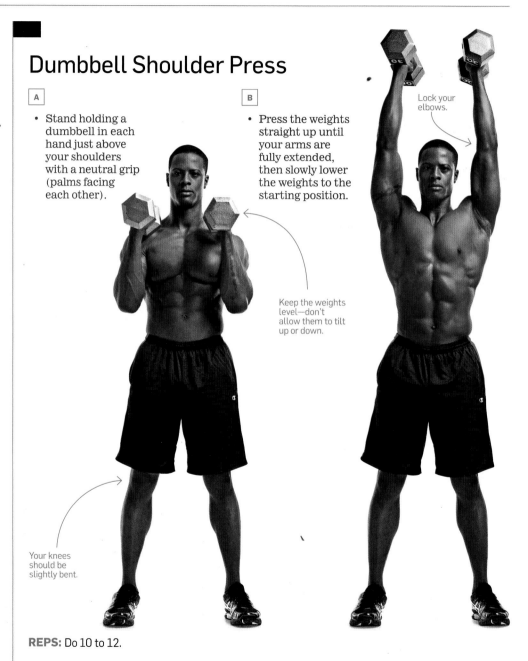

Dumbbell Shoulder Press

A

- Stand holding a dumbbell in each hand just above your shoulders with a neutral grip (palms facing each other).

B

- Press the weights straight up until your arms are fully extended, then slowly lower the weights to the starting position.

Lock your elbows.

Keep the weights level—don't allow them to tilt up or down.

Your knees should be slightly bent.

REPS: Do 10 to 12.

Dumbbell Front Raise

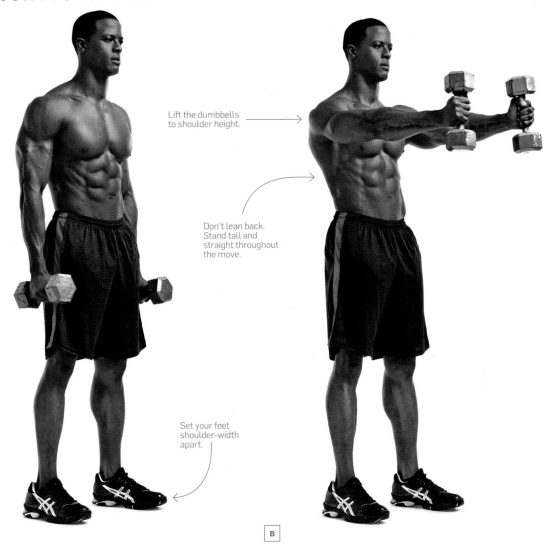

Lift the dumbbells to shoulder height.

Don't lean back. Stand tall and straight throughout the move.

Set your feet shoulder-width apart.

A

- Stand holding a pair of light dumbbells at arm's length with a neutral grip.

REPS: Do 10 to 12.

B

- Keeping your arms straight, slowly raise the weights in front of you until your arms are parallel to the floor.
- Pause, then slowly lower the weights.

Shoulders and Arms Combo Workout 2

Cable Reverse Fly

A

- Stand between the weight stacks of a cable station with your arms crossed in front of you and grab a handle from each low pulley.
- Bend forward at the waist until your torso is almost parallel to the floor, arms beneath your shoulders.

Your back should be flat and nearly parallel to the floor.

Raise your arms until they're parallel to the floor.

B

- Pull your shoulder blades back, then raise your arms out to your sides.
- Lower and repeat.

REPS: Do 10 to 12.

Dumbbell Cuban Press

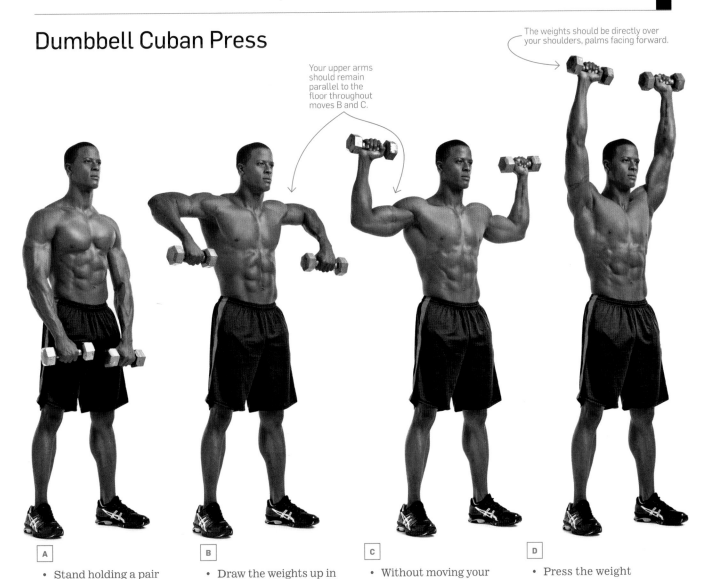

The weights should be directly over your shoulders, palms facing forward.

Your upper arms should remain parallel to the floor throughout moves B and C.

A

- Stand holding a pair of light dumbbells in front of your thighs with an overhand grip.

REPS: Do 10 to 12.

B

- Draw the weights up in front of your body, keeping them close to your torso and bending your elbows, until your upper arms are parallel to the floor.

C

- Without moving your upper arms or elbows, rotate your forearms until they point upward.

D

- Press the weight overhead.
- Slowly reverse the move, returning to the starting position.

Shoulders and Arms Combo Workout 3

START HERE:
START HERE:
Perform two
sets of each
exercise
before moving
on to the
next lift.
Rest for 60 to
90 seconds
between sets.

Seated Shoulder Tug

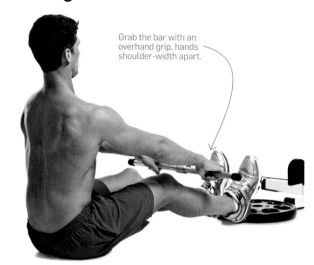

A

- Sit at a rowing station with a straight-bar handle and grab the bar with both hands.
- Keep your arms straight and lean back until your back is perpendicular to the floor.

Grab the bar with an overhand grip, hands shoulder-width apart.

B

- Without bending your elbows to pull the bar toward you, slowly draw your shoulder blades back as far as possible.
- Pause, then allow your arms to move forward again.

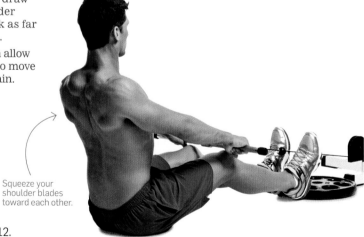

Squeeze your shoulder blades toward each other.

REPS: Do 8 to 12.

Incline L Raise

A

- Lie facedown on a bench that's set at a 45-degree incline and hold a light dumbbell in each hand with an overhand grip.

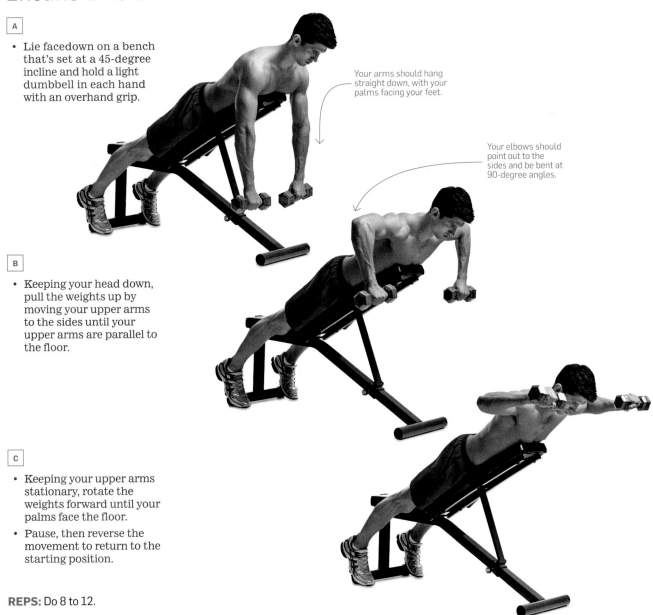

Your arms should hang straight down, with your palms facing your feet.

Your elbows should point out to the sides and be bent at 90-degree angles.

B

- Keeping your head down, pull the weights up by moving your upper arms to the sides until your upper arms are parallel to the floor.

C

- Keeping your upper arms stationary, rotate the weights forward until your palms face the floor.

- Pause, then reverse the movement to return to the starting position.

REPS: Do 8 to 12.

Shoulders and Arms Combo Workout 3

Javorek Complex

NOTE: *This series of moves is based on the time-saving training philosophy of Istvan "The Dumbbell King" Javorek, a former Romanian Olympic coach and, later, a coach at Texas A&M.*

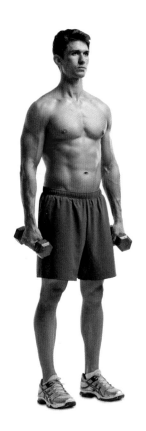

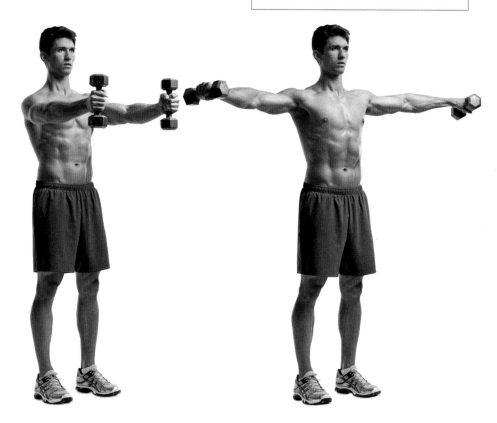

A

- Stand holding a pair of dumbbells, arms at your sides, palms facing each other.

B

- Raise your arms in front of you until they're parallel to the floor.
- Lower the weights and repeat for a total of 6 reps.

C

- Now raise your arms out from your sides until they're parallel to the floor, then lower them. Again, complete 6 reps.

REPS: Do 6 of each move for a total of 30.

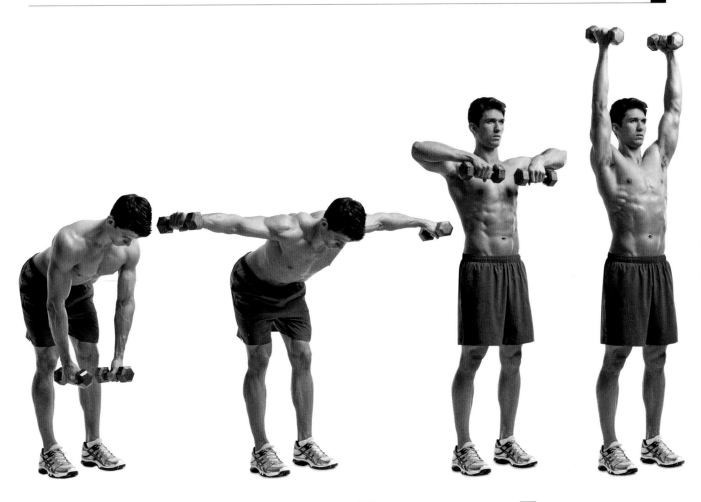

D
- Next, bend forward at the waist until your torso is almost parallel to the floor.

E
- Raise your arms out to your sides, lower them, and repeat for a total of 6 reps.

F
- Stand up and place your hands in front of your thighs, palms toward you.
- Pull both weights up until they're just below your chin.
- Lower and repeat for 6 reps.

G
- Finally, turn your palms so they face each other, curl the weights up to your shoulders, and press them overhead.
- Reverse the move and repeat for 6 reps.

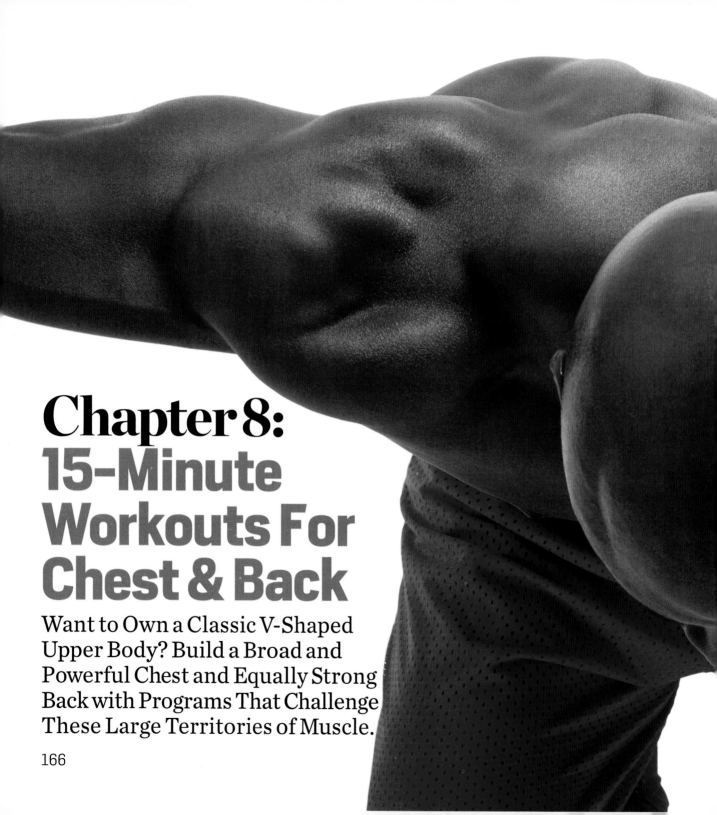

Chapter 8:
15-Minute Workouts For Chest & Back

Want to Own a Classic V-Shaped Upper Body? Build a Broad and Powerful Chest and Equally Strong Back with Programs That Challenge These Large Territories of Muscle.

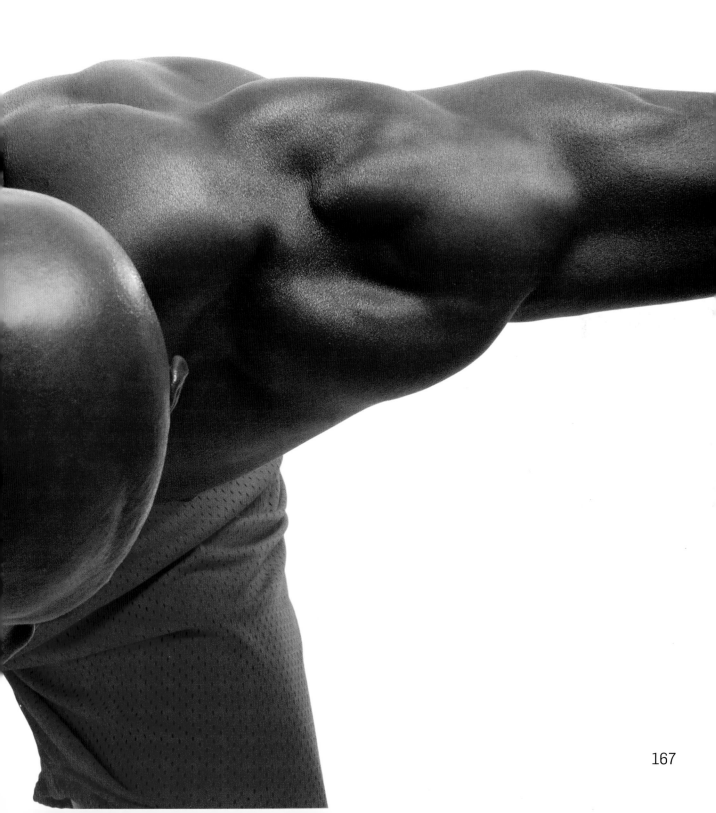

Superfast Chest & Back Workouts

Building a bigger, stronger chest and back adds size to your shoulders and triceps, widening the top of your body. The larger you are on top, the smaller your waistline appears, creating the classic V-shaped torso. So even if your diet has been lagging, building a larger upper body will create the illusion of a thinner midsection. Adding muscle to these two vast expanses of real estate will help you fry belly fat, too, because the more muscle you have, the more calories you burn even at rest. A strong chest and back offer two more key benefits: power for sports moves like setting picks in basketball, pushing off in football, and slamming the ball across the court in tennis; and better posture. By building your back, you balance out the larger muscles of your chest, pulling your shoulders back so you stand tall.

Begin with the basics...

There are two approaches to building impressive chest and back muscles. The classic method is to isolate the pectoral, trapezius, and lat muscles and minimize the involvement of other, secondary muscles. A smarter plan for strength and power is to use compound exercises to force your chest, shoulders, back, and other upper-body muscles to work together. The programs found in this chapter offer both exercises that isolate your chest and back muscles for size and exercises that integrate your shoulders and triceps and biceps for strength. There's lots to choose from, so try rotating through the workouts each week and see which work best for you. Do the prescribed number of sets and reps for each exercise, using a weight at which you can barely squeeze out the last rep of your final set with spot-on form.

Find It Quick: Your 15-Minute Circuit Plan for a V-shaped Torso

MAKE IT HARDER

Want to make pushups more challenging? Do them on a stability ball. Place your hands shoulder-width apart on the ball. Assume a plank position with your toes on the floor and your back straight. Trying to maintain balance as you lower your chest to the ball and press back up challenges more muscle fibers than regular pushups do.

Chest Pound Workout 1

The best chest-building program takes advantage of the versatility of your upper-body muscles by working your pecs and all their buddies, using every angle and rep range. With this strategy, you can end up with more beef in your back, shoulders, and arms, *and* in your chest than you'd ever see with a steady diet of bench presses.

START HERE: Do one set of these exercises as a circuit without resting between moves. Recover for 60 seconds after the final rep. Then repeat the circuit once more.

Parallel Bar Dip

A

- Grab parallel dip bars and lift yourself so your arms are straight.

B

- Keeping your elbows tucked close to your body, slowly lower yourself by bending your elbows until your upper arms are parallel to the floor.
- Pause, then push yourself up to the starting position.

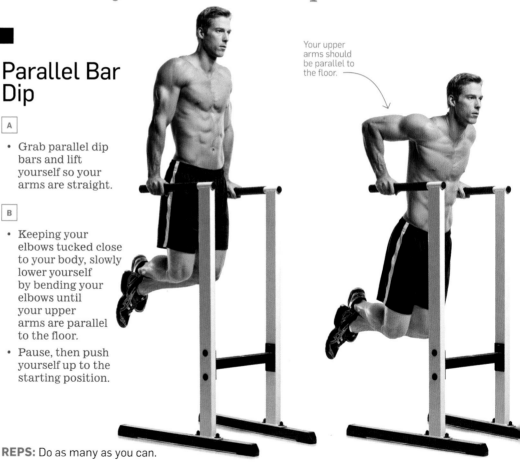

Your upper arms should be parallel to the floor.

REPS: Do as many as you can.

Barbell Bench Press

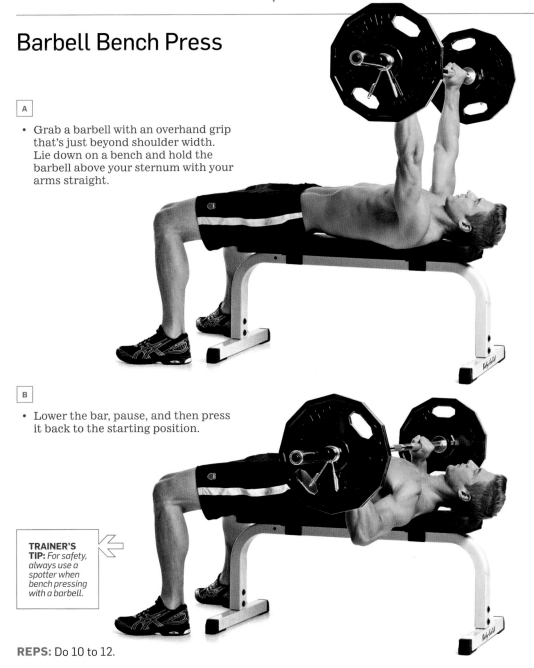

A

- Grab a barbell with an overhand grip that's just beyond shoulder width. Lie down on a bench and hold the barbell above your sternum with your arms straight.

B

- Lower the bar, pause, and then press it back to the starting position.

TRAINER'S TIP: *For safety, always use a spotter when bench pressing with a barbell.*

REPS: Do 10 to 12.

GET MORE OUT OF YOUR BENCH PRESS

Just before you lift the bar off the rack, squeeze the metal as if you are trying to crush it with your bare hands. "You will 'lock up' proximally, meaning that the center of your body will reflexively activate to give you more trunk stability," says Eric Cressey, CSCS, a Boston-based strength and conditioning coach who works with many pro athletes. This, in turn, will help you lift more weight. Maintain your clench throughout the set.

Chest Pound Workout 1

Incline Dumbbell Fly

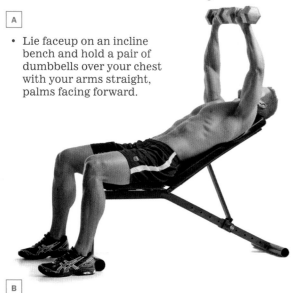

A

- Lie faceup on an incline bench and hold a pair of dumbbells over your chest with your arms straight, palms facing forward.

B

- Keeping your palms forward and bending your elbows, slowly sweep your arms down and out to your sides until the weights are level with your chest.
- Pause, then reverse the motion until the weights are once again above you.

Lower the dumbbells down and slightly back.

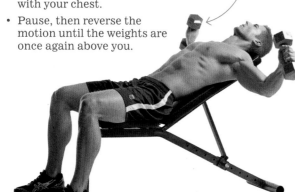

REPS: Do 10 to 12.

Seated Single-Arm External Rotation

A

- Sit on a bench with your right foot flat on one end, that knee bent, and your other foot on the floor.
- Hold a light dumbbell in your right hand and rest your right elbow on your right knee.
- Bend your right arm 90 degrees and allow the weight to hang down next to your right leg.

This move works your rotator cuff, so use a very light weight.

B

- Keeping your elbow in place, slowly rotate your right arm upward.
- Pause when your forearm points to the ceiling, then reverse the motion until the weight is again in the starting position.

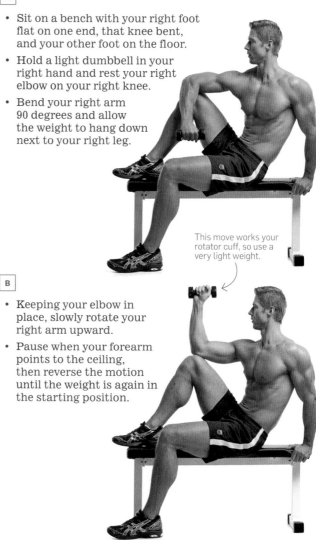

REPS: Do 10 to 12, then repeat with your left arm.

Single-Arm Dumbbell Row

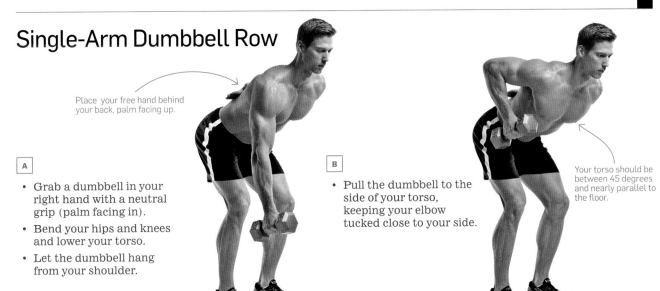

Place your free hand behind your back, palm facing up.

A

- Grab a dumbbell in your right hand with a neutral grip (palm facing in).
- Bend your hips and knees and lower your torso.
- Let the dumbbell hang from your shoulder.

B

- Pull the dumbbell to the side of your torso, keeping your elbow tucked close to your side.

Your torso should be between 45 degrees and nearly parallel to the floor.

REPS: Perform 15 with each arm.

Weighted Pushup

A

- Assume the standard pushup position, with your hands beneath your shoulders.
- Ask your workout partner to place a weight plate on your back, between your shoulder blades.

B

- Keeping your body straight, lower yourself by bending your elbows until your chest nearly touches the floor.
- Pause, then push yourself back up.

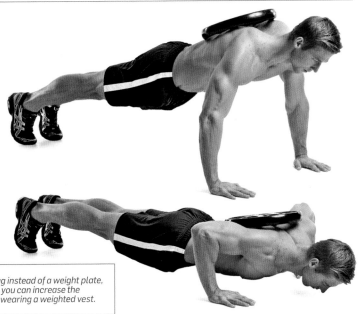

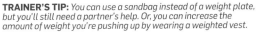
TRAINER'S TIP: You can use a sandbag instead of a weight plate, but you'll still need a partner's help. Or, you can increase the amount of weight you're pushing up by wearing a weighted vest.

REPS: Do 10 to 12.

Chest Pound Workout 2

Single-Arm Dumbbell Bench Press

A

- Lie on your back on a bench with a heavy dumbbell in one hand along the side of your chest, palm facing in.
- Hold your opposite arm along the bench or straight out to the side for balance.

B

- Push the weight up so your arm is straight above your chest.
- Pause, then slowly lower the weight to the starting position.

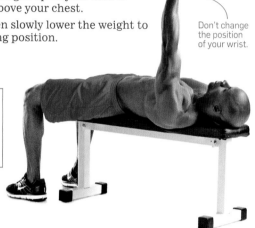

Don't change the position of your wrist.

TRAINER'S TIP: *Using just one dumbbell creates imbalance, which forces your core to work harder.*

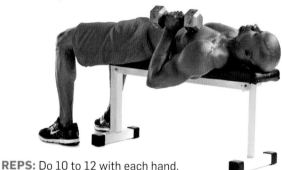

REPS: Do 10 to 12 with each hand.

Side-Lying Single-Arm External Rotation

A

- Lie on your left side with your left arm bent and your head resting on your left hand.
- Holding a light dumbbell in your right hand, bend your right arm 90 degrees and tuck your upper arm against your right side.
- Let the weight hang in front of your midsection.

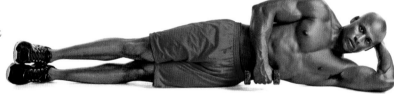

B

- Keeping your upper arm stationary, slowly rotate your forearm until it points toward the ceiling.
- Rotate your forearm back to the starting position.

Use a very light dumbbell; 1 to 5 pounds is enough to work the muscles of your rotator cuff.

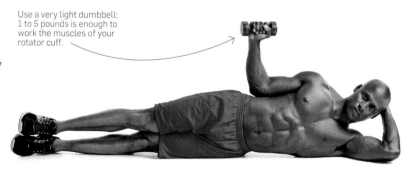

REPS: Perform 10 to 12 with each arm.

Dumbbell Incline Bench Press

A

- Lie faceup on an incline bench and hold a pair of heavy dumbbells along the outsides of your chest with a neutral grip (palms facing in).

B

- Slowly press the weights straight above your chest.
- Pause, then lower them to the starting position.

REPS: Perform 10 to 12.

Lying Cable Fly

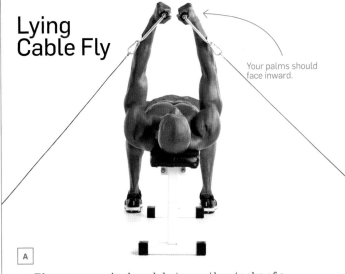

Your palms should face inward.

A

- Place an exercise bench between the stacks of a cable crossover station and attach stirrup handles to the low-pulley cables.
- Grab a handle with each hand and lie faceup on the bench with your feet flat on the floor.
- Hold your arms straight above your chest, palms facing each other.

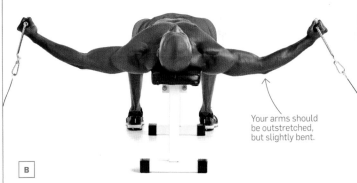

Your arms should be outstretched, but slightly bent.

B

- Keeping your elbows slightly bent, lower your hands out to your sides in an arc, then reverse the motion to return to the starting position.

REPS: Do 10 to 12.

Chest Pound Workout 2

Dip

3,989

Most parallel-bar dips ever done in 1 hour.

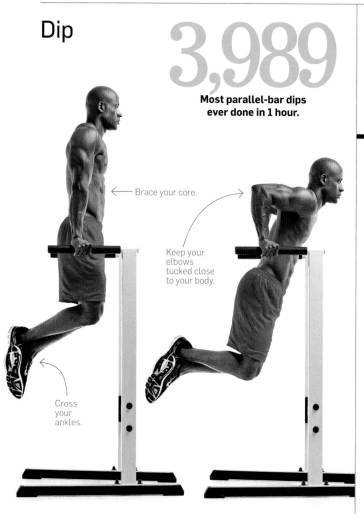

← Brace your core. →

Keep your elbows tucked close to your body.

Cross your ankles.

A

- Grab the bars of a dip station and lift yourself until your arms are completely straight.

REPS: Do as many as you can.

B

- Slowly lower yourself by bending your elbows until your upper arms dip just below your elbows.
- Pause, and then push back up to the starting position.

Pullup

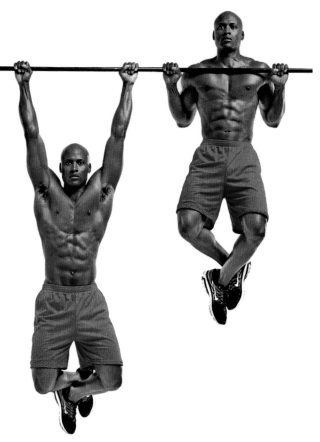

A

- Grab a pullup bar with a shoulder-width overhand grip and hang at arm's length.

REPS: Do as many as you can.

B

- Pull your chest up to the bar.
- Pause.
- Lower back to the starting position and repeat.

Overhead Triceps Extension

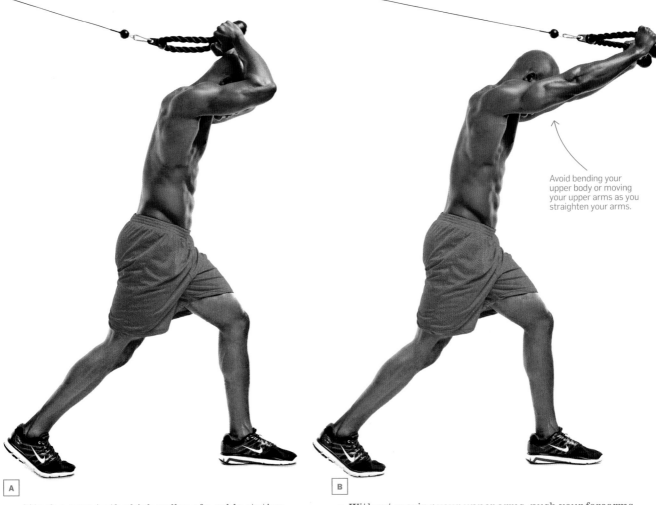

Avoid bending your upper body or moving your upper arms as you straighten your arms.

A

- Attach a rope to the high pulley of a cable station and face away from it.
- Grab an end of the rope in each hand and stagger your stance.

REPS: Do 10 to 12.

B

- Without moving your upper arms, push your forearms forward, pause, and return.

The Back Attack Workout

Unlike your chest, your back is made up of more than just one major muscle group—it has lots of them. In fact, this hard-to-see part of your upper body houses a complex system of muscles, from your lats (latissimus dorsi) to your rotator cuffs to your upper, middle, and lower traps (trapeziuses), with each performing a variety of functions. That's why sculpting a V-shaped torso isn't as simple as doing "back" exercises, such as lat pulldowns. You need specialized exercises that zero in on the often-ignored muscles. You'll know which ones they are because they'll be sore tomorrow.

1,005
Heaviest weight, in pounds, lifted in the bench press.

START HERE:
Do the exercises in the order shown, using the heaviest weight that allows you to complete the prescribed number of reps. Do these moves one after another with no rest in between. Recover for 60 seconds after the final move. Then repeat the circuit for a total of two times.

Thoracic Rotation

A
- Kneel down, place your right hand behind your head, and point your elbow out to the side.
- Brace your core and rotate your right shoulder toward your left arm.

B
- Follow your elbow with your eyes as you reverse the movement until your right elbow points toward the ceiling. That's 1 rep.

REPS: Do 20 with each arm.

Dumbbell Bench Press

A
- Lie on your back on a bench with a dumbbell in each hand held along the sides of your chest, palms facing in.

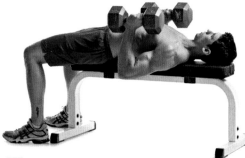

B
- Push the weights up so your arms are straight above your chest.
- Pause, then slowly lower the weights to the starting position.

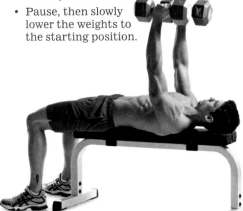

REPS: Do 10 to 12.

The Back Attack Workout

Rack Pull

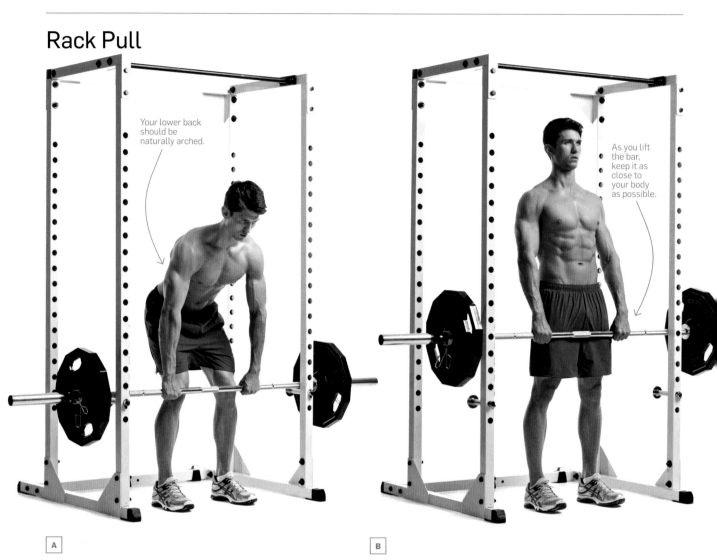

Your lower back should be naturally arched.

As you lift the bar, keep it as close to your body as possible.

A

- Set a barbell at knee level in a squat rack.
- Assume a shortstop stance—your hips back, knees slightly bent and against the bar.
- Bend over to grab the bar with an overhand grip, your hands just outside your legs.

REPS: Do 10 to 12.

B

- Stand up by pushing your hips forward.

TRAINER'S TIP: *Begin with no weight until the exercise feels natural, and then start adding weight. Once the exercise becomes easy from the rack, lift the barbell from the floor using the same form.*

Two-Part Dumbbell Row

Shrug your shoulders and pull your shoulder blades together, and pause.

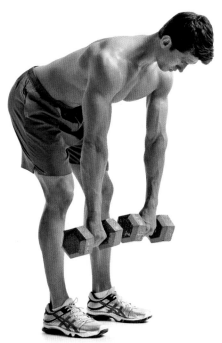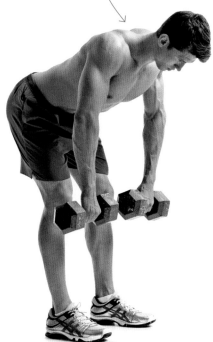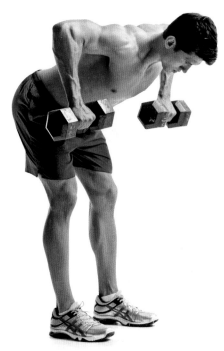

A

- Grab a pair of dumbbells, bend at your hips and knees, and lower your torso until it's almost parallel to the floor.
- Allow the weights to hang at arm's length from your shoulders, palms facing you.

REPS: Do 10 to 12.

B

- Shrug your shoulders and pull your shoulder blades together. Hold that position for two counts before rowing the weight.

C

- Bend your elbows and raise them out to the sides as you pull the weights to the sides of your torso. Continue to squeeze your shoulder blades together toward your spine.
- Lower the weights to the starting position and repeat.

The Back Attack Workout

Pullup Hold

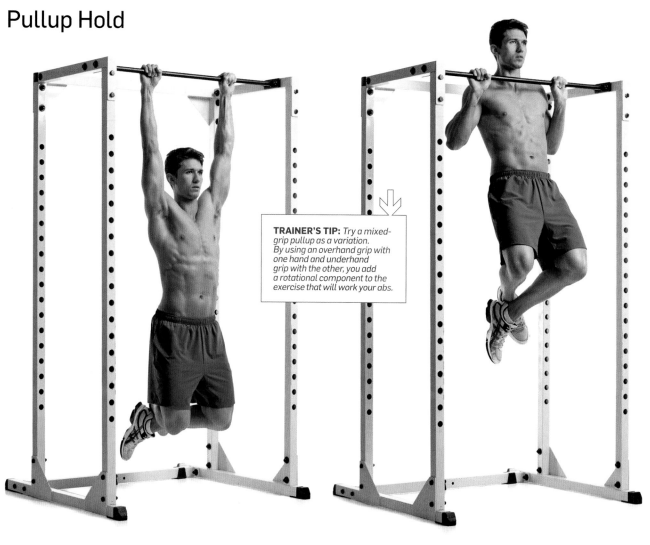

TRAINER'S TIP: *Try a mixed-grip pullup as a variation. By using an overhand grip with one hand and underhand grip with the other, you add a rotational component to the exercise that will work your abs.*

A

- Hang from a pullup bar with an overhand grip, your hands at the exact width you use when you do a bench press.

REPS: Do 5.

B

- Pull your chest up to the bar and hold for 10 to 20 seconds.
- Once you can do more than 5 reps, add resistance with a weighted vest or a dumbbell held between your feet.

Alternating Dumbbell Shoulder Press

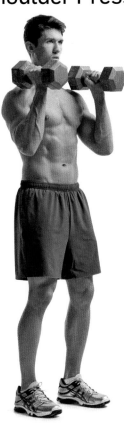

A

- Hold a pair of dumbbells just outside your shoulders, your arms bent and your palms facing each other.
- Set your feet shoulder-width apart and bend your knees slightly.

REPS: Do 10 to 12.

B

- Press one dumbbell up until your arm is straight.
- As you lower that dumbbell, press the other one up, in an alternating fashion. That's 1 rep.

Cable Diagonal Raise

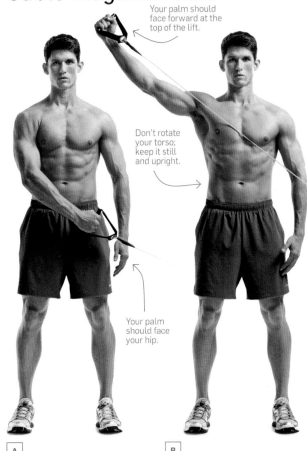

Your palm should face forward at the top of the lift.

Don't rotate your torso; keep it still and upright.

Your palm should face your hip.

A

- Attach a handle to the low pulley of a cable station.
- Standing with your left side toward the pulley, grab the handle with your right hand in front of your left hip and bend your elbow slightly.

REPS: Do 10 to 12 with each arm.

B

- Pull the handle up and across your body until your hand is over your head and your thumb is pointing up (a Statue of Liberty pose).
- Return to the starting position and repeat.

Strong and Steady

This routine is designed to improve the endurance as well as the strength of your stabilizing muscles. You'll work your lateral stabilizer muscles, which are crucial for supporting your spine, as well as your lower and middle back extensors. As a result, you'll stand taller and straighter and have a strong foundation for lifting heavier weights.

START HERE: Do these exercises as a circuit, without resting between moves. Recover for 60 seconds, then repeat the circuit two more times.

Cat-Camel

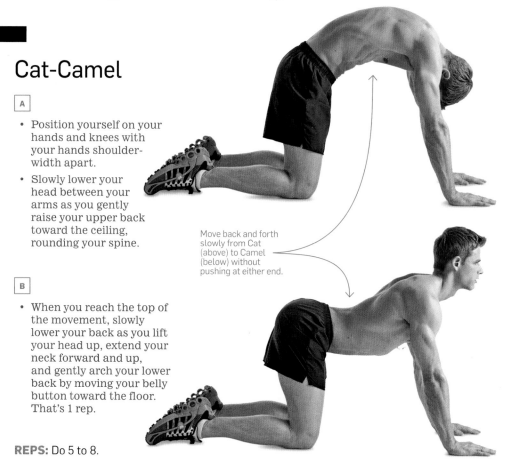

A

- Position yourself on your hands and knees with your hands shoulder-width apart.
- Slowly lower your head between your arms as you gently raise your upper back toward the ceiling, rounding your spine.

Move back and forth slowly from Cat (above) to Camel (below) without pushing at either end.

B

- When you reach the top of the movement, slowly lower your back as you lift your head up, extend your neck forward and up, and gently arch your lower back by moving your belly button toward the floor. That's 1 rep.

REPS: Do 5 to 8.

Curl-Up

A

- Lie faceup on the floor with your left leg straight and flat on the floor. Your right knee should be bent and your right foot flat.

- Place your palms on the floor under the natural arch in your lower back.

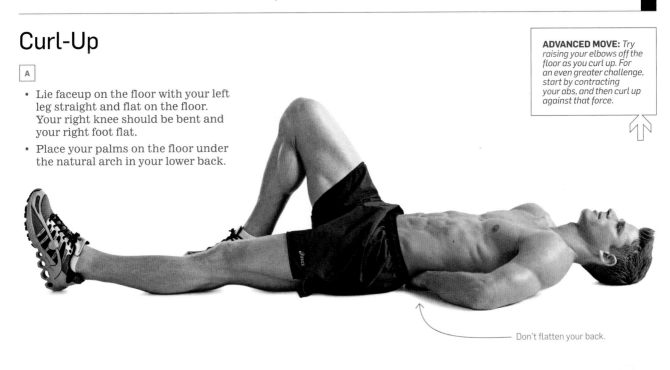

ADVANCED MOVE: *Try raising your elbows off the floor as you curl up. For an even greater challenge, start by contracting your abs, and then curl up against that force.*

Don't flatten your back.

B

- Slowly raise your head and shoulders off the floor without bending your lower back or spine.

- Hold this position for 7 to 8 seconds, breathing deeply the entire time. That's 1 rep.

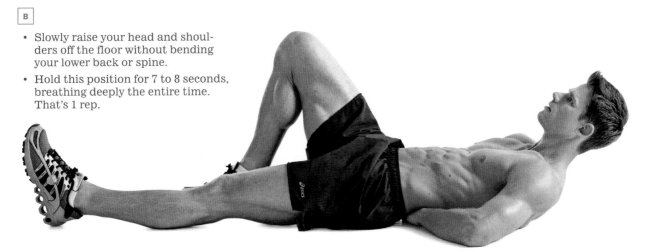

REPS: Do 4, then switch legs and do 4 more.

Strong and Steady

Side Bridge

A

- Lie on your left side with your legs straight and your upper body propped up on your left elbow and forearm.

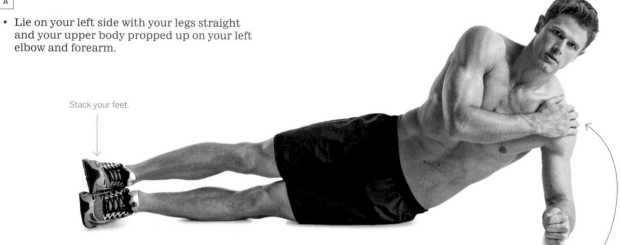

Stack your feet.

Place your right hand on your left shoulder or your right hip.

B

- Brace your core and raise your hips until your body forms a straight line from your ankles to your shoulders.
- Hold this position for 7 to 8 seconds, breathing deeply the entire time. That's 1 rep.

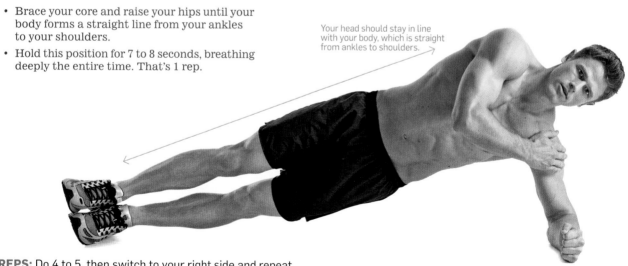

Your head should stay in line with your body, which is straight from ankles to shoulders.

REPS: Do 4 to 5, then switch to your right side and repeat.

Bird Dog

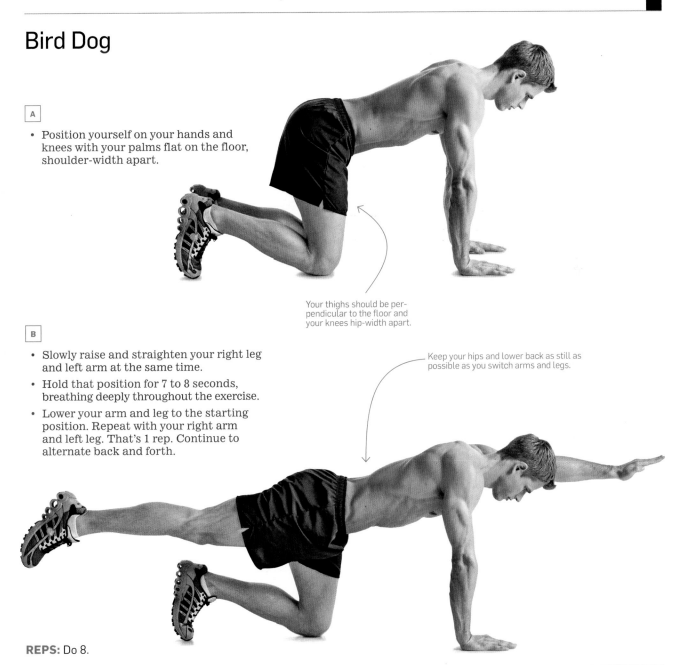

A

- Position yourself on your hands and knees with your palms flat on the floor, shoulder-width apart.

Your thighs should be perpendicular to the floor and your knees hip-width apart.

B

- Slowly raise and straighten your right leg and left arm at the same time.
- Hold that position for 7 to 8 seconds, breathing deeply throughout the exercise.
- Lower your arm and leg to the starting position. Repeat with your right arm and left leg. That's 1 rep. Continue to alternate back and forth.

Keep your hips and lower back as still as possible as you switch arms and legs.

REPS: Do 8.

Chest and Back Combo

This heavy-hitting combo platter challenges your A and B sides in one effective circuit. As a bonus, you'll work your upper back's scapular muscles and the rotator cuff muscles of your shoulders. Collectively, these muscles, which tend to be weak in most men, are the key to stable, healthy shoulders and a strong upper body.

START HERE:
Do one set of each exercise in the circuit without resting between moves. After completing the circuit, recover for 60 seconds. Then repeat twice more for a total of three circuits.

Cable Face Pull with External Rotation

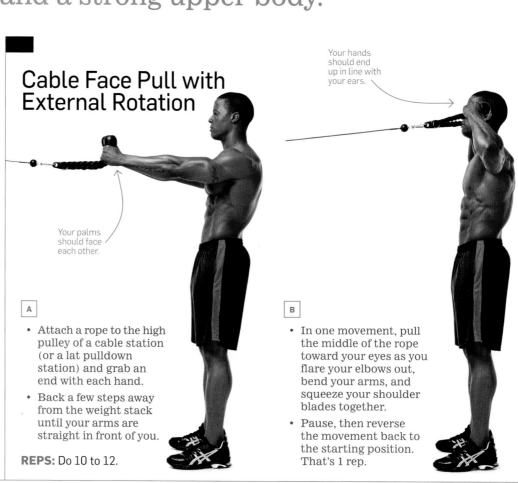

Your palms should face each other.

Your hands should end up in line with your ears.

A
- Attach a rope to the high pulley of a cable station (or a lat pulldown station) and grab an end with each hand.
- Back a few steps away from the weight stack until your arms are straight in front of you.

REPS: Do 10 to 12.

B
- In one movement, pull the middle of the rope toward your eyes as you flare your elbows out, bend your arms, and squeeze your shoulder blades together.
- Pause, then reverse the movement back to the starting position. That's 1 rep.

Alternating Dumbbell Chest Press

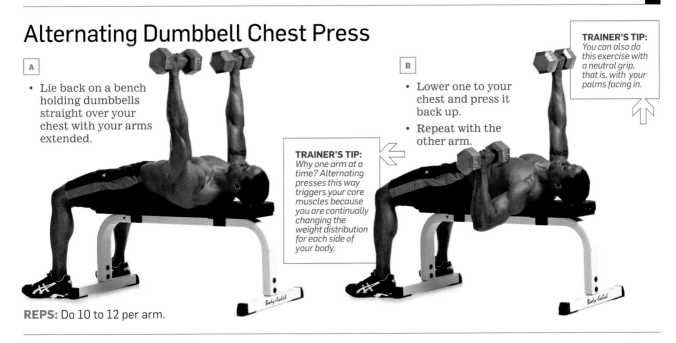

A

- Lie back on a bench holding dumbbells straight over your chest with your arms extended.

TRAINER'S TIP:
Why one arm at a time? Alternating presses this way triggers your core muscles because you are continually changing the weight distribution for each side of your body.

B

- Lower one to your chest and press it back up.
- Repeat with the other arm.

TRAINER'S TIP:
You can also do this exercise with a neutral grip, that is, with your palms facing in.

REPS: Do 10 to 12 per arm.

EZ-Curl Bar Triceps Extension

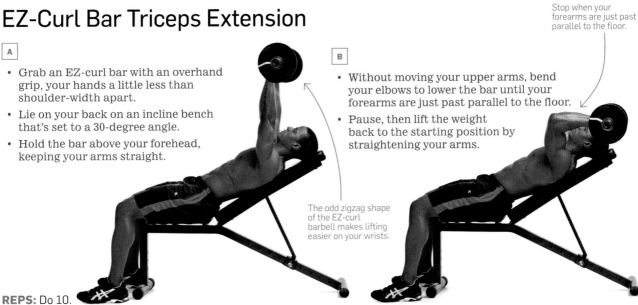

A

- Grab an EZ-curl bar with an overhand grip, your hands a little less than shoulder-width apart.
- Lie on your back on an incline bench that's set to a 30-degree angle.
- Hold the bar above your forehead, keeping your arms straight.

B

- Without moving your upper arms, bend your elbows to lower the bar until your forearms are just past parallel to the floor.
- Pause, then lift the weight back to the starting position by straightening your arms.

Stop when your forearms are just past parallel to the floor.

The odd zigzag shape of the EZ-curl barbell makes lifting easier on your wrists.

REPS: Do 10.

Chest and Back Combo

Underhand-Grip Inverted Row

TRAINER'S TIP: *Focus on pulling your shoulder blades together. This move trains your trapeziuses, rhomboideus, rear deltoids, and rotator cuff muscles, all of which help stabilize your shoulders.*

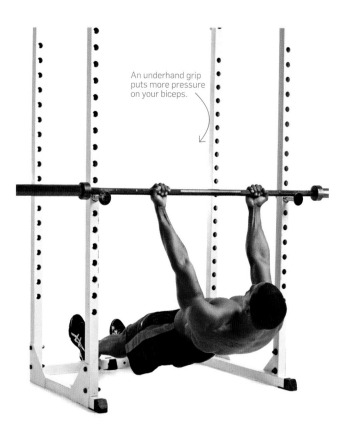

An underhand grip puts more pressure on your biceps.

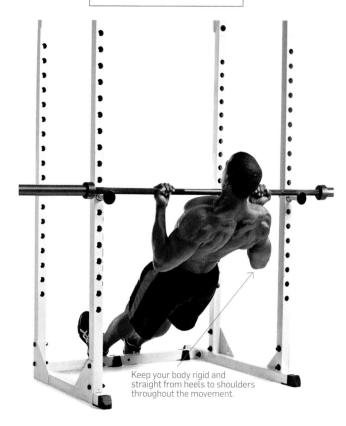

Keep your body rigid and straight from heels to shoulders throughout the movement.

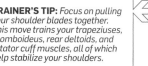

A

- Set a bar at hip height in a Smith machine or squat rack.
- Lie on the floor underneath the bar with your legs outstretched and your heels on the floor. Grab the bar using an underhand grip (palms facing you). Hang with your arms completely straight.

REPS: Do 10 to 12.

B

- Begin the lift by pulling your shoulder blades back, then continue the pull with your arms to lift your chest to the bar.
- Pause, then slowly lower yourself until your arms are straight.

Lean-Away Pulldown

Leaning back increases the involvement of your middle and upper back muscles and decreases the demand on your lats.

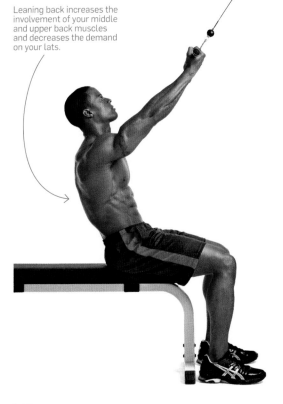

Don't rock back to change the angle of your torso as you pull the bar to your chest.

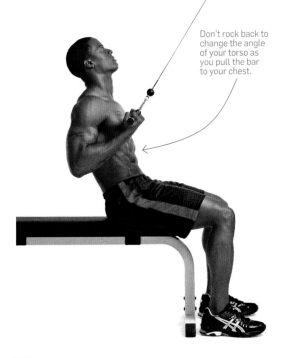

 A

- Sit in a lat pulldown machine and grab the bar using a shoulder-width, underhand grip.
- Lean back until your body forms a 30- to 45-degree angle with the floor. Hold this position for the entire exercise.

REPS: Do 10 to 12.

 B

- Without moving your torso, pull the bar down to your chest.
- Pause, and slowly return to the starting position.

The Perfect Pushup Circuits Workout 1

There is no more perfect exercise than the pushup. It's simple, requires no equipment, and can develop your size, strength, and endurance. More versatile than machines or free weights, pushups allow you to alter arm placement and body orientation and to use equipment—such as steps, balls, and benches—to provide an infinite array of exercises.

START HERE:
Complete one set of each pushup in workout 1. Rest between pushups only if you need to. Do three circuits of workout 1, resting 60 seconds after each circuit. Follow this pattern for workouts 2 and 3 as well.

Diamond Pushup

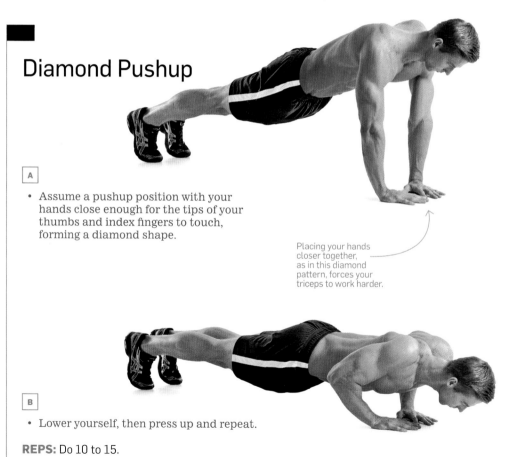

A
- Assume a pushup position with your hands close enough for the tips of your thumbs and index fingers to touch, forming a diamond shape.

Placing your hands closer together, as in this diamond pattern, forces your triceps to work harder.

B
- Lower yourself, then press up and repeat.

REPS: Do 10 to 15.

Alternating Shuffle Pushup

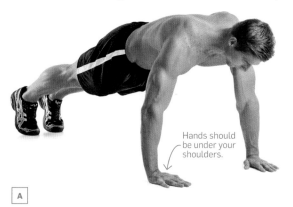

A

Hands should be under your shoulders.

- Assume a pushup position and do 1 pushup.

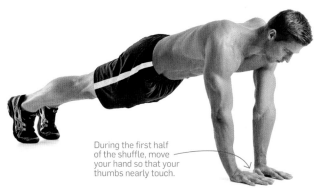

During the first half of the shuffle, move your hand so that your thumbs nearly touch.

B

- Now move your right hand to the left until both hands are next to each other. Then, slide your left hand farther left until your hands are shoulder-width apart again.
- Do another pushup.
- Now move your left hand to your right and your right farther right.
- Do a pushup and continue alternating this way. Each pushup is 1 rep.

REPS: Do 10 to 15.

Suspended Pushup

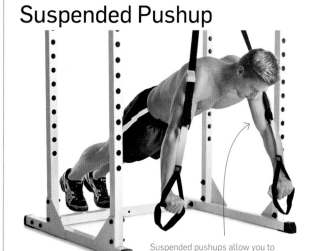

A

Suspended pushups allow you to lower yourself through a greater range of motion than floor pushups do.

- Loop Blast Straps or TRX Suspension Training straps around a chinup bar or rack so that the handles hang a few inches off the floor.
- Assume a pushup position with your arms straight and your hands grasping the handles, so that only your feet touch the floor.

Keep your forearms perpendicular to the floor as you lower your torso.

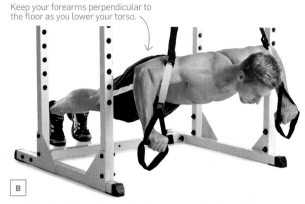

B

- Bend at the elbows to lower your body until your upper arms are parallel to the floor, then push yourself up.

REPS: Do 10 to 15.

The Perfect Pushup Circuits Workout 2

Crossover Box Pushup

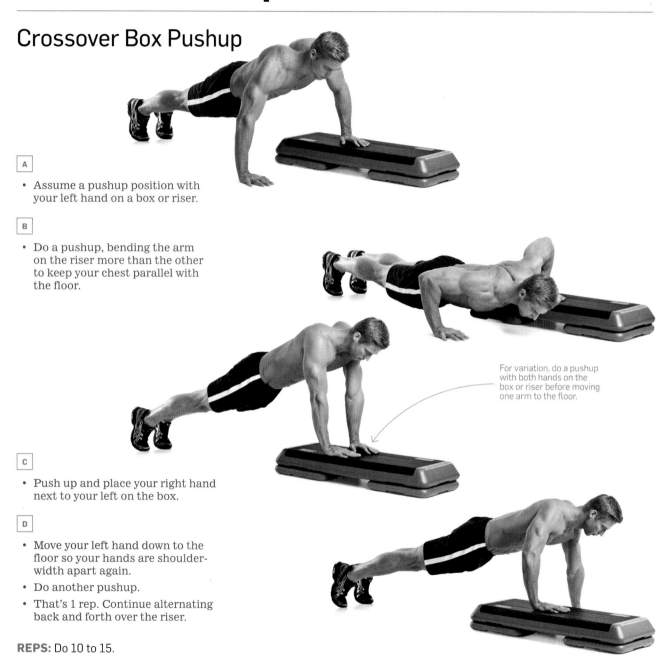

A

- Assume a pushup position with your left hand on a box or riser.

B

- Do a pushup, bending the arm on the riser more than the other to keep your chest parallel with the floor.

For variation, do a pushup with both hands on the box or riser before moving one arm to the floor.

C

- Push up and place your right hand next to your left on the box.

D

- Move your left hand down to the floor so your hands are shoulder-width apart again.
- Do another pushup.
- That's 1 rep. Continue alternating back and forth over the riser.

REPS: Do 10 to 15.

One-Arm Pushup

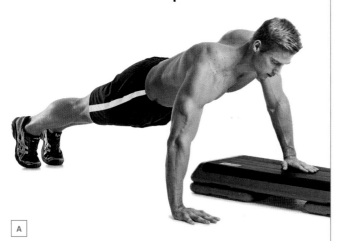

- Assume a pushup position with your hands spread slightly more than shoulder-width apart, one hand on a box or riser that's about 6 inches high and the other on the floor.

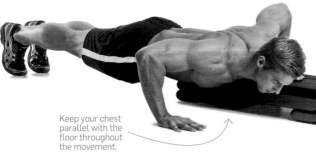

Keep your chest parallel with the floor throughout the movement.

- Lower your body until your chest touches the box. Complete all the reps, then place your right hand on the box and your left on the floor, and repeat.

REPS: Do 10 to 15 with each hand on the box.

Medicine Ball Rolling Pushup

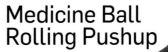

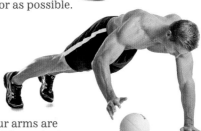

- Assume a pushup position with your right hand on top of a medicine ball and your left hand on the floor.

- Bend your arms to lower yourself until your chest is as close to the floor as possible.

- Press up so your arms are straight again. Then, placing your weight on your left hand, roll the ball toward your left hand.

- When your right palm hits the floor, lift your left and place it on the ball to stop its roll.
- Do another pushup, then roll the ball back to the right. That's 1 rep.

REPS: Do 5 to 10, moving quickly.

The Perfect Pushup Circuits Workout 3

Bosu Pushup

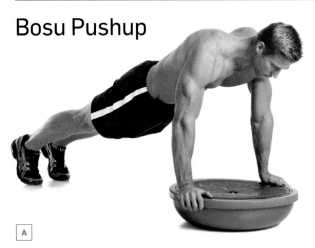

A

- Place a Bosu on the floor with the rounded, inflated side down.
- Assume a pushup position with your arms straight and hands holding the sides of the Bosu directly under your shoulders.

TRAINER'S TIP: *The Bosu half ball creates instability, which forces your arms and chest to engage more muscle fibers in order to balance.*

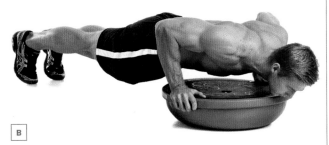

B

- Slowly bend your elbows to lower your body until your chin touches the edge of the Bosu.
- Straighten your arms to press your body to the starting position. Repeat.

REPS: Do 10 to 20.

Single-Leg Decline Pushup

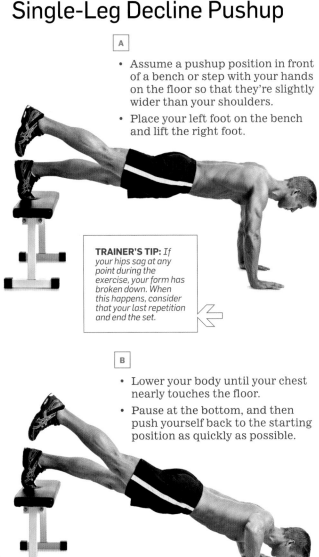

A

- Assume a pushup position in front of a bench or step with your hands on the floor so that they're slightly wider than your shoulders.
- Place your left foot on the bench and lift the right foot.

TRAINER'S TIP: *If your hips sag at any point during the exercise, your form has broken down. When this happens, consider that your last repetition and end the set.*

B

- Lower your body until your chest nearly touches the floor.
- Pause at the bottom, and then push yourself back to the starting position as quickly as possible.

REPS: Do 10, then repeat with your right foot on the bench and your left foot elevated.

Dynamic Box Pushup

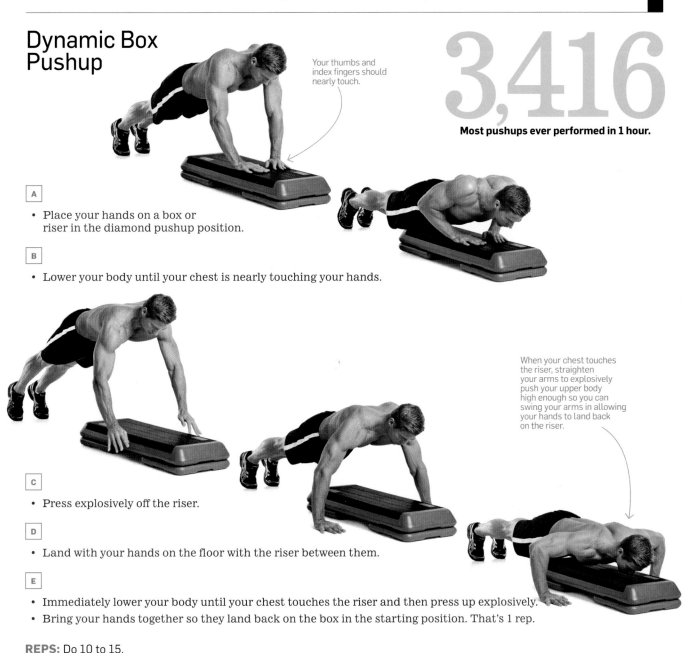

Your thumbs and index fingers should nearly touch.

3,416

Most pushups ever performed in 1 hour.

When your chest touches the riser, straighten your arms to explosively push your upper body high enough so you can swing your arms in allowing your hands to land back on the riser.

A
- Place your hands on a box or riser in the diamond pushup position.

B
- Lower your body until your chest is nearly touching your hands.

C
- Press explosively off the riser.

D
- Land with your hands on the floor with the riser between them.

E
- Immediately lower your body until your chest touches the riser and then press up explosively.
- Bring your hands together so they land back on the box in the starting position. That's 1 rep.

REPS: Do 10 to 15.

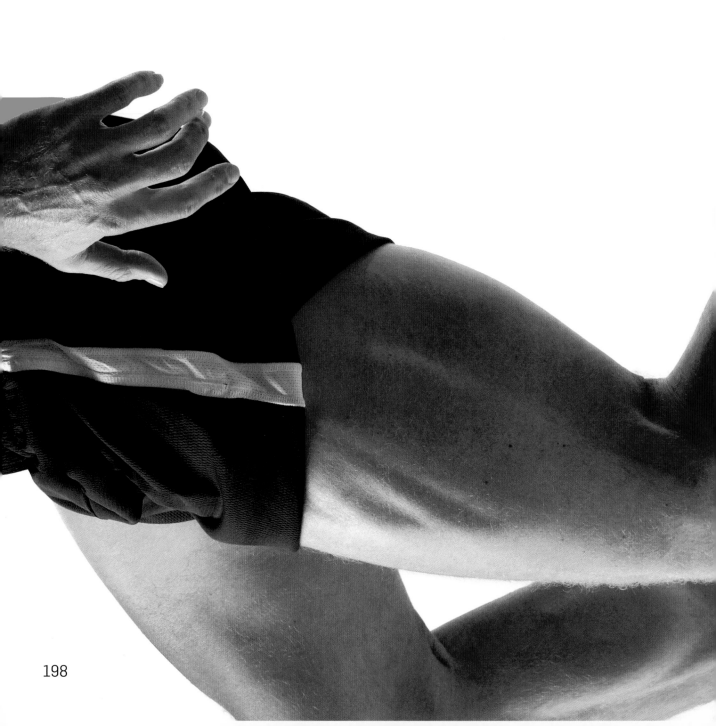

198

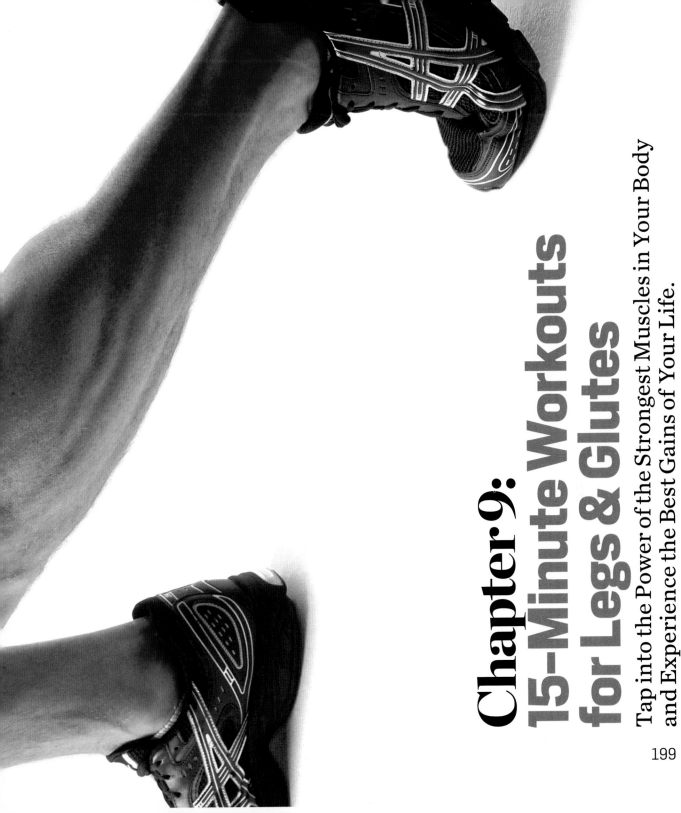

Chapter 9:
15-Minute Workouts for Legs & Glutes

Tap into the Power of the Strongest Muscles in Your Body and Experience the Best Gains of Your Life.

Superfast Lower-Body Workouts

Take a look around the typical weight room and you'll see a lot of guys with big chests and massive biceps but scrawny chicken legs who treat their lower halves solely as vehicles to get from the bench press to the preacher curl. That's a mistake. Neglect your wheels and you can end up cartoonishly out of proportion. A balanced body not only fills out your suit, but is also better suited for weekend basketball, tackling hills on your bike, and running those 5Ks. Plus, a strong butt does more than look good in your Levis, it also protects your back. Consider Olympic weight lifters: In the most basic measure of raw athletic ability—the vertical jump—they excel above all others. Don't ignore your legs. It only takes 15 minutes to give them some love.

In this chapter...

You'll find routines to address all of your lower-body muscles. For the best results, do one (or more) of the leg workouts 2 days a week. You can do more, but just be sure to leave a day of rest between workouts so your muscles can recover. (And you can always piggyback any of these routines on to another 15-minute workout for an über body blast.) Do the prescribed number of sets and reps for each exercise, opting for a weight at which you can barely eke out the last rep of your final set with perfect form. These workouts will give you a strong, solid lower half in as little as 3 to 4 weeks.

Find It Quick: Your 15-Minute Lower-Body Workout Plan

p.202

THE FLAT BUTT FIX
Front Lunge Push Off
1 and ¼ Barbell Squat
Hip Bridge and Heel Drag
Alternate-Leg Deadlift
Dumbbell Stepup Press Back
Glute Bridge March

p.206

THE IRON GLUTE WORKOUT
Rotation Lunge
Reverse Lunge Single-Arm Press
Hydrant Extension
Lateral Shuffle
Wide Squat with Ball
45-Degree Lunge
Static Squat with Front Raise

p.210

READY FOR LIFTOFF
SUPERSET 1
Dynamic Forward Lunge
Dynamic Side Lunge
SUPERSET 2
Single-Leg Deadlift Reach
Hack Squat

p.214

THE TOTAL LOWER-BODY BLAST
Alternate-Leg Deadlift
Prone Hip Extension
Good Morning Bend
Stability Lunge
Skater's Stepup
Single-Leg Plank

p.218

LOWER-BODY LEAPS AND BOUNDS
Standing Jump and Reach
Hip Twist and Ankle Hop
Front Cone Hop
Lateral Cone Hop
Alternating Box Pushoff
Squat Depth Jump

p.224

PROTECT YOUR ASSETS
Bench Hip Raise
Clamshell
Single-Leg Bench Get Up

GO EXPLOSIVE

Plyometric jumps can be used as substitutes for strength exercises when you don't have access to weight, but they also make terrific quick warmups for lower-body workouts. Explosive movements develop coordination as you boost your heart rate and warm up your muscles. Try this mogul jump plyometric to prime your limbs for a routine focusing on your legs.

The Mogul Jump:
Stand about 12 inches away from a curb (or a 6- to 8-inch-high step), with your right side facing the step. Rest your arms at your sides, hands in light fists. Jump sideways so both feet land on the curb at the same time, while bending your right arm and raising your right fist to shoulder height without moving your upper arm (as in a hammer curl). Jump down to the left with your feet together, raising your left fist. That's 1 rep. Perform 30 to 50, rest for 15 seconds, then repeat on the other side.

The Flat Butt Fix

If you rolled a quarter off the back of your head, would it hit anything on the way down? If not, you have a flat butt, which is more than a cosmetic concern. Strong glutes protect the lower back and provide explosive power for sports. Round out your rear view with moves for the beefy gluteus maximus and the oft-overlooked medius and minimus.

START HERE: Do these moves one after another with no rest between them. Then repeat the circuit for a total of two times.

Front Lunge Push Off

A

- Grab a pair of 10- to 15-pound dumbbells and stand with your feet together and your arms at your sides. This is the starting position.
- Leading first with your left foot, lunge forward and lower your hips until both knees form 90-degree angles.

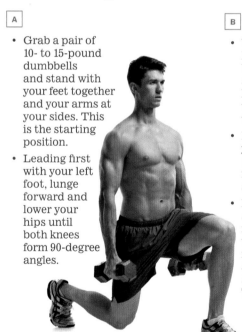

REPS: Do 5 to 6.

B

- With your right leg, pull yourself back to standing as you raise your left leg until your thigh is parallel to the floor.
- Balance on your right leg for 1 second, then return to the starting position.
- Repeat the lunge and balance movement, this time with your right leg in the lead, and return to the starting position. That's 1 rep.

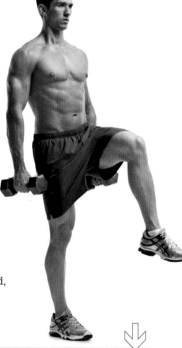

TRAINER'S TIP: *Contract your glutes and look straight ahead to maintain your balance.*

1 and ¼ Barbell Squat

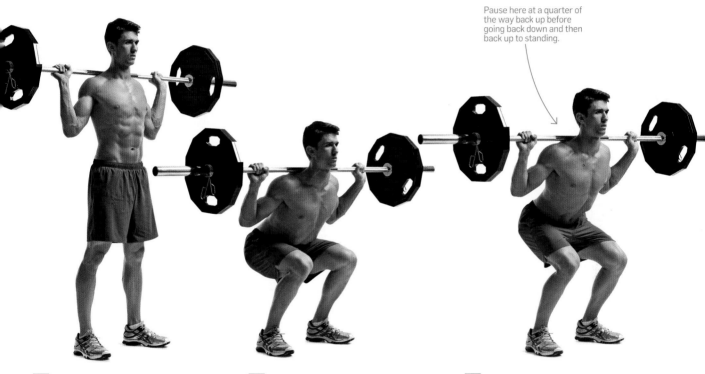

Pause here at a quarter of the way back up before going back down and then back up to standing.

A

- Place a barbell across your upper back and stand with your feet hip-width apart.

B

- Lower your hips by bending at the knees until your thighs are parallel to the floor.

C

- Push back up a quarter of the way, then pause before going back down to parallel.
- Pause, then return to the starting position. That's 1 rep.

REPS: Do 10 to 12.

The Flat Butt Fix

Hip Bridge and Heel Drag

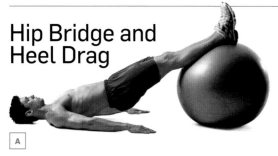

A

- Lie on your back with your lower legs on a stability ball.
- Raise your hips until they're aligned with your feet and shoulders.

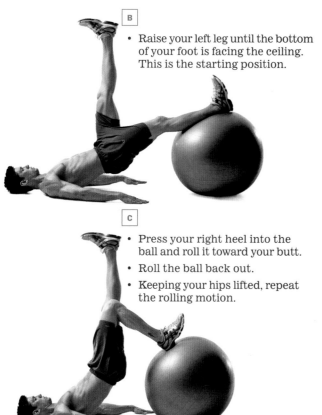

B

- Raise your left leg until the bottom of your foot is facing the ceiling. This is the starting position.

C

- Press your right heel into the ball and roll it toward your butt.
- Roll the ball back out.
- Keeping your hips lifted, repeat the rolling motion.

REPS: Do 10 to 12, then repeat with your other leg.

Alternate-Leg Deadlift

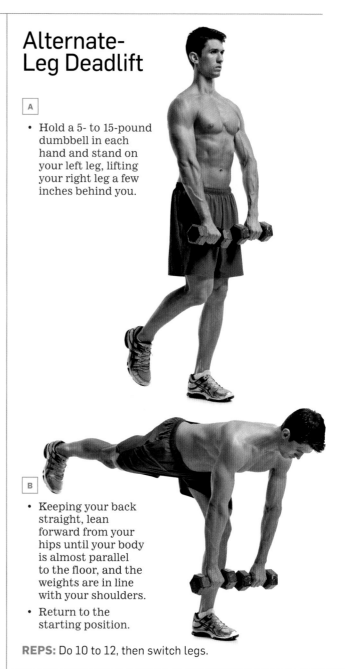

A

- Hold a 5- to 15-pound dumbbell in each hand and stand on your left leg, lifting your right leg a few inches behind you.

B

- Keeping your back straight, lean forward from your hips until your body is almost parallel to the floor, and the weights are in line with your shoulders.
- Return to the starting position.

REPS: Do 10 to 12, then switch legs.

Dumbbell Stepup Press Back

A

- Grab a pair of 5- to 10-pound dumbbells, stand in front of a bench or step, and place your left foot firmly on the step.

B

- Press down with your left heel and push your body up until your left leg is straight.
- Slowly lower yourself back to the starting position.
- That's 1 rep.

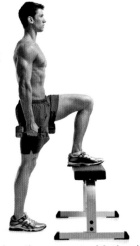
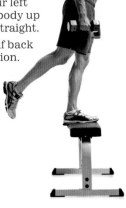

REPS: Do 10 to 12 with the left leg, then repeat with the right.

Glute Bridge March

Lifting the knee forces you to use your glutes to raise your hips.

A

- Lie on your back with your knees bent and your feet flat on the floor.
- Rest your arms on the floor, palms up, at shoulder level.
- Raise your hips so your body forms a straight line from your shoulders to your knees.

B

- Brace your abs and lift your right knee toward your chest.
- Hold for 2 counts, then lower your right foot.
- Repeat with the other leg. That's 1 rep.

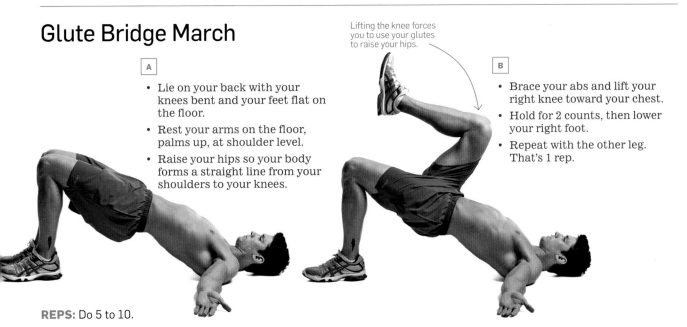

REPS: Do 5 to 10.

The Iron Glute Workout

Sitting for hours a day at your job can cause your glutes to forget how to fire. That makes you weak in one of the body's largest muscles. What's more, weak glutes can cause your pelvis to tilt forward, which pushes your lower abdomen outward, making your belly stick out—even if you don't have an ounce of fat.

START HERE:
Do these moves one after another with no rest in between. Then repeat the circuit once more.

Rotation Lunge

A

- Hold a 5- to 15-pound dumbbell by the ends with both hands.
- Stand with your feet hip-width apart and your arms straight out.

B

- Take a big step forward with your right foot and, bracing your abs, twist your torso to the right as you bend your knees and lower your body until both of your legs form 90-degree angles.
- Twist back to the center, push off your right foot, and stand back up. Repeat on the other leg. That's 1 rep.

REPS: Do 10 to 15.

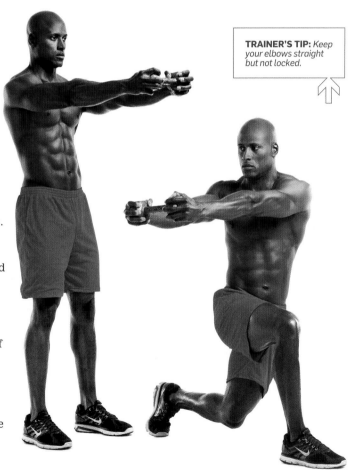

TRAINER'S TIP: *Keep your elbows straight but not locked.*

Reverse Lunge Single-Arm Press

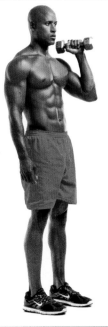

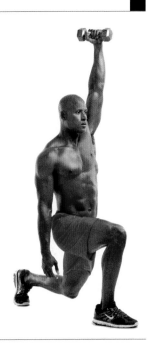

A

- Grab a dumbbell in your left hand and hold it up next to your left shoulder, palm facing in.

REPS: Do 10 to 15, then switch sides.

B

- Step backward with your left foot and lower your body until your knees are bent 90 degrees (your left knee should nearly touch the floor) while pressing the dumbbell directly over your shoulder without bending or leaning at the waist.
- Lower the weight back to the starting position as you push quickly back to standing. That's 1 rep.

Hydrant Extension

Keep your lower back as still as possible throughout the exercise.

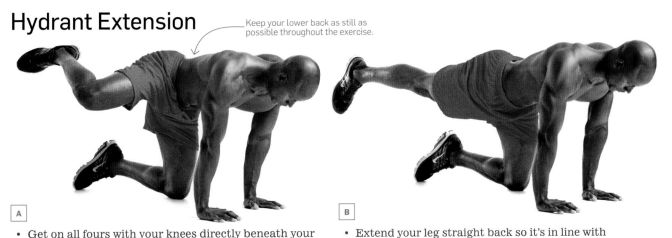

A

- Get on all fours with your knees directly beneath your hips and your hands under your shoulders.
- Keeping your knee bent, lift your right leg up and out to the side as high as possible.

REPS: Do 12 to 15.

B

- Extend your leg straight back so it's in line with your torso.
- Pause, then bring it back to the starting position. Repeat with your left leg. That's 1 rep.

The Iron Glute Workout

Lateral Shuffle

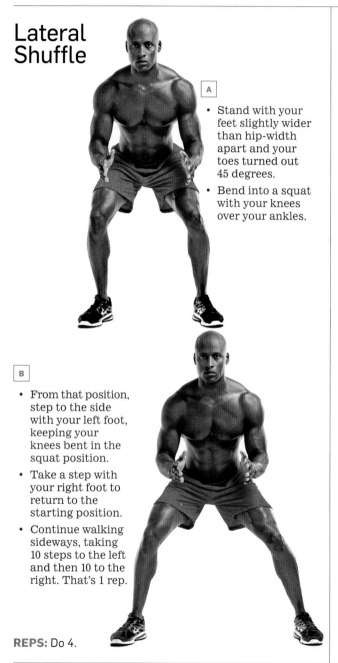

A
- Stand with your feet slightly wider than hip-width apart and your toes turned out 45 degrees.
- Bend into a squat with your knees over your ankles.

B
- From that position, step to the side with your left foot, keeping your knees bent in the squat position.
- Take a step with your right foot to return to the starting position.
- Continue walking sideways, taking 10 steps to the left and then 10 to the right. That's 1 rep.

REPS: Do 4.

Wide Squat with Ball

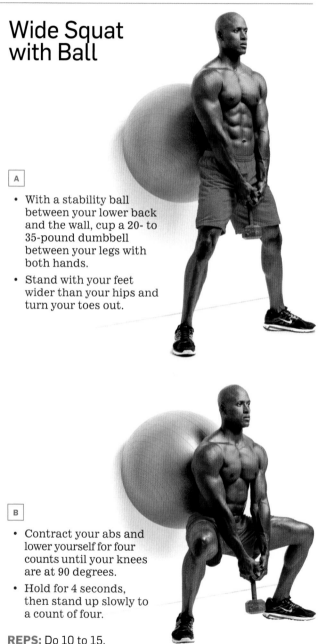

A
- With a stability ball between your lower back and the wall, cup a 20- to 35-pound dumbbell between your legs with both hands.
- Stand with your feet wider than your hips and turn your toes out.

B
- Contract your abs and lower yourself for four counts until your knees are at 90 degrees.
- Hold for 4 seconds, then stand up slowly to a count of four.

REPS: Do 10 to 15.

45-Degree Lunge

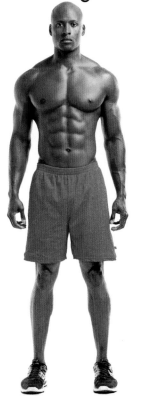
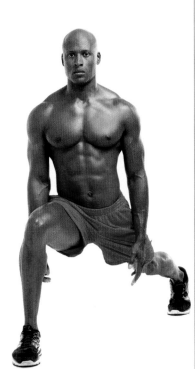

Static Squat with Front Raise

A

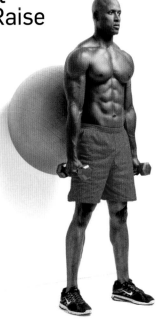

- With a stability ball between your lower back and the wall, hold a 5- to 10-pound dumbbell in each hand.
- Step forward with your feet hip-width apart and lean back into the ball.

A

- Stand with your feet hip-width apart, your arms at your sides.

B

- Lunge 45 degrees to the right, keeping your hips facing forward and your left leg straight.
- Pause, then return to the starting position. That's 1 rep.

B

- Contract your abs and glutes, then lower your hips until your knees are at 90 degrees.
- In this position, slowly raise your arms in front of your body to shoulder height 8 times.
- Rise to the starting position.

REPS: Do 10 to 12. Then repeat on your left side.

REPS: Do 2 to 4.

Ready for Liftoff

Add power to your legs with this hard-core hurdle workout. It creatively uses a barbell as a barrier to step over to force you to activate your leg muscles and build more muscle in less time. The hurdle corrects a mistake that most men make as they do lunges—not stepping out far enough and pushing off sluggishly rather than explosively.

START HERE:
Perform the sets within each superset without rest, but rest 60 seconds after you've done both sets. Do Superset 1 three times, and then move on to Superset 2, which you'll also do three times.

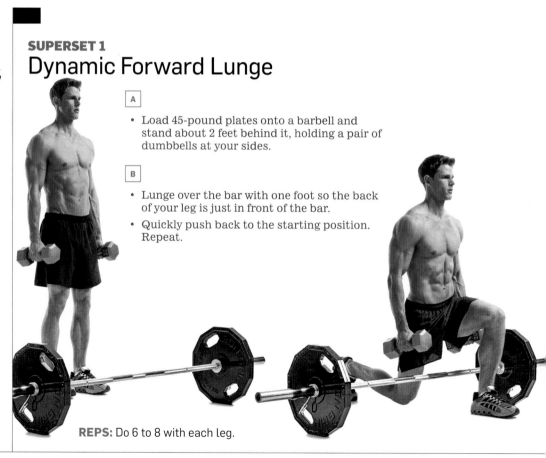

SUPERSET 1
Dynamic Forward Lunge

A
- Load 45-pound plates onto a barbell and stand about 2 feet behind it, holding a pair of dumbbells at your sides.

B
- Lunge over the bar with one foot so the back of your leg is just in front of the bar.
- Quickly push back to the starting position. Repeat.

REPS: Do 6 to 8 with each leg.

Dynamic Side Lunge

A

- Stand to the right of the loaded barbell while still holding the dumbbells.

B

- Lift your left leg over the bar.
- Bend your left knee and lower your body as far as you can.
- Then push back up explosively.

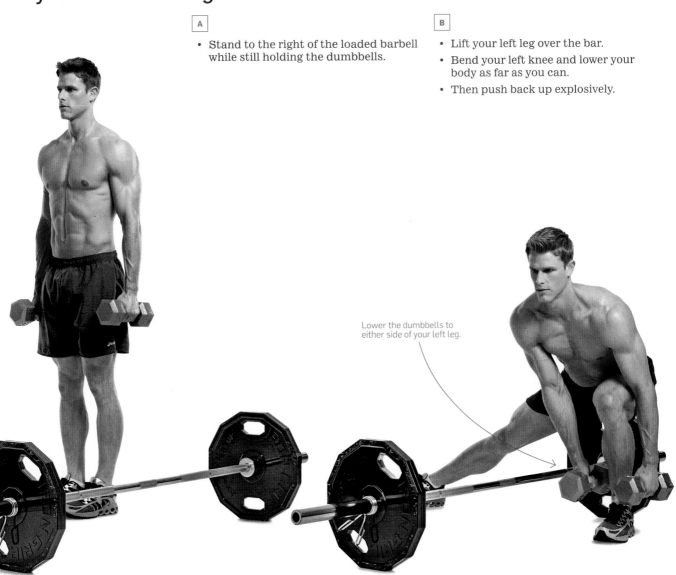

Lower the dumbbells to either side of your left leg.

REPS: Do 6 to 8 with each leg.

Ready for Liftoff

Single-Leg Deadlift Reach

A

- Place a loaded bar on the floor 18 inches in front of you.
- Stand on your left leg and hold a dumbbell in your right hand.

B

- Keeping your back naturally arched, push your hips back and allow your right leg to swing behind you as you lower the weight toward the barbell.
- Touch the bar with the weight, then return to the starting position.
- Complete all reps, then hold the dumbbell in your left hand and repeat.

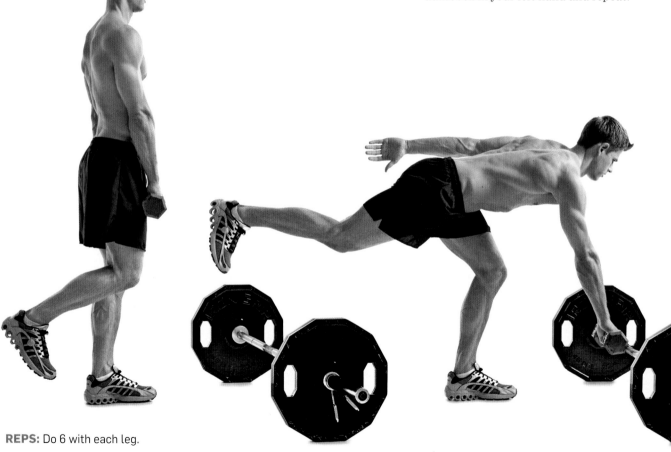

REPS: Do 6 with each leg.

Hack Squat

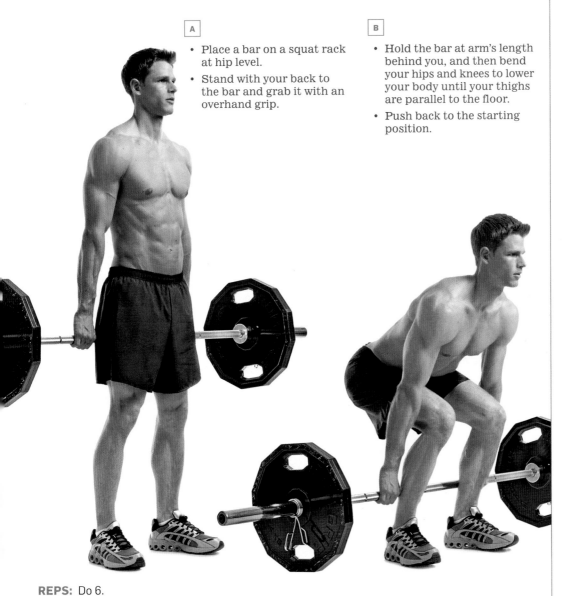

A
- Place a bar on a squat rack at hip level.
- Stand with your back to the bar and grab it with an overhand grip.

B
- Hold the bar at arm's length behind you, and then bend your hips and knees to lower your body until your thighs are parallel to the floor.
- Push back to the starting position.

SQUAT TO PREVENT KNEE INJURIES

Weak glutes can make your knees collapse inward, causing muscle strains and tears. Give your glutes and hamstrings top billing in your training routine; working your butt and the backs of your legs will help keep the knees stable.

REPS: Do 6.

The Total Lower-Body Blast

It's always good to mix up your workouts so your muscles don't get too comfortable doing any one routine. Here's one to add variety. It'll firm your butt, strengthen your thighs, tighten your core, and zap your love handles. In short, it'll help you pare down your middle and firm up and fill out your favorite denim.

START HERE:
Do these moves one after another with no rest in between. Then repeat the circuit for a total of two times.

Alternate-Leg Deadlift

A
- Hold a 15- to 20-pound dumbbell in each hand and stand with your feet hip-width apart.

B
- Lean forward and push your right leg back until your back and leg are nearly parallel to the floor.
- Stand up and repeat this move, this time with your left leg back. That's 1 rep.

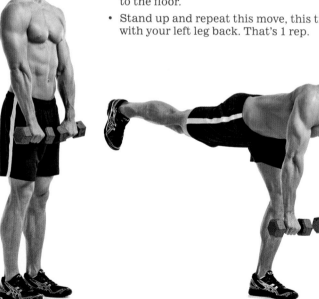

REPS: Do 10 to 12.

Prone Hip Extension

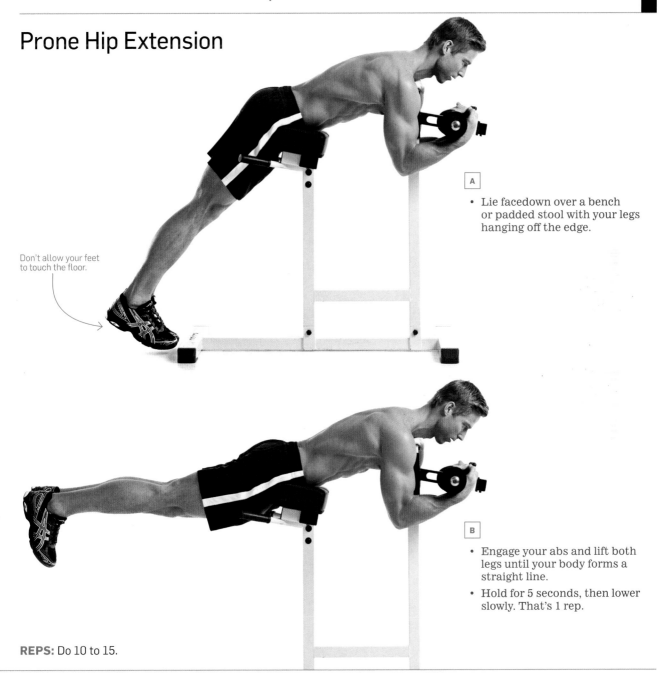

Don't allow your feet to touch the floor.

A

- Lie facedown over a bench or padded stool with your legs hanging off the edge.

B

- Engage your abs and lift both legs until your body forms a straight line.
- Hold for 5 seconds, then lower slowly. That's 1 rep.

REPS: Do 10 to 15.

The Total Lower-Body Blast

Good Morning Bend

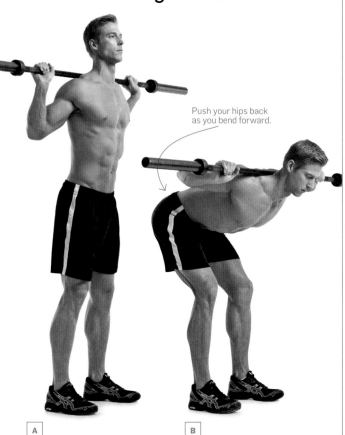

Push your hips back as you bend forward.

A
- Stand with your feet shoulder-width apart and hold a light barbell across your upper back, palms facing forward.

B
- Keeping your knees slightly bent and your torso straight, slowly bend from your hips until your upper body is parallel to the floor.
- Hold for 5 seconds and return to the starting position. That's 1 rep.

REPS: Do 8 to 10.

Stability Lunge

Balance for 5 seconds before lunging forward.

A
- Stand with your feet shoulder-width apart and your arms at your sides.
- Lift your right knee until your thigh is parallel to the floor and raise your arms overhead, palms together.
- Hold for 5 seconds.

B
- Keeping your knee bent, slowly drop your right foot into a front lunge.
- Bring your left leg forward and return to standing. That's 1 rep.

REPS: Do 10 to 12 on each leg, alternating sides.

Skater's Stepup

A

- Hold a pair of 10- to 25-pound dumbbells at hip level and stand facing a step with your right foot planted on the step.

- Leaning your chest forward slightly, lunge backward with your left leg, bending your right knee 90 degrees.

B

- From that position, bring your left foot up to meet the right on the step; squat and hold for 2 seconds.

- Stand and return to the starting position. That's 1 rep.

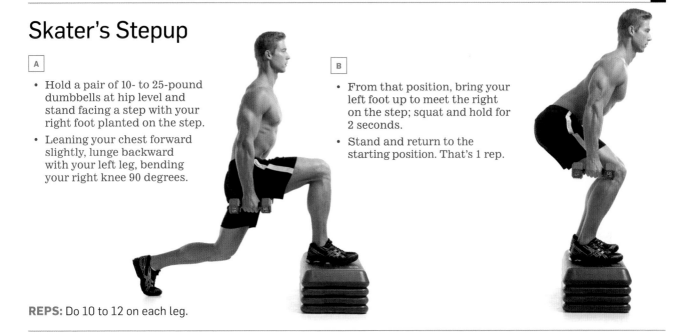

REPS: Do 10 to 12 on each leg.

Single-Leg Plank

A

- Assume a plank position by propping yourself up on your forearms with your elbows directly under your shoulders and your toes flexed underneath you.

B

- Brace your abs and lift your right leg up about 10 inches.

- Balance your body weight on your forearms and the stabilizing leg.

- Hold for up to 60 seconds.

- Switch legs and repeat on the other side.

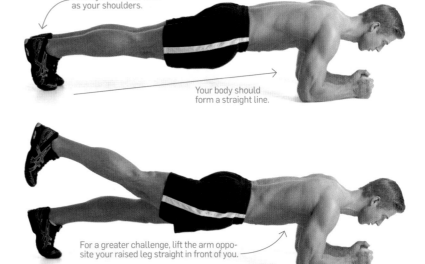

Place your feet as wide as your shoulders.

Your body should form a straight line.

For a greater challenge, lift the arm opposite your raised leg straight in front of you.

REPS: Do 1 with each leg elevated. Hold for 60 seconds each.

Lower-Body Leaps and Bounds

Whether you play basketball or racquet sports, or run or cycle, adding plyometric exercises to your workout can have a huge impact on your performance. How? By building explosive leg power and endurance using moves that simulate how your muscles work in action. Here are six that will get your heart pumping, too.

START HERE:
Do these six plyometric moves as a circuit. Catch your breath while setting up the cones and boxes needed for the last three exercises in the circuit. Rest for 60 to 90 seconds after the final exercise, then repeat the circuit once or twice more.

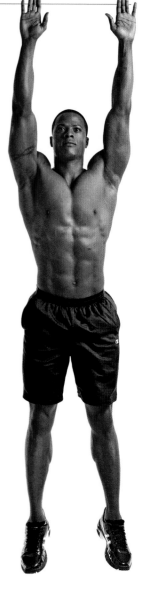

Standing Jump and Reach

A

- Squat slightly with your feet shoulder-width apart and your arms down at your sides.

B

- Quickly explode upward, lifting both arms overhead.
- Land with soft knees, then explode up again.

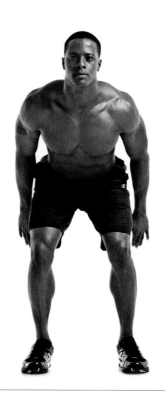

REPS: Do 8 to 10.

Hip Twist and Ankle Hop

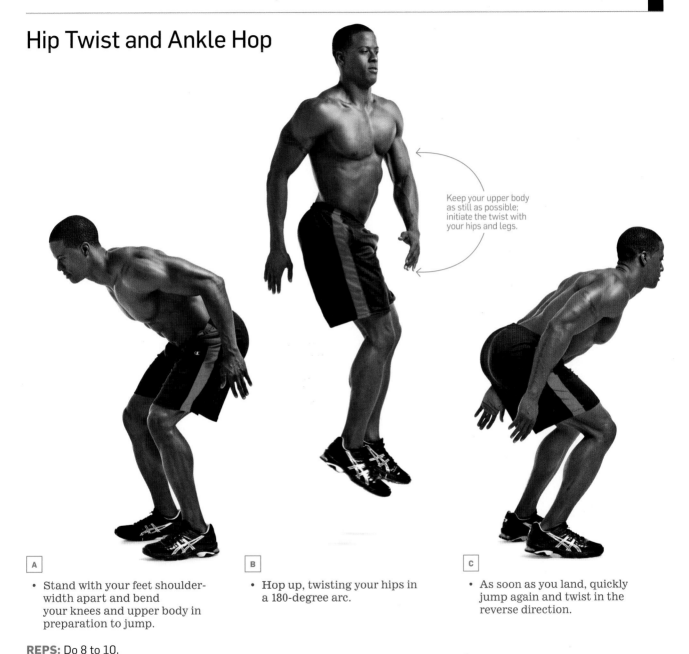

Keep your upper body as still as possible; initiate the twist with your hips and legs.

A

- Stand with your feet shoulder-width apart and bend your knees and upper body in preparation to jump.

REPS: Do 8 to 10.

B

- Hop up, twisting your hips in a 180-degree arc.

C

- As soon as you land, quickly jump again and twist in the reverse direction.

Lower-Body Leaps and Bounds

Front Cone Hop

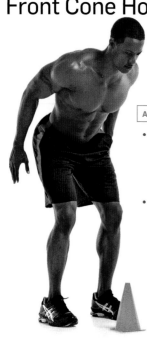

A

- Set 6 to 10 small cones or barriers that are approximately a foot tall in a straight line, about 2 feet apart.
- Stand at one end of the row with your feet shoulder-width apart and your arms at your sides.

B

- Hop forward over the first cone, swinging your arms to help with your forward momentum.

C

- Land with both feet together.
- Immediately repeat until you've completed the entire row of cones. That's 1 rep.

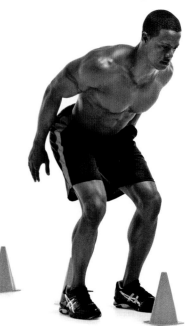

REPS: Do 5.

Lateral Cone Hop

A

- Stand next to a cone or box that's about a foot tall, with your arms at your sides and your feet shoulder-width apart.

- Jump sideways over the cone and land with both feet together.

B

- Upon landing, immediately jump back over the cone. That's 1 rep.

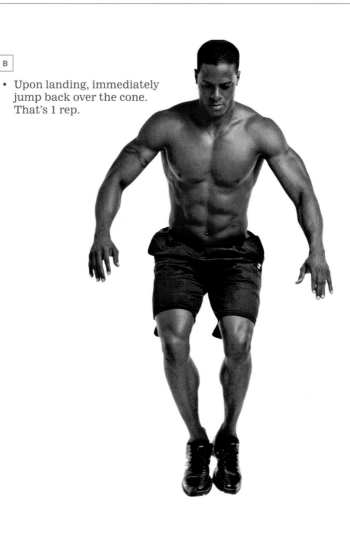

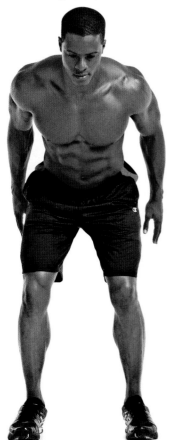

REPS: Do 8 to 10.

FIT FACT

The most basic measure of raw athletic ability is the height of the vertical jump.

221

Lower-Body Leaps and Bounds

Alternating Box Pushoff

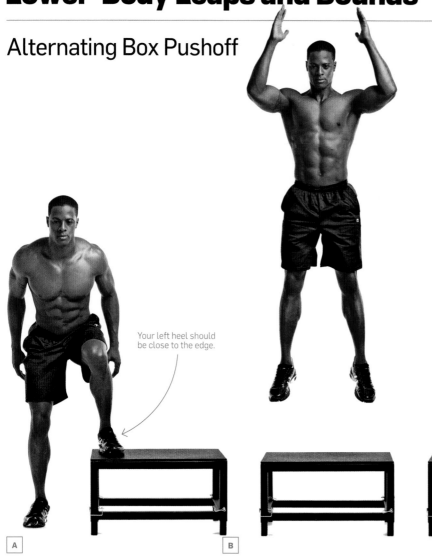

Your left heel should be close to the edge.

A

- Stand with your right foot on the floor and your left on a box that's about a foot tall.

B

- Push off your left foot and jump as high as possible, swinging your arms upward to help you catch more air.

C

- Switch legs in midair and land on the other side of the box with your feet reversed, your right on the box and your left on the ground.
- Immediately jump and reverse sides again.

REPS: Do 4 to 6 with each leg.

Squat Depth Jump

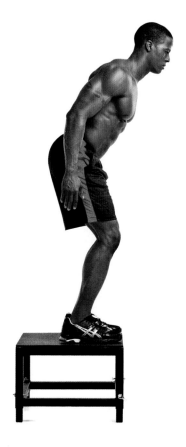

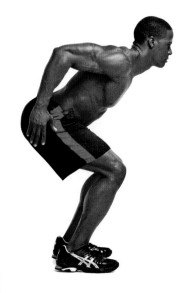

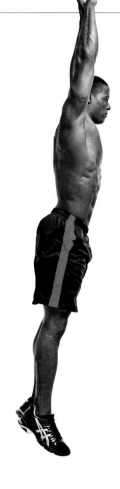

A
- Stand on a sturdy box that's 1 to 2 feet tall.
- Bend into a quarter- to half-squat position, with your toes close to the edge of the box.

REPS: Do 8 to 10.

B
- Hop off and land softly. Dip into a quarter squat.

C
- Immediately jump again, reaching as high as possible with your outstretched arms.

Protect Your Assets

If you routinely suffer from bouts of knee and back pain, chances are your glutes are not pulling their weight in stabilizing your pelvis when you walk, run, and play sports. This routine designed by Bill Hartman, PT, CSCS, will improve your hip and glute functioning, activating muscles that have been ignored (or sat upon) for too long.

START HERE: Perform three sets of each move before moving on to the next exercise. Rest for 30 to 60 seconds between sets.

Bench Hip Raise

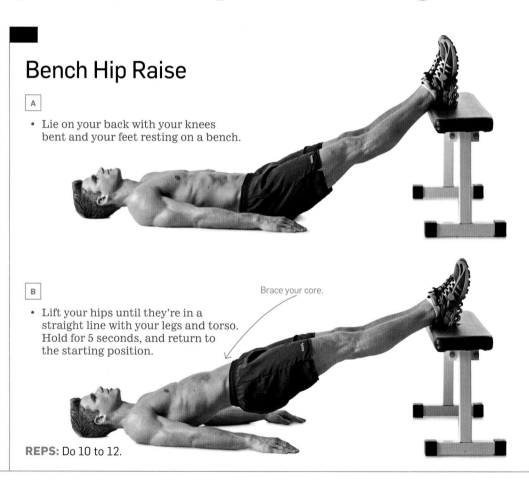

A

- Lie on your back with your knees bent and your feet resting on a bench.

B

Brace your core.

- Lift your hips until they're in a straight line with your legs and torso. Hold for 5 seconds, and return to the starting position.

REPS: Do 10 to 12.

Clamshell

A

- Slip your legs through a tight exercise band and position it just above your knees. Lie on your side with your knees bent 90 degrees and your heels together and in line with your butt.

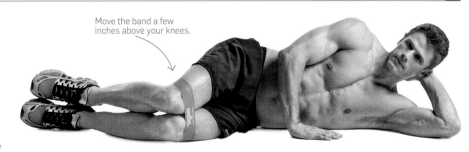

Move the band a few inches above your knees.

B

- Open your knees as far as you can without rotating your pelvis or back.
- Pause; return to the starting position.

REPS: Do 10 to 12 with each leg.

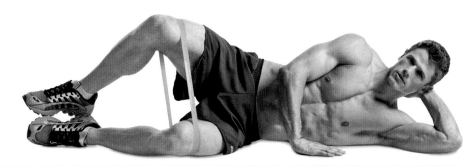

Single-Leg Bench Get Up

A

- Sit on an exercise bench with your left foot flat on the floor and your right foot raised.
- Extend your arms so that they are parallel with the floor.

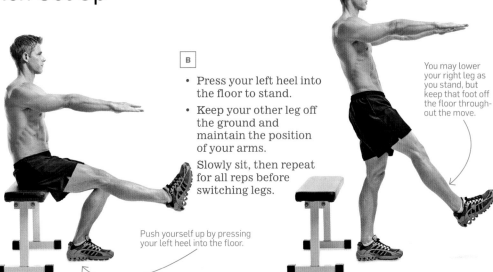

B

- Press your left heel into the floor to stand.
- Keep your other leg off the ground and maintain the position of your arms.

  Slowly sit, then repeat for all reps before switching legs.

You may lower your right leg as you stand, but keep that foot off the floor throughout the move.

Push yourself up by pressing your left heel into the floor.

REPS: Do 5 with each leg.

Chapter 10:
15-Minute Cardio Interval Training Workouts

High-Intensity Interval Training, or HIIT,
Is Your Weekly Weapon for
Losing Weight and Strengthening Your Heart.

This chapter

about cardiovascular exercise asks you to make a paradigm shift. Instead of logging miles and meters—the traditional measures of running, cycling, and swimming workouts—you'll track your workout progress in seconds, speed, and level of effort (determined, in large part, by how difficult you find it to breathe!) These are serious workouts. Done properly, they are very challenging. You'll understand and appreciate the secret benefits of high-intensity interval training the first time you try one; your body will feel as though you've been exercising for nearly an hour when only 15 minutes has passed. Our prediction: These will fast become your favorite workouts in this Big Book.

Superfast Cardio HIIT Workouts

The next time you're in the gym, look at the dashboard of your treadmill (or elliptical or stationary bike). You see that colored bar chart about what your heart rate should be to put you in the "fat-burning zone?" Ever wonder why reaching that rate was so easy (or why it seemed to take an endless amount of time to burn a decent amount of calories)? That type of training, where you slog along slowly for hours on end in the hopes of burning stored fat, is like cooking a roast in a slow cooker—it's great if you have all day to do it, but it's nowhere near as efficient as firing up the grill and searing the sucker. And that's exactly what you'll be doing to your fat with our superfast cardio workouts, which rely on HIIT, or high-intensity interval training.

Find It Quick: Your 15-Minute High Intensity Interval Training Plan

SPRINT AWAY FROM DIABETES

A study in Norway found that a high-intensity interval exercise program can reverse metabolic syndrome, the precursor to type 2 diabetes. Researchers compared 45 minutes of moderate exercise with an interval training program in which participants performed four 4-minute bouts at 90 percent of their maximum heart rate, and found that HIIT workouts are more beneficial than the longer, slower exercise routines at preventing obesity, diabetes, and cardiovascular problems.

As you learned in Chapter 1, HIIT workouts are built for speed. So they tap into every single muscle fiber, scorch tons of calories, and rev up your metabolism for hours (even days) afterward. With these workouts, you'll be burning fat almost from the get-go by going faster and harder than your normal cardio rate. Sound intimidating? Don't worry. You'll only be doing these "sprints" briefly, for 30 seconds to 2 minutes. Then you'll slow down to a normal speed. It's an incredibly efficient way to get rid of extra pounds, explains Jason Talanian, PhD, who researched HIIT training at the University of Guelph, Ontario. "HIIT elicits rapid skeletal muscle remodeling and increases your total exercise capacity—the ability to use oxygen and burn fat—in a fraction of the time than if you work out less intensely," he says. That means you also make more muscle tissue and generate more fat-burning enzymes and hormone.

We've taken the HIIT principles and applied them to all your favorite forms of cardio to create this group of superfast workouts. Do one a week as the plan (see page 19) recommends. If you're inspired, you can do more; but remember, these workouts are strong medicine, so cap them at three times a week, allowing a day of recovery between them. During each exercise, alternate between short, high-intensity bursts, when you're exerting yourself at say, level 8 or 9 on a one to 10 scale; and longer, medium-intensity sessions, when your effort will be more like a 6 on that same scale.

Treadmill Workouts

There are two ways to turn up the intensity on the treadmill—push the pace or jack up the incline. Here are two HIIT workouts to get it done whichever way you like best.

Workout 1: The Speed Demon

The Speed Demon uses sprints to fry fat, but we still recommend putting the incline at 1 (when it's 0, it's like you're running down hill.) As you get fitter, you can increase the speed even more to make the workout harder, or add a percent or two to the incline. If you're a beginner, you can lower the speeds by 1 mph, or as far as you need to stay within the recommended effort range.

TIME	ACTIVITY	SPEED (MPH)	EFFORT (1-10)
0:00 – 3:00	Warmup walk	3.5 – 3.8	4 – 5
3:00 – 3:45	Sprint!	8+	9 – 10
3:45 – 4:30	Brisk jog	5.5 – 6.5	7
4:30 – 5:30	Sprint!	8+	9 – 10
5:30 – 7:00	Brisk jog	5.5 – 6.5	7
7:00 – 8:15	Sprint!	8+	9 – 10
8:15 – 9:15	Brisk jog	5.5 – 6.5	7
9:15 – 10:15	Sprint!	8+	9 – 10
10:15 – 11:15	Brisk jog	5.5 – 6.5	7
11:15 – 12:00	Sprint!	8+	9 – 10
12:00 – 12:45	Brisk jog	5.5 – 6.5	7
12:45 – 15:00	Cooldown walk	3 – 3.5	4 – 5

Workout 2: HIIT the Hills

This workout uses the treadmill's incline to simulate the challenge of hills. If you find it a little too high to start, simply take each down by 1%. As you become fitter and stronger, crank up the incline to conquer mountains (of calories!).

TIME	ACTIVITY/EFFORT (1-10)	SPEED (MPH)	INCLINE %
0:00 – 3:00	Warmup walk (4 – 5)	3.5–3.8	1
3:00 – 4:00	Small hill jog (8 – 9)	4–5	5 – 6
4:00 – 6:00	Brisk flat jog (7)	5.5–6.5	0
6:00 – 7:00	Medium hill jog (9)	4–5	7
7:00 – 9:00	Brisk flat jog (7)	5.5–6.5	0
9:00 – 10:00	Big hill jog (10)	4–5 (if possible)	8 – 9
10:00 – 12:00	Brisk flat jog (7)	5.5–6.5	0
12:00 – 13:00	Peak! (10)	4 to 5 (if possible)	10 – 12
13:00 – 15:00	Cooldown jog to walk (4 – 5)	3.5–3.8	1

Running Workouts

When you run long distances, your body actually becomes more efficient, so you burn fewer calories. These hard-hitting workouts help you shed pounds with minimal mileage by forcing your body out of its comfort zone and making it work in ways it rarely does. It not only boosts your speed and fitness, it takes a quarter of the time! These workouts are designed to be done on a track (try your local high school or college).

Workout 1: Dash It Off

Two-hundred meters (that's halfway around the track) is the perfect leg-searing distance because you don't have to hold back to finish. It's just flat-out full throttle the whole time, followed by a recovery jog for 1 lap. Seasoned runners will be a little quicker; novice runners may take a little longer.

TIME	SPEED	DISTANCE
0:00 – 5:00	Easy jog to warm up	@2 laps
5:00 – 5:30	Dash!	Aim for ¼ to ½ lap
5:30 – 7:00	Jog	Aim for about 1 lap
7:00 – 7:30	Dash!	Aim for ¼ to ½ lap
7:30 – 10:00	Jog	Aim for about 1 lap
10:00 – 10:30	Dash!	Aim for ¼ to ½ lap
10:30 – 13:00	Jog	Aim for about 1 lap
13:00 – 13:30	Dash!	Aim for ¼ to ½ lap
13:30 – 15:00	Cooldown jog to walk	

MISERY LOVES COMPANY

If you're finding that HIIT workouts are a real pain in the butt, recruit some friends. Researchers at the University of Oxford found that people who train in groups have better pain tolerance than those who exercise alone. The scientists speculate that group dynamics during workouts may contribute to an underlying endorphin surge. We think people feed off the energy of others, which may be the same thing.

Workout 2: Flying Laps

These 1-lap wonders will challenge all your energy systems to the max. Unlike the half-laps, when you're going full steam from the get-go, keep just enough energy in reserve that you don't find yourself flagging at the end of the interval, but rather can finish a little stronger than you started. Seasoned runners will be a little quicker; novice runners may take a little longer.

TIME	SPEED	DISTANCE
0:00 – 5:00	Easy jog to warm up	@2 laps
5:00 – 7:00	Dash!	Aim for about 1 lap
7:00 – 8:00	Easy Jog	Aim for about ½ a lap
8:00 – 10:00	Dash!	Aim for about 1 lap
10:00 – 11:00	Easy jog	Aim for about ½ a lap
11:00 –13:00	Dash!	Aim for about 1 lap
13:00 – 15:00	Jog easy to cool down	

Cycling Workouts

Whether you ride indoors or out, a bike is the perfect tool for superfast fat burning since there's no pounding on your joints, just pure, unabated, lactic-acid-building effort. These workouts are designed for a road, spin, or stationary bike. On a spin or stationary bike you'll just be increasing the resistance, while on a road bike you'll be shifting into a larger gear.

Workout 1: The Lance Armstrong

These workouts get your calorie-burning motor running by becoming progressively harder until you're at your ceiling (then you just hang on!). Gauge your intensity on a scale of 1 to 10. If you're outside, you can use the average speeds as a guide. More-experienced riders may pedal faster.

TIME	ACTIVITY	LEVEL (1-10)	APPRX. SPEED
0:00 – 3:00	Warmup	6	10 – 15 mph
3:00- 5:00	Fast pedaling	8	16 – 17 mph
5:00 – 6:00	Chase pace	9	18 – 19 mph
6:00 – 6:30	Sprint!	10	20+ mph
6:30 – 9:30	Easy pedaling	6	10 – 15 mph
9:30 – 11:30	Fast pedaling	8	16 – 17 mph
11:30 – 12:30	Chase pace	9	18 – 19 mph
12:30 – 13:00	Sprint!	10	20+ mph
13:00 – 15:00	Cool down	6	10 – 15 mph

Workout 2: Rolling Hills

If you're outside and there are hills, ride up them for the prescribed amount of time and then cruise down and continue with the next segment of the workout. If you're using a stationary bike, simply click into a bigger gear to increase resistance. The goal is to make those pedals hard to turn. Pedal smoothly. Your speed will drop as the resistance increases, but you should be able to keep your pedal stroke fluid, not choppy. When the workout calls for a standing climb, rise off the seat for the duration of the interval. For seated climbs, stay in the saddle and increase your pace to pedal as quickly as you can.

TIME	ACTIVITY	LEVEL/GEAR	INCLINE/RESISTANCE
0:00 – 3:00	Warmup	6	0 – 3%/light
3:00 – 4:00	Fast seated climb	7	4 – 6%/medium
4:00 – 5:30	Seated climb	8	6 – 8%/hard
5:30 – 6:00	Standing climb	9	8 – 10%/very hard
6:00 – 8:00	Fast and flat	6	0 – 3%/light
8:00 – 9:00	Fast seated climb	7	4 – 6%/medium
9:00 – 10:30	Seated climb	8	6 – 8%/hard
10:30 – 11:00	Standing climb	9	8 – 10%/very hard
11:00 – 13:00	Fast and flat	7	0 – 3%/light
13:00 – 15:00	Cool down	6	0 – 3%/light

Elliptical Workout

This perennial favorite gym machine provides a sweat-breaking, impact-free platform for high-intensity intervals. The following workout will push you through the machine's toughest settings for a full-body burn. You'll be increasing your speed, measured by the strides-per-minute indicator on the machine's dashboard, and ratcheting up the resistance at the same time, getting a little faster and tougher with each effort until you are maxed out. Remember, don't hold onto the rails; instead, pump your arms to keep your feet turning over as quickly as you can. If you have a machine with an incline feature, add intensity by simulating hill climbs. Just use the HIIT the Hills workout on page 231.

NOT A WALK IN THE PARK

While the elliptical has always been known as a great tool for injury rehab, lately it has developed an unfair reputation as the machine for those who would rather read than sweat. True, you can take it easy on this device by hanging onto the handrails and allowing pedal momentum to do the work, but used properly, it can kick your metabolism into high gear. A new study from the University of Nebraska found that exercising on an elliptical trainer burned as many calories as running on a treadmill at the same level of effort. Oxygen consumption was also equivalent on the machines, but people's average heart rates were actually higher when working out on the elliptical, possibly because the newness of the motion required their muscles to do more balancing work. To keep your body guessing, alternate between the two cardio machines.

The Boredom Beater

During the sprint stages, don't allow momentum to work for you. Make sure you feel your legs pushing the ramp down on each revolution.

TIME	ACTIVITY	SPM*/EXERTION(1-10)	RESISTANCE
0:00 – 2:00	Warmup	130 – 140 (5-6)	3 – 5
2:00 – 4:00	Ramp (medium pace)	150 – 180 (7-8)	7 – 8
4:00 – 5:00	Sprint!	190 (9-10)	8 – 9
5:00 – 6:00	Steady	150 (6-7)	7
6:00 – 8:00	Ramp (medium pace)	160 – 190 (7-8)	7 – 8
8:00 – 9:00	Sprint!	200 (10)	9 – 10
9:00 – 10:00	Steady	150 (6-7)	7
10:00 – 12:00	Ramp (medium pace)	170 – 200 (7-8)	7 – 8
12:00 – 13:00	Sprint!	210 (10)	9 – 10
13:00 – 15:00	Cool down	130 – 140 (5-6)	3 – 5

*SPM = Strides Per Minute

Swimming Workout

Water is 800 times denser than air, so sprinting across a pool burns fat like nothing else. This workout will shed inches off your body. Do the interval program as prescribed, swimming the recommended stroke for the prescribed number of lengths and at the level of effort specified from 1 to 10. Note: The workout is based on a standard 25-meter lap pool; Olympic-size pools are 50 meters. One length is across the pool. One lap is across the pool and back.

A STROKE OF GENIUS

To get the most from your swimming intervals, build a more efficient (longer and faster) stroke. Try this drill: Take two strokes with your right arm, one with your left, one with your right, and then two with your left. Next, take one stroke with your right and left and two with your right and left. Continue this pattern for 5 minutes. This helps you even out your stroke and find a good rhythm, says Keith Bell, PhD, of the American Swimming Association.

FREESTYLE POINTERS

Better form means a better workout. Practice these fine points when learning to crawl.

1. Look at the bottom of the pool. Lifting your head causes your hips to drop and slows you down.

2. Be a fish. Swim smooth and quiet without slapping water, a sign of wasted energy.

3. When extending your leading hand, let it sink 8 inches before starting your pull. Imagine you're wrapping your arm over a barrel and pushing it behind you.

4. Roll, baby, roll. Developing good body roll allows you to use your strong lats, core, and back muscles to drive your stroke, and it helps you cut through the water efficiently. And breathing becomes easier. To learn proper rotation, practice kicking on your side with a pair of flippers and one arm stretched in front of you.

Interval Medley

TIME	STROKE	LENGTH	EFFORT
0:00 – 3:00	Freestyle/mixed kicking	About 2 laps	4 – 5
3:00 – 5:00	Freestyle	About 2 laps	6 – 7
5:00 – 5:45	Freestyle	About 1 lap	9
5:45 – 7:00	Freestyle/mixed kicking	About 1 lap	6
7:00 – 7:45	Freestyle	About 1 lap	9
7:45 – 9:00	Freestyle/mixed kicking	About 1 lap	6
9:00 – 9:45	Freestyle	About 1 lap	9
9:45 – 11:00	Freestyle/mixed kicking	About 1 lap	6
11:00 – 11:30	Breast	About 1 length	8 – 9
11:30 – 13:00	Freestyle	1 lap + 1 length	8 – 9
13:00 – 15:00	Back/mixed kicking	About 1 lap	4 – 5

Jump Rope Workout

Ever notice that most boxers and mixed martial arts fighters never seem to have an ounce of fat on their bodies? Maybe it has something to do with all the rope jumping they do in training. The jump rope forces your body to work hard and burn calories. This interval workout mixes pace and jumping style in quick bursts. Try to jump about 2 inches off the floor—just enough to allow the rope to skim the floor beneath your feet. Keep your elbows close to your body while you're swinging the rope, and stay on the balls of your feet.

PICK UP YOUR PACE

Strengthening the muscles in your feet can help prevent injury to your ankles, hips, and back when you run or jump rope. One of the best exercises is the Marble Pickup: Sit in a chair with marbles spread out on the floor in front of you. With bare feet, use your toes to grasp as many marbles as you can, lift your leg up, and drop the marbles into a cup. Repeat two or three times, then exercise your other foot. This exercise strengthens your arch, reducing pronation. To bolster your ankles, balance on one leg while standing barefoot on a pillow or sofa cushion. Make it harder by closing your eyes or holding a medicine ball and moving it in clockwise and counterclockwise circles. To strengthen the tendons and ligaments of the underside of your foot, do the toe walk: Lift your toes off the floor and walk around on the balls of your feet, maintaining a slow pace. Do these exercises for a couple of minutes 2 or 3 times a week for a couple of months and your dogs will be stronger and feel awesome.

The Skipper 2

If this jump rope HIIT workout is too taxing, work up to it by reducing your speed or by splitting it in two: At the 6-minute mark do 30 seconds of fast double jumping, then stop and rest for a minute or so before resuming with the two-foot jumps.

TIME	JUMP STYLE	SPEED	EFFORT
0:00 – 1:00	Two-foot jump	Moderate	5 – 6
1:00 – 1:30	Single-foot hop	Moderate	7
1:30 – 2:30	Two-foot jump	Moderate	5 – 6
2:30 – 3:00	Single-foot hop	Moderate	7
3:00 – 5:00	Two-foot jump	Fast	8 – 9
5:00 – 6:00	Two-foot jump	Moderate	5 – 6
6:00 – 7:30	Double jump*	Fast	9 – 10
7:30 – 8:30	Two-foot jump	Moderate	5 – 6
8:30 – 10:30	Jumping jacks**	Moderate to fast	8
10:30 – 11:30	Two-foot jump	Moderate	5 – 6
11:30 – 13:30	Run through***	Moderate to fast	8 – 9
13:30 – 15:00	Two-foot jump	Moderate	5 – 6

Jump high enough to pass the rope under your feet twice before landing.

** *Jump over the rope and land with feet wide apart. Then, on the next jump, land with feet together.*

*** *Run in place while swinging the rope up and around.*

Chapter 11:
The 15-Minute Plan to Fight Fat with Food

Eating Healthy Starts with Being Prepared with
the Right Ingredients, the Best Tools, and Delicious Recipes.
You'll Find It All in This Chapter.

Generally

speaking, when it comes to nutrition, speed compromises health. But there are ways to feed yourself fast other than by heading for the nearest drive-thru. In Chapter 3, you learned the ins and outs of the Superfast Weight-Loss System. But knowing what to eat and applying it to the meals you actually put on your plate can be two different things. That's why we've added this chapter on how to fight fat with food—the chapter will actually tell you how and what to eat. Having the right tools, counter layout, and, of course, meal plans in place will go a long way toward speeding up your success.

The Superfast Kitchen Overhaul

For most men who are scheduled to the gills, time is a precious commodity. To whip up the lightning-quick meals in this chapter, you need a kitchen set up for NASCAR-level speed. That means all the right tools in all the right places. Here's a two-step, 15-minute kitchen makeover that will have you prepared for healthy cooking in less time than it takes to call for take out.

Clean House

The first step in your 15-Minute Kitchen Overhaul is a clean sweep of your fridge, cabinets, and pantry. We're asking you to be ruthless, to toss out perfectly good food (that's bad for you), whether you've opened it or not. The key is to get rid of all of your temptations. Because if the Cheetos aren't there, you can't eat them in a moment of salt-craving weakness. So grab a large trash bag and let's get started: Take all the sweets and treats like candy and cookies and toss them. If you just can't bear to trash those $30 gourmet chocolates, then at least hide them from plain view where they can't be easily reached. Even better, place them in opaque containers before you hide them. Researchers have found that men and women eat far fewer sweets when they're stored in containers that obscure what's inside than when they're in clear jars. In fact, in one study from the University of Illinois, office workers ate 25 percent fewer Hershey's Kisses when they were placed inside a slightly inconvenient spot out of sight, like inside a desk drawer, than when they were within arm's reach in plain view.

Did you get rid of the snack cakes and baked goods? Good. Next, sniff out the white bread, white rice and pasta, boxed and canned pasta meals, and other highly processed foods. The nonperishable stuff can be donated to a local food bank, including juices and sodas. Banish all sugary beverages from your home. Remember, if it's not there, you can't drink it or eat it. Out of sight, out of mind, out of mouth, out of belly.

Get Ready for Action

Okay, your trash bag is full and your cupboard is bare, but you still have 5 minutes left in your 15-Minute Kitchen Overhaul. Now focus on your tools. You can't make quick meals if you have to spend 10 minutes fumbling through your junk drawer for a measuring spoon. Take the time right now to dig out the following items and place them prominently on your countertops or in easy-to-grab spaces in your cupboards, so you have quick access to your food-prep tools any time of day.

Cutting boards: For chopping fruits and vegetables, slicing meats, and general food prep.

Knives: At least one good chef's knife is a must. And make sure it's sharp! All good chefs know that dull knives are dangerous knives. Round out your knife arsenal with a serrated version and a paring knife.

Measuring cups and spoons: They help keep portions (and pounds) in check.

Colander: For rinsing vegetables.

Blender/food processor: To crush ice for smoothies, purée raw ingredients into silky-smooth soups or sauces, and grind meat or chop nuts.

Shredder: For cheese, of course, but also for shredding ginger and other flavorings. (We also recommend a grater or zester—think tinier teeth—for grating spices and making citrus zest.)

Oven mitts: For handling HOT pots and pans.

Flexible nylon food turner: Because they won't scratch your nonstick pans.

Tongs: A stainless steel model, as well as one with nylon-covered tips for those nonstick pans.

A wooden spoon: For stirring sauces and sneaking tastes.

A pepper mill: Because there's nothing like having fresh ground peppercorns to spice up a meal.

JUST ADD WATER

Replace your can of diet whatever with ice cold water. Researchers at the University of Utah found that volunteers who drank 8 to 12 8-ounce glasses of water per day had higher metabolic rates than those who sipped only 4 glasses. Your body may burn a few calories heating the cold water to your core temperature, says Madelyn Fernstrom, PhD, founder and director of the University of Pittsburgh Medical Center Weight Management Center. Though the extra calories you burn drinking a single glass is pretty small, making it a habit can add up to pounds lost with essentially zero additional effort.

YOUR STAPLES: Restock your refrigerator and pantry with these mainstays of healthy eating

HIGH-QUALITY PROTEINS	LOW-STARCH VEGETABLES*		NATURAL FATS
Beef	Artichokes	Mushrooms	Avocados
Cheese	Asparagus	Onions	Butter
Eggs	Bok choy	Peppers	Coconut
Fish	Broccoli	Radishes	Cream
Pork	Brussels sprouts	Salad greens	Nuts and seeds
Poultry	Carrots	Spinach	Olives, olive oil, and canola oil
Soy	Cauliflower	Tomatoes	Full-fat salad dressings
Whey and casein proteins	Celery	Turnips	
	Cucumbers	Zucchini	

Any vegetables besides potatoes, peas, and corn are fair game.

245

15 Delicious Muscle-Building, Fat-Fighting Meals You Can Make in 15 Minutes or Less

Let's get something straight: The following recipes won't turn you into the next Food Network star. But they will help you to eat better for good health and weight loss. And they won't keep you kitchen-bound for hours up to your elbows in wheat grass. Oh yeah, most important: These meals taste great. That's a promise.

In the spirit of this book—simplicity and quarter-hour speed—we've compiled recipes for 15 nutrient-dense meals that you can make in 15 minutes or less. When you tire of these meals or for days when you have more time to spend in the kitchen, grab a copy of *The New Abs Diet Cookbook*, also from *Men's Health*. It's packed with more than 200 recipes utilizing the same healthy ingredients recommended in this book. Meanwhile, grab a plate and try these.

BREAKFAST

GREEN EGGS OMELET

2   large eggs
2   egg whites
1   tablespoon milk
1   teaspoon butter
¾ cup baby spinach, washed
¼ cup reduced fat shredded
     Cheddar cheese
     ground black pepper

- Beat the eggs and milk together in a bowl.
- Melt the butter in a skillet over medium heat. Add the eggs and cook until it begins to set.
- Add the spinach and shredded cheese on top and cook for another minute; then, using a spatula or nylon food turner, fold into an omelet.
- Cook until the eggs are thoroughly set.
- Season with salt and pepper and serve.

Makes 1 serving.

Per serving: 260 calories, 23 g protein, 4 g carbohydrates, 15 g fat (7 saturated), 1 g fiber

SUPERFAST HUNGER BUSTER

¼ cup cottage cheese
½ cup fresh blueberries
1   tablespoon crushed walnuts

- Mix all together in a bowl.

Makes 1 serving.

Per serving: 198 calories, 10 g protein, 14 g carbohydrates, 12.5 g fat (2.5 g saturated), 3 g fiber

NUKED OATMEAL

1   cup rolled oats
1   cup low-fat milk
½ cup frozen strawberries
     dash of salt
     teaspoon of sugar (optional)
     dash ground cinnamon
1   scoop vanilla whey protein powder

- Combine the oats and milk in a microwavable bowl.
- Microwave for 1 minute, stir, and then microwave for 1 more minute.
- Allow to cool for a minute before mixing in the protein powder, salt, cinnamon, and sugar.

Makes 1 serving.

Per serving: 585 calories, 43 g protein, 80 g carbohydrates, 11 g fat (3.6 g saturated), 10 g fiber

PROTEIN MAKES A MEAL

Building every meal around protein helps build and maintain lean muscle mass. Muscle burns more calories than fat does, even at rest, says Donald Layman, PhD, professor of nutrition at the University of Illinois. Aim for about 30 grams of protein—the equivalent of about 1 cup of low-fat cottage cheese or a 4-ounce boneless chicken breast—at each meal.

15-Minute Plan to Fight Fat With Food

10 WAYS TO SNEAK FIBER INTO YOUR DIET

The golden number for daily grams of dietary fiber is between 20 and 35, according to the USDA. But few of us consume that much. To get more of the belly-filling, cholesterol-lowering, metabolism-boosting good stuff, try these tricks:

1. Sprinkle garbanzo beans into your salad. A half-cup delivers up to 6 grams of extra fiber.

2. Drop a handful of berries to add flavor to plain or vanilla yogurt. Half a cup provides 4 grams of fiber.

3. Eat the skin of your next baked potato for 2 extra grams of fiber.

4. Add fiber to chips and salsa by dumping some black or kidney beans into jarred salsa.

5. Crunch on 1 ounce (about a handful) of almonds, peanuts or sunflower seeds for 2 to 4 grams of fiber.

LUNCHES, SNACKS

A LITTLE ITALY

2 Wasa Crispbreads
4 thin slices prosciutto
6 basil or baby spinach leaves
2 slices ripe red tomato
2 slices part-skim mozzarella cheese (about 2 ounces)
1 teaspoon extra virgin olive oil
Cracked black pepper to taste

- Top each crisp with 2 slices of prosciutto, 3 basil leaves, 1 tomato slice, and 1 mozzarella slice.
- Drizzle with olive oil and grind some black pepper on top.

Makes 1 serving.

Per serving: 409 calories, 23 g protein, 15.5 g carbohydrates, 26.5 g fat (5.3 g saturated), 3 g fiber

SPICY TUNA SANDWICH

⅛ cup mayonnaise
¼ teaspoon wasabi paste
4 ounces canned tuna
4 slices whole-wheat bread
2 thin slices red onion
2 thin rings red bell pepper, seeded
½ cup avocado, sliced
¼ cup pickled ginger, sliced
4 romaine lettuce leaves

- In a small bowl, mix the mayonnaise and wasabi paste. Fork the tuna into the bowl and mix well.
- Spread an equal amount of the spicy tuna on 2 slices of bread.
- Top the tuna with an onion slice, pepper ring, avocado, some ginger, and 2 lettuce leaves. Then add the second slice of bread.

Makes 2 servings.

Per serving: 315 calories, 22 g protein, 35 g carbohydrates, 10 g fat (2.3 g saturated), 7 g fiber

ZIPPY PITA PIZZA

¼ cup chunky salsa
1 whole-wheat pita pocket
¼ cup cooked ham, diced
¼ cup mozzarella cheese, shredded

- Using a spoon, spread the salsa over one side of the pita.
- Top with the diced ham and shredded mozzarella.
- Place on a microwave-safe plate and microwave for a few seconds until the cheese melts.

Makes 1 serving.

Per serving: 360 calories, 23 g protein, 39 g carbohydrate, 13 g fat (5.5 g saturated), 5 g fiber

ZIPPY NO-DOUGH PIZZA

1 large Portobello mushroom cap
1 tablespoon thick spaghetti sauce
½ cup mozzarella cheese
5 thin slices pepperoni

- Preheat an oven to 400 degrees.
- If the stem is still attached to the mushroom, remove it. Also cut some of the gills out of the inside of the cap to make more room for the sauce and cheese.
- Place the mushroom cap side down on an oiled baking sheet and bake in the preheated oven for 4 minutes to remove some of the moisture.
- Take the baking sheet out of the oven and top the mushroom with spaghetti sauce, shredded mozzarella, and pepperoni slices.
- Bake for another 10 minutes or until the cheese has melted.

Makes 1 serving.

Per serving: 235 calories, 10.6 g carbohydrates, 19 g protein, 13.6 g fat (6.6 g saturated), 2.3 g fiber

SMOOTHIES

ANTIOXIDANT POWER PUNCH

1 green tea bag
1 teaspoon honey
1½ cups frozen blueberries
½ ripe banana
¾ cup vanilla soymilk

- Brew a cup of tea using boiling water and the tea bag. Remove the bag and stir in honey.
- Allow to cool. Add 5 tablespoons of the tea, blueberries, banana, and soy milk to a blender on a "chop" or "crush" setting.
- Blend until smooth.

Makes 2 servings.

Per serving: 151 calories, 5 g protein, 30 g carbohydrates, 1 g fat (0 g saturated), 3 g fiber

VIRGIN CABO DAIQUIRI

½ cup 1 percent milk
2 tablespoons low-fat plain yogurt
¼ cup frozen orange juice concentrate
½ ripe banana
¼ cup strawberries
½ cup cubed mango
2 teaspoons vanilla whey protein powder
3 ice cubes

- In a blender, puree the milk, yogurt, juice concentrate, banana, strawberries, mango, protein powder, and ice cubes.

Makes 2 servings.

Per serving: 154 calories, 7 g protein, 31 g carbohydrates, 1 g fat (0.5 g saturated), 2 g fiber

(From The New Abs Diet Cookbook.)

6. Bite an apple, spread on some almond butter, bite again and repeat.

7. Add lentils to soups. One-quarter cup of these tiny legumes is crammed with 11 g of fiber.

8. Munch on 2 cups of low-fat popcorn for 2 grams of fiber.

9. Drop a whole orange into the blender to flavor your morning smoothie. (Uh, peel it first.) One orange has nearly 3 grams more fiber than even the pulpiest orange juice.

10. Doctor your favorite jarred pasta sauce with ½ cup of frozen chopped spinach. The spinach will adopt the flavor of the sauce and pad the fiber count by more than 2 grams.

DINNERS

CORNED BEEF AND CABBAGE

It cooks in a slow cooker while you're at work. Prep takes less than 15 minutes.

8   small red potatoes (keep skin on)
4   medium carrots cut in half
3   cloves garlic
1   tablespoon brown sugar
1   bay leaf
3   pounds corned beef brisket
3   cups water
1   bottle Guinness beer
1   medium green cabbage cut into quarters

- Combine potatoes, carrots (not the cabbage), garlic, sugar, and bay leaf in a slow cooker.
- Add the brisket on top of the vegetables and pour the water and beer over the beef.
- Cover and cook on low for up to 10 hours.
- An hour before serving, add the cabbage.
- Remove the beef and vegetables from the cooker and place on a large platter.
- Discard the bay leaf. Serve with mustard and horseradish.

Makes 8 servings.

Per serving: 350 calories, 19 g protein, 23 g carbohydrates, 17 g fat (6 g saturated), 4 g fiber

STUFFED CHEESE LAMB BURGER

1   pound ground lamb
¼   pound smoked mozzarella cheese
4   large romaine lettuce leaves
    Salt and pepper to taste

- Cut the mozzarella into quarters.
- Form four burger patties by dividing the ground lamb evenly and molding each around a hunk of the cheese.
- Grill for about 4 minutes per side over high heat.
- Wrap each burger in a romaine leaf to serve.

Makes 4 servings.

Per serving: 397 calories, 26 g protein, 2 g carbohydrates, 31 g fat (14.5 g saturated), 1 g fiber

GRILLED TUNA KEBABS WITH ASIAN SAUCE

For the Asian sauce (make beforehand)

¼   cup low-sodium soy sauce
½   cup hoisin sauce
½   teaspoon sesame oil
½   teaspoon sugar
2   garlic cloves, minced
1   teaspoon fresh ginger, minced

- Combine all ingredients in a saucepan. Cook over medium heat until bubbly.
- Cool and store in a covered glass jar in refrigerator for up to 2 weeks.

For the kebabs

1   pound tuna steak
12 white button mushrooms
12 cherry tomatoes
6   scallions cut into 2-inch pieces
4   bamboo or wooden skewers

- Soak the skewers for 30 minutes.
- Cut the tuna into cubes a little larger than bite-sized.
- Divide the tuna cubes and vegetables into four even groups and thread the pieces alternately onto each skewer.
- Brush with the Asian sauce to cover. Grill or broil for 6 minutes, turning once, and brushing with the remaining dressing after 2 minutes of cooking.

Makes 4 servings.

Per serving: 220 calories, 30 g protein, 14 g carbohydrate, 5 g fat (0.5 g saturated), 2 g fiber

ROAST RATATOUILLE

1   medium eggplant, peeled and cut into ½-inch pieces

1   large zucchini, cut into ½-inch pieces

1   medium red onion, chopped

1   red bell pepper, seeded and cut into large 2-inch pieces

1   yellow bell pepper, seeded and cut into large 2-inch pieces

½   medium fennel bulb, cored and thinly sliced

1   can (15 ounces) diced tomatoes

1   tablespoon olive oil

1½ teaspoons oregano

½   teaspoon coarse kosher or sea salt

¼   teaspoon freshly ground black pepper

• Preheat an oven to 500 degrees.

• Coat a large roasting pan with cooking spray.

• Place eggplant, zucchini, onion, peppers, fennel, and tomatoes in the roasting pan.

• Toss with olive oil, oregano, salt, and pepper to coat.

• Roast, stirring occasionally, for about 15 minutes or until vegetables are tender.

Makes 4 servings.

Per serving: 127 calories, 3.5 g protein, 19 g carbohydrates, 4 g fat (1 g saturated), 7 g fiber

SALAD FOR DINNER

This salad is loaded with muscle-building protein and quality carbs, plus fats that will satisfy your hunger, roughly 30 grams of each. Made with leftover grilled skirt steak, it can be built in just minutes.

4   ounces grilled skirt or hanger steak, sliced thinly against the grain

2   cups chopped romaine lettuce

1   hard-boiled egg, halved

6   cherry tomatoes, halved

¼   avocado, sliced

1   tablespoon blue cheese, crumbled

1   cup sugar snap peas, steamed and halved

1   tablespoon extra-virgin olive oil

1   strip pre-cooked bacon, heated

• Toss all ingredients together and serve.

Makes 1 serving.

Per serving: 650 calories, 49 g protein, 32 g carbohydrates, 35 g fat (13.5 g saturated), 8 g fiber

HEALTHY OPTION: *Trim extra calories by eating half of this salad with a bowl of soup and saving the rest for tomorrow's lunch.*

A SIDE OF LEMONY SPROUTS

1   16-ounce package frozen petite Brussels sprouts

1   tablespoon butter

1   teaspoon extra-virgin olive oil

½   teaspoon lemon zest

1   teaspoon lemon juice
Salt and ground pepper to taste

• Toss the Brussels sprouts into a large pan with ¼ cup of water. Bring to a boil, cover, reduce heat, and simmer for 10 minutes or until tender.

• While the sprouts are cooking, heat 1 tablespoon of butter in a small saucepan until almost melted.

• Stir in the olive oil, finely grated lemon zest and lemon juice.

• Drain the sprouts and toss with the lemon-butter. Season with salt and fresh ground pepper.

Makes 4 servings.

Per serving: 187 calories, 3 g protein, 8 g carbohydrates, 16 g fat (8 g saturated), 3 g fiber

RECHARGE WITH MILK

Milk is the new post-workout drink. And it helps torch fat. In a study in the journal *Medicine and Science in Sports and Exercise,* people who drank skim milk after exercising lost 3.5 pounds of fat in 12 weeks. Those who sipped sports drinks after working out actually gained weight. Milk's protein improves the body's ability to burn calories and build muscle.

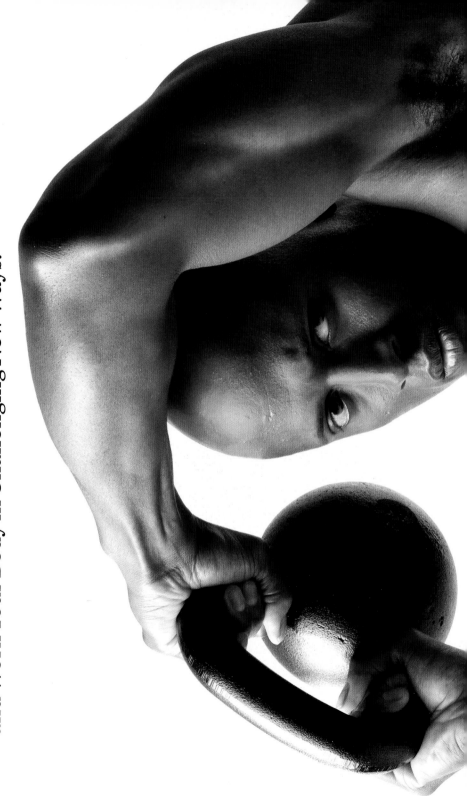

Chapter 12:
15-Minute Workouts For Special Gear

Balls, Bars, Bands, and Kettlebells Make Workouts Fun and Work Your Body in Challenging New Ways.

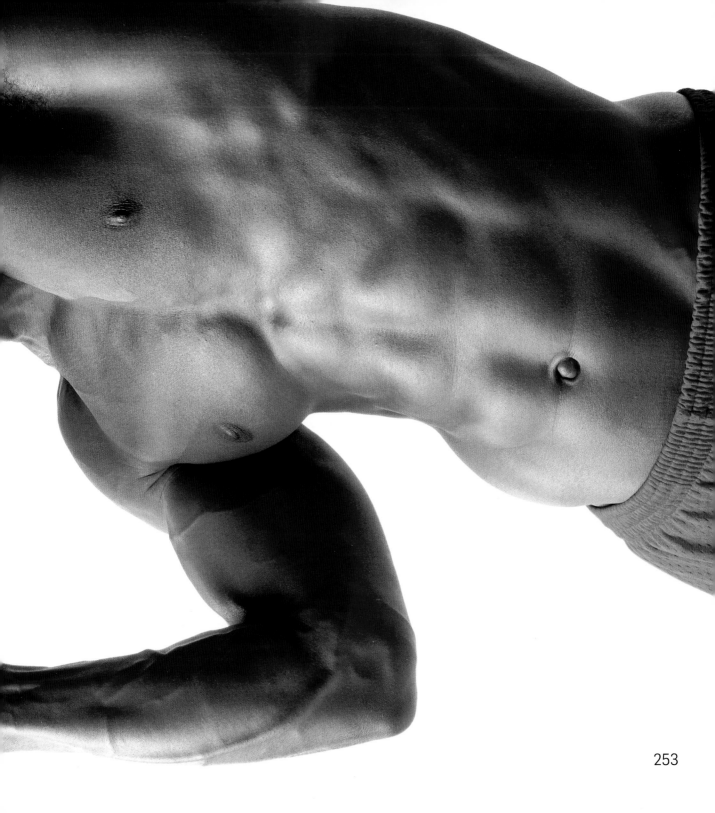

Superfast Workouts for Special Fitness Gear

I love gear. Balls, bands, foam rollers, and bells are like spices. You can use them to add pizzazz to your usual routine or you can build an entire workout around them. If you've been avoiding trying new workout gear and just settling for the tried-and-true barbells and dumbbells, expand your horizons. The beauty of exercise bands, kettlebells, and stability balls is that each item lets you work your muscles in a fresh way, activating new fibers and taking your fitness and strength to another level. After all, that's why the stuff got invented in the first place.

Begin with the basics...

In this chapter you'll find 51 moves using five pieces of unique equipment. Gear workouts, particularly kettlebell, can be a little tougher than your standard strength-training routines. If you're just starting a fitness routine, work up to these gradually. On the other hand, the fresh challenge these routines present makes them excellent options to jump-start the benefits for seasoned gym rats who may have hit a plateau. So grab your gear and let's go.

Find It Quick: Your 15-Minute Gear-Specific Circuit Plan

NEVER MISS A WORKOUT

Work travel can really mess up your ability to stick with an exercise program even if you're staying at a hotel with a gym. It's just a hassle to get down there sometimes. Exercise bands, which stow easily in a suitcase and can be used in your room, eliminate that excuse. Another packable piece of special gear to consider taking along a suspension training system like the TRX, which consists of two nylon straps with a loop at one end. The straps anchor to something sturdy, such as a door frame, for many different bodyweight exercises: dips, pullups, triceps presses, shoulder extensions, and more.

Kettlebell Workout 1

Kick up your metabolism with kettlebells. Working out with these asymmetrical cannonball-like weights absolutely scorches calories. Researchers from the University of Wisconsin found that doing kettlebell swings (a move where you simply squat and swing the bell, like the move on page 258) burns 20 calories a minute. That's more than spinning, rowing, elliptical training, stair stepping, or swimming! The two 15-minute kettlebell workouts here can burn close to 300 calories each. And that's just for starters. Factor in the muscle-building impact and the afterburn (the calories you burn after you exercise as your body repairs itself), and the total energy expenditure could shoot up by 50 percent.

Anatomy of a Kettlebell

The sculpting power of the kettlebell comes from its unique shape. The weight is asymmetrical, so your muscles have to work harder to balance and move it. That's why you should start with a light weight (no more than 20 pounds) until you get used to the unwieldy shape and master ideal form.

HANDLE: For most moves, you hold onto the handle, so you can swing the bell and pass it from hand to hand.

HORNS: The sides of the handle are called the horns. For some moves, especially if you're holding the bell upside down, you'll hold on here.

BASE (OR BELL): This is the main part of the weight, which is round with a flat base.

START HERE:

Do these moves one after another with no rest in between. Rest for 60 seconds at the end. Then repeat the circuit twice more.

Around the Body Pass

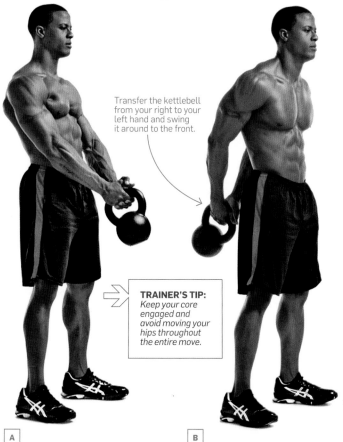

Transfer the kettlebell from your right to your left hand and swing it around to the front.

TRAINER'S TIP:
Keep your core engaged and avoid moving your hips throughout the entire move.

A

- Hold the kettlebell with both hands in front of your torso and stand with your feet hip-width apart.

REPS: Do 10, then switch directions and repeat without stopping to rest.

B

- Release the kettlebell into your right hand and move both arms behind your back. Grab the bell with your left hand and bring it back to the front (completing a full circle around your body). That's 1 rep.

DO WHAT YOU LOVE

The bottom line to being fit for life: Find what you really enjoy and what gets you going, says Kristen Dieffenbach, PhD, an assistant professor of athletic coaching education at West Virginia University. "Try as many classes, running paths, and exercise machines as you can. Somewhere between swimming and spinning, you will click with an activity or two." Spend your workout hours doing these types of exercise and you'll find excuses to get out more often rather than to skip sessions.

Kettlebell Workout 1

Swing

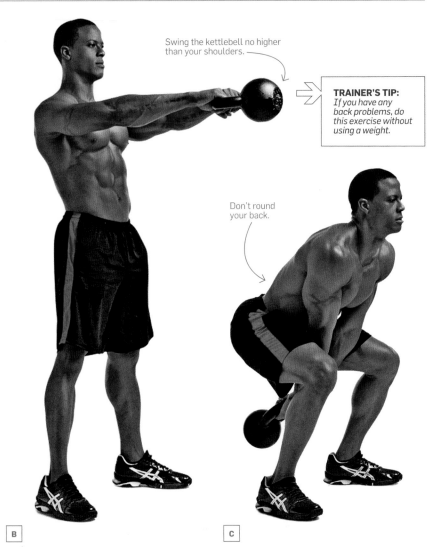

Swing the kettlebell no higher than your shoulders.

TRAINER'S TIP:
If you have any back problems, do this exercise without using a weight.

Don't round your back.

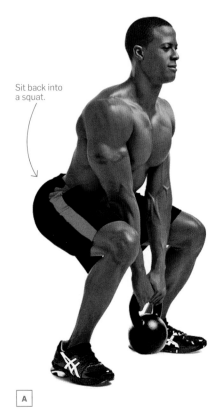

Sit back into a squat.

A

- Grab a kettlebell with both hands and stand with your feet wider than hip-width apart.
- Squat down until your thighs are nearly parallel to the floor.

REPS: Do 15 to 20.

B

- Immediately stand and swing the kettlebell up to shoulder height, keeping your arms extended.

C

- As the kettlebell begins to arc back down, bend your knees and squat, swinging the kettlebell between your legs. That's 1 rep.

Dead Lift

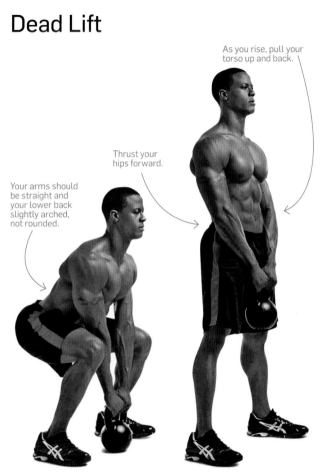

Your arms should be straight and your lower back slightly arched, not rounded.

Thrust your hips forward.

As you rise, pull your torso up and back.

A

- Stand with your feet hip-width apart, the kettlebell on the floor between your feet.
- Squat down and grab the handle with both hands, keeping your back flat.

B

- Brace your abs, squeeze your glutes, and slowly push down into your heels as you stand up, keeping your arms extended. That's 1 rep.

REPS: Do 10 to 12.

Halo

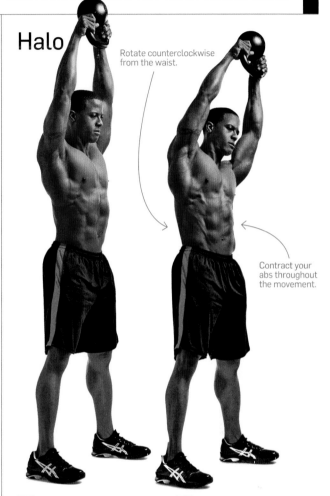

Rotate counterclockwise from the waist.

Contract your abs throughout the movement.

A

- Hold the kettlebell upside down by the horns with both hands, arms extended overhead.

B

- Keeping your shoulders down, chest forward, and abs tight, rotate your torso from the waist in a circle to the left.
- The kettlebell should make a small, controlled halo overhead.

REPS: Repeat for 6 circles, then switch directions.

Kettlebell Workout 2

Here are four more kettlebell exercises that take advantage of the weight's unique grip and unbalanced design. You can alternate this circuit with workout 1 for more variety.

START HERE:

Do these exercises one after another with no rest in between. Rest for 60 seconds at the end of the circuit. Then repeat the circuit twice more.

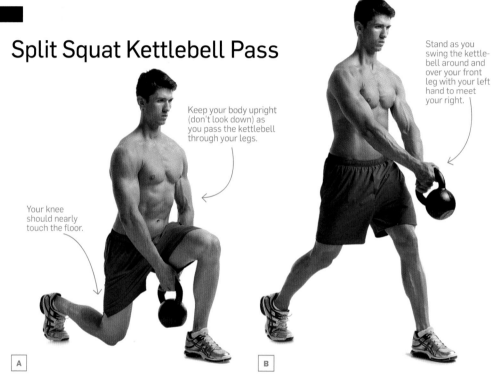

Split Squat Kettlebell Pass

Keep your body upright (don't look down) as you pass the kettlebell through your legs.

Your knee should nearly touch the floor.

Stand as you swing the kettlebell around and over your front leg with your left hand to meet your right.

A

- Hold a kettlebell by the handle in your right hand, arms at your sides, palms facing in. Stand with your left foot 2 to 3 feet in front of your right, toes pointing forward, back heel off the floor.
- Bend your knees, lowering your hips toward the floor, as you pass the bell under your front leg to your left hand.

B

- Take the kettlebell in your left hand and pass it over your leg to your right hand as you straighten your legs
- Continue for 8 clockwise circles, then reverse the direction for 8 counterclockwise circles.
- Next, repeat the exercise with your right leg forward.

REPS: Do 16 under each leg, switching directions after 8 reps.

Figure 8

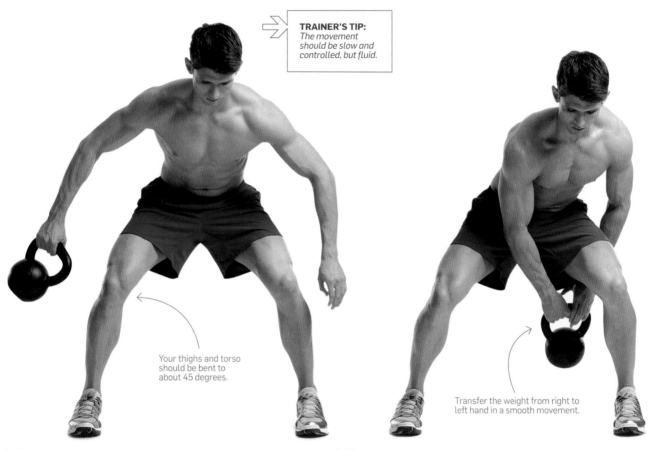

TRAINER'S TIP:
The movement should be slow and controlled, but fluid.

Your thighs and torso should be bent to about 45 degrees.

Transfer the weight from right to left hand in a smooth movement.

A

B

- Stand with your feet wider than hip-width apart, knees bent into a quarter-squat position, back straight, and chest up.
- Grab the kettlebell with your right hand and swing it in front of your right leg, between your legs, and behind your left leg.

REPS: Do 10.

- Grab the bell with your left hand, let go of it with your right hand, and swing the weight around your left leg and then between your legs, where you then grab it with your right hand behind your right calf. That's 1 rep.

Kettlebell Workout 2

Half Get-Up

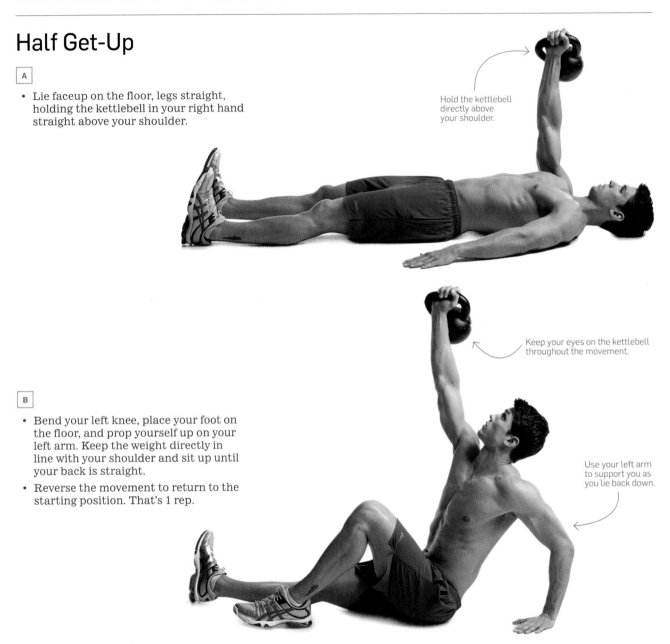

A

- Lie faceup on the floor, legs straight, holding the kettlebell in your right hand straight above your shoulder.

Hold the kettlebell directly above your shoulder.

Keep your eyes on the kettlebell throughout the movement.

B

- Bend your left knee, place your foot on the floor, and prop yourself up on your left arm. Keep the weight directly in line with your shoulder and sit up until your back is straight.

- Reverse the movement to return to the starting position. That's 1 rep.

Use your left arm to support you as you lie back down.

REPS: Do 5, then repeat on the other side.

Snatch, Pull, and Push Press

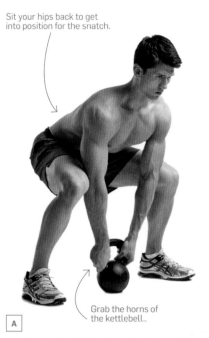

Sit your hips back to get into position for the snatch.

Grab the horns of the kettlebell..

A

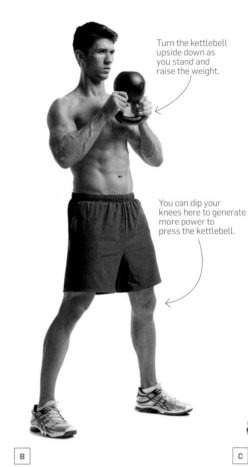

Turn the kettlebell upside down as you stand and raise the weight.

You can dip your knees here to generate more power to press the kettlebell.

B

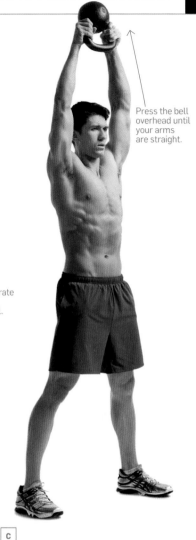

Press the bell overhead until your arms are straight.

C

- Grab a kettlebell and stand with your feet shoulder-width apart, toes turned out about 45 degrees.
- Place the kettlebell on the floor between your feet.

REPS: Do 10.

- Stand up forcefully and bend your arms to lift the weight to your chest.

- Explosively push the kettlebell straight overhead.
- Lower the weight to your chest, then sit back into a squat to return the kettlebell right side up to the floor. That's 1 rep.

Exercise Band Workout 1

It's easy to dismiss exercise bands or tubes as workout tools for lightweights. Nothing could be further from the truth. Despite their pretty colors and featherweight feel, exercise bands challenge your muscles with constant tension through a full range of motion, targeting parts that are often missed with free weights. And you can buy both the band style and the rubber tube style in different resistance strengths to vary your exercise. The result is a powerful workout that you can take anywhere.

The first few times you do band exercises, you may feel more wobbly than usual. That's because unlike free-weight lifting, where the resistance is toughest in midlift and easier in both the starting and final positions, a band's resistance becomes progressively more difficult from beginning to end. Concentrate on keeping your movements slow, smooth, and controlled.

START HERE:

Do one set of each exercise in order without resting between moves. When you complete the last exercise, rest for 30 seconds, then repeat the entire circuit two more times.

Resistance Pushup

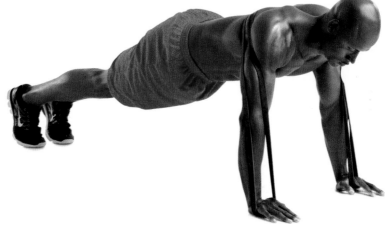

A

- Start in a pushup position, with your legs extended straight behind you and your hands shoulder-width apart.
- Position an exercise strap or band across your shoulder blades with tight resistance, each end tucked under a hand.

> **TRAINER'S TIP:** *If this move is too easy, use a thicker band or add a second band.*

B

- Lower your body until your upper arms are parallel to the floor) then push back to the starting position. That's 1 rep.

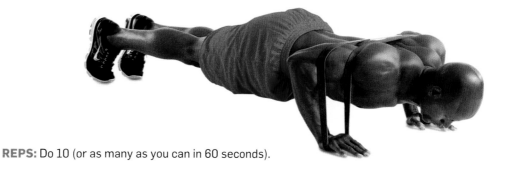

REPS: Do 10 (or as many as you can in 60 seconds).

Exercise Band Workout 1

Squat with Side Kick

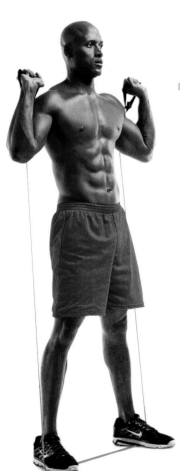

TRAINER'S TIP: *Use long exercise tubing with handles for this exercise.*

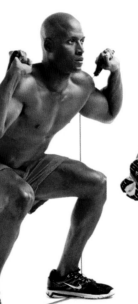

Lift your leg out to the side as you stand.

A

- Stand with your feet hip-width apart, your abs tight, and a band under both feet. Grasp the ends and raise your hands to shoulder height.

REPS: Do 10 to 12.

B

- Bend your knees and hips and sit back as though you're sitting in a chair, keeping your knees in line with your ankles.

C

- Push through your heels and return to the starting position, immediately lifting the right leg out to the side as you stand. Squat again, then do a side kick with the left leg. That's 1 rep.

Seated Row

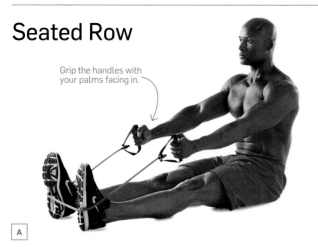

Grip the handles with your palms facing in.

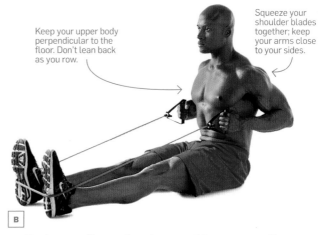

Keep your upper body perpendicular to the floor. Don't lean back as you row.

Squeeze your shoulder blades together; keep your arms close to your sides.

A

B

- Sit on the floor with your legs straight and loop the resistance band securely under the bottoms of your feet. Hold an end in each hand, arms extended in front of you. Keep your back straight and shoulders square.

REPS: Do 10 to 12.

- Tuck your elbows close to your sides as you pull the band to the sides of your torso, squeezing your shoulder blades together.
- Pause, then slowly return to the starting position. That's 1 rep.

Frog Press

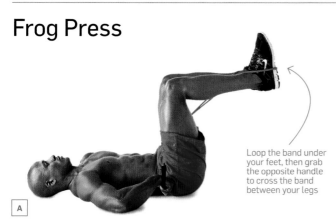

Loop the band under your feet, then grab the opposite handle to cross the band between your legs

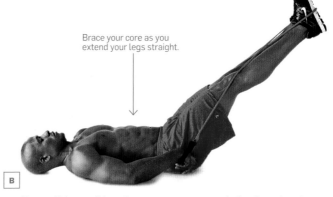

Brace your core as you extend your legs straight.

A

B

- Lie faceup, bend your hips and knees 90 degrees, and loop the band around your feet, crossing the band to create an X.
- Hold an end in each hand just above your hips or shoulders depending on the length of the band.

REPS: Do 10 to 12.

- From this position, brace your core and slowly extend your legs into the air straight in front of you.
- Pause, then return to the starting position. Don't let your feet touch the floor. That's 1 rep.

Exercise Band Workout 2

For variety, alternate Exercise Band Workout 1 with this challenging total-body circuit, which employs a Superband, exercise tubing with handles and an anchor, and a flat loop band.

START HERE:

Move from one exercise to the next without resting. When you complete the last move, rest for 30 seconds, then repeat the entire circuit two more times.

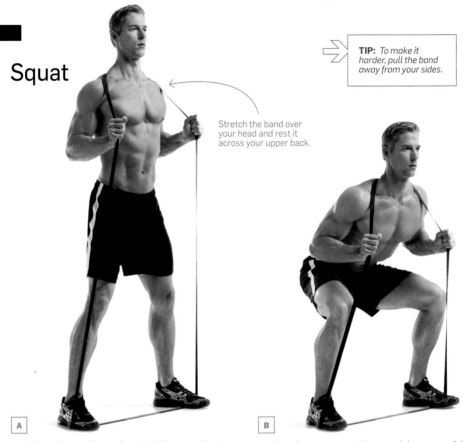

Squat

Stretch the band over your head and rest it across your upper back.

TIP: *To make it harder, pull the band away from your sides.*

A

- Stand on a Superband with your feet shoulder-width apart.
- Stretch the band up and over your head and place it on your shoulders and across your upper back.

REPS: Do 10 to 12.

B

- Perform a squat by pushing your hips back and lowering your body until your thighs are at least parallel to the floor.
- Push back up to the starting position.

Standing Incline Fly

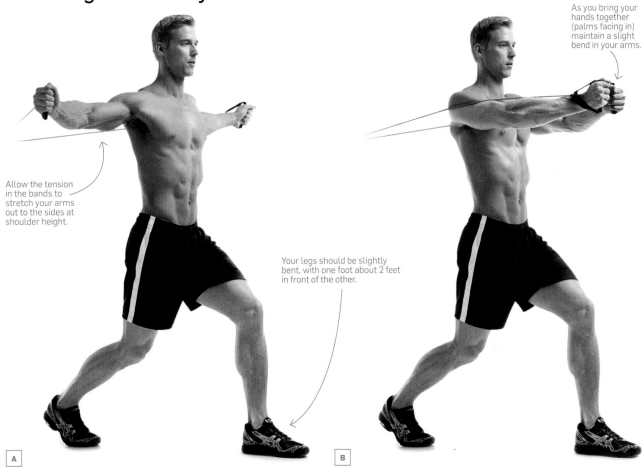

As you bring your hands together (palms facing in) maintain a slight bend in your arms.

Allow the tension in the bands to stretch your arms out to the sides at shoulder height.

Your legs should be slightly bent, with one foot about 2 feet in front of the other.

A

B

- Using an exercise tube anchor, attach the band to a door.
- Turn your back to the door and grasp the handles of the bands, extending your arms out to the sides at about shoulder level, keeping your elbows soft.
- Step forward until the band is taut.
- Maintain a staggered stance, with your arms slightly bent.

REPS: Do 10 to 12.

- Without changing the angle of your elbows, pull your hands together in front of your body.
- Return to the starting position.

Exercise Band Workout 2

Resisted Supine Lying Crunch

A

- Attach the exercise tubes securely to the lowest hinge on a door using the anchor.
- Lie faceup on the floor with your head closest to the door and your feet farthest from it, your knees bent, and your feet flat on the floor.
- Grasp the handles of the tubes with your palms facing in. Form right angles with your arms, your upper arms perpendicular to the floor. Shimmy away from the door until there is tension in the tubes.

Secure the tubes to the low hinge of a door.

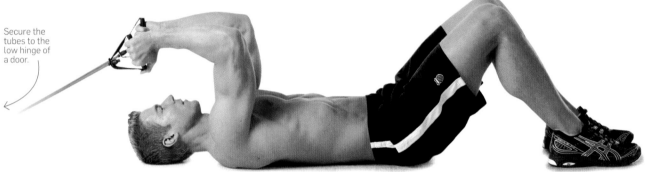

B

- Contract your abs and raise your torso as high as you can off the floor without moving the position of your arms.
- Lower yourself back to the starting position and repeat.
- Perform the exercise as quickly as possible.

Your upper arms should remain perpendicular to your upper body as you curl.

REPS: Do 10 to 12.

Rubber Band Sidesteps

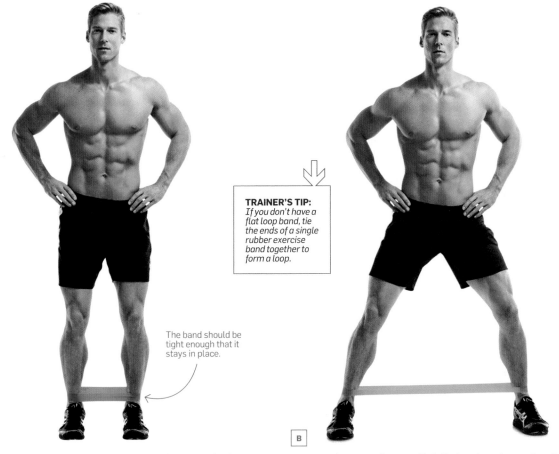

TRAINER'S TIP:
If you don't have a flat loop band, tie the ends of a single rubber exercise band together to form a loop.

The band should be tight enough that it stays in place.

A

- Step into a flat rubber loop band with both feet and position your legs about hip-width apart.
- Position the band just above your ankles.
- Stand up straight and place your hands on your hips.

B

- Keeping your knees slightly bent and your back straight, take a giant step with your right foot to the right side.
- Then take a step to the right with your left foot, returning your feet to about hip-width apart, and keeping tension on the band.
- Then take a giant step with your left foot to the left, and a step to the left with your right. That constitutes 1 rep.

REPS: Do 10 to 12.

Medicine Ball Workout 1

The medicine ball may be the most functional piece of workout gear going because it allows your arms, legs, and core to move fluidly in a wide range of motion, mimicking the moves of swimming, tennis and other sports. Tossing and catching these classic weighted balls also stimulates your central nervous system. The old-school medicine balls were sand- or bead-filled and covered with thick leather. Today's models are made of rugged rubberlike materials and come in all shapes and sizes. And a dozen cool colors, too, to coordinate with your gym shorts, we suppose. The two workouts on the following pages are inspired by strength and conditioning programs used by University of North Carolina Tar Heels athletes.

START HERE:

Do one set of each exercise and move to the next without resting in between. After finishing the circuit, rest for 60 seconds, then repeat twice for a total of three circuits.

Wood Chopper

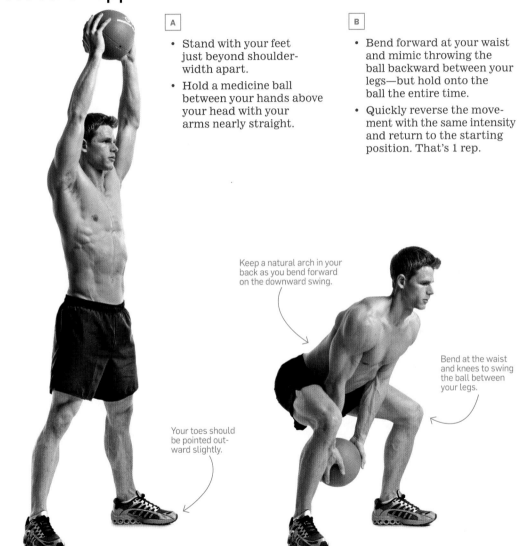

A
- Stand with your feet just beyond shoulder-width apart.
- Hold a medicine ball between your hands above your head with your arms nearly straight.

B
- Bend forward at your waist and mimic throwing the ball backward between your legs—but hold onto the ball the entire time.
- Quickly reverse the movement with the same intensity and return to the starting position. That's 1 rep.

Keep a natural arch in your back as you bend forward on the downward swing.

Bend at the waist and knees to swing the ball between your legs.

Your toes should be pointed outward slightly.

REPS: Do 15 to 20.

Medicine Ball Workout 1

Step and Extend

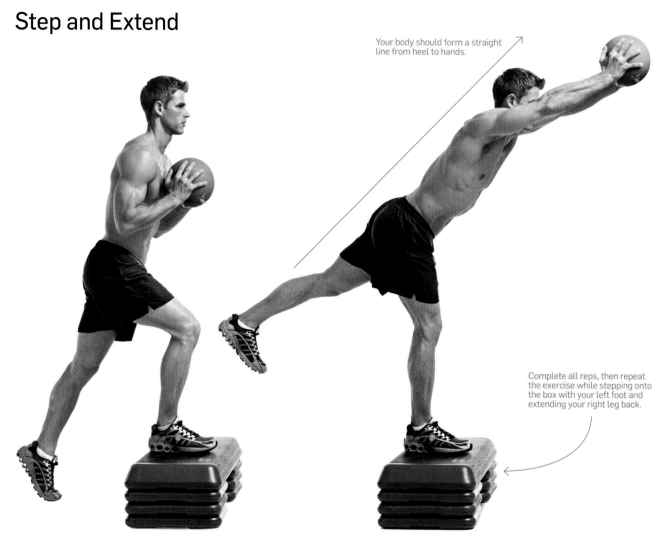

Your body should form a straight line from heel to hands.

Complete all reps, then repeat the exercise while stepping onto the box with your left foot and extending your right leg back.

A

- Stand about a foot away from a sturdy box or step, holding a medicine ball at chest height in front of you.
- Step onto the box with your right foot.

REPS: Do 10 to 12 with each leg.

B

- Press the ball above your head as you straighten your right leg, bend slightly at the waist, and extend your left leg behind you.
- Pause, then reverse the motion, stepping back down to the floor. Do all reps, then switch legs.

Big Circles

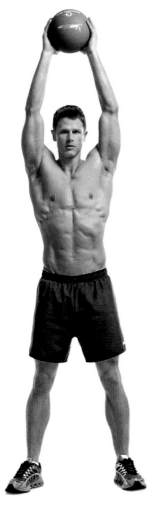

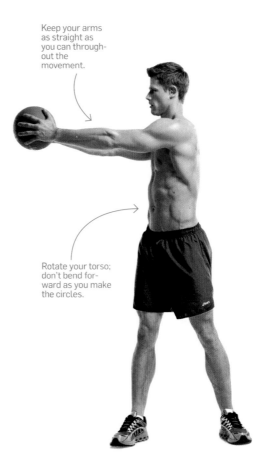

Keep your arms as straight as you can throughout the movement.

Rotate your torso; don't bend forward as you make the circles.

A

- Stand with your feet shoulder-width apart and your knees slightly bent, and hold the ball with your arms extended above your head.

REPS: Do 10 in each direction.

B

- Without bending your elbows, rotate your arms clockwise, using the ball to draw large circles in front of your body.

- After completing all the reps, repeat making the circles in a counterclockwise direction.

Medicine Ball Workout 1

Squat to Press

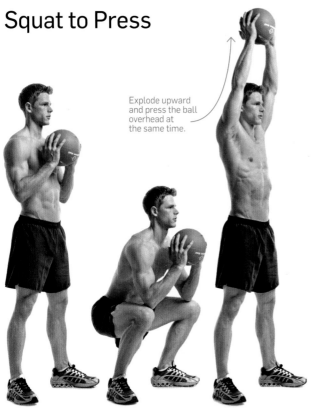

Explode upward and press the ball overhead at the same time.

A

- Stand holding the medicine ball close to your chest with both hands, your feet just beyond shoulder-width apart.

B

- Push your hips back, bend your knees, and lower your body until the tops of your thighs are at least parallel to the floor.

C

- Then simultaneously drive your heels into the floor and push back to the standing position while pressing the ball overhead.
- Lower the ball back to the starting position. That's 1 rep.

REPS: Do 15 to 20.

Standing Russian Twist

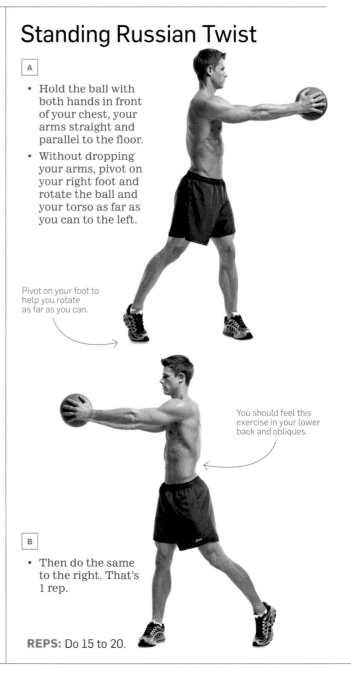

A

- Hold the ball with both hands in front of your chest, your arms straight and parallel to the floor.
- Without dropping your arms, pivot on your right foot and rotate the ball and your torso as far as you can to the left.

Pivot on your foot to help you rotate as far as you can.

You should feel this exercise in your lower back and obliques.

B

- Then do the same to the right. That's 1 rep.

REPS: Do 15 to 20.

Circle Crunches

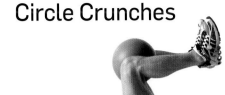
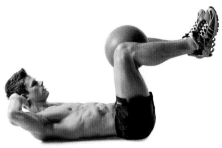
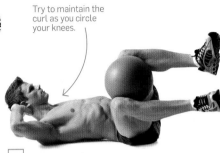

Try to maintain the curl as you circle your knees.

A

- Squeeze a ball between your knees and lie on your back with your legs bent so your thighs are perpendicular and your calves are parallel to the floor.
- Hold your hands behind your head with your elbows out to the sides.

REPS: Do 10 (5 to the right, 5 to the left).

B

- Contract your abs and raise your upper back, shoulders, and head off the floor about 30 degrees.

C

- Slowly move your knees in a circular motion starting to the right. Repeat for half a set (about 5 circles).
- Pause. Then slowly move your knees 5 times in a circular motion starting to the left.

Situp

A

- Grab the ball with both hands and lie on your back. Bend your knees 90 degrees, place your feet flat on the floor, and hold the medicine ball against your chest.

B

- Perform a classic situp by raising your torso into a sitting position.
- Lower back to the start. That's 1 rep.

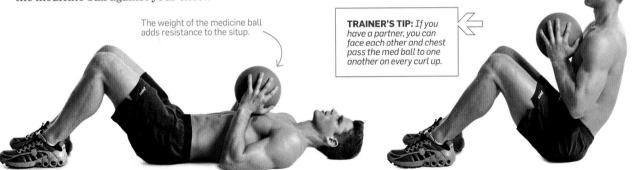

The weight of the medicine ball adds resistance to the situp.

TRAINER'S TIP: *If you have a partner, you can face each other and chest pass the med ball to one another on every curl up.*

REPS: Do 15 to 20.

Medicine Ball Workout 2

Here's another "med ball" workout for variety. If you like the range-of-motion benefits of this piece of gear, supplement your 6-pound, 8-inch, general-use ball with lighter and heavier models.

START HERE: ▬

Starting with the first move, complete each exercise back-to-back without resting. Rest for 60 seconds, then repeat the circuit twice more for a total of three circuits.

Rising and Setting Sun

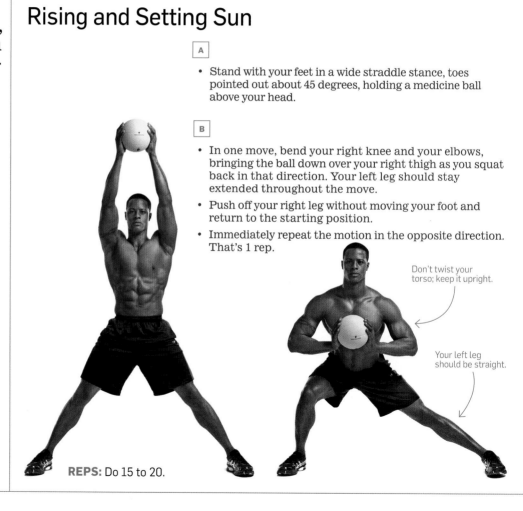

A

- Stand with your feet in a wide straddle stance, toes pointed out about 45 degrees, holding a medicine ball above your head.

B

- In one move, bend your right knee and your elbows, bringing the ball down over your right thigh as you squat back in that direction. Your left leg should stay extended throughout the move.
- Push off your right leg without moving your foot and return to the starting position.
- Immediately repeat the motion in the opposite direction. That's 1 rep.

Don't twist your torso; keep it upright.

Your left leg should be straight.

REPS: Do 15 to 20.

Walking Lunge

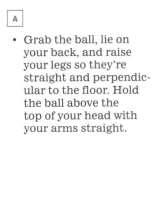

A

- Grab a medium-weight medicine ball and stand with your feet shoulder-width apart, holding the ball in front of your chest.

B

- Step forward with your left leg and lower into a lunge, so your left thigh is parallel to the floor.
- Twist from your waist as far as you can to the right.
- Press into your left heel to rise to the starting position and bring the ball back to center. Repeat with your right leg to complete 1 rep.

REPS: Do 10 to 12, alternating sides.

Toe Touch

A

- Grab the ball, lie on your back, and raise your legs so they're straight and perpendicular to the floor. Hold the ball above the top of your head with your arms straight.

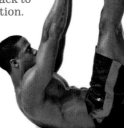

B

- Without moving your legs or bending your elbows, simultaneously lift your arms and torso until the ball touches your toes.
- Lower yourself back to the starting position. That's 1 rep.

REPS: Do 10 to 20.

PERFECT THE LUNGE

When a move is part of your workout stable, it's essential that your form be spot on. One such move many of us get a bit wrong is the lunge. What goes awry? We sometimes lean forward, causing our front heel to rise. Fix it by narrowing your stance, says Gray Cook, author of *Athletic Body in Balance*. The closer your feet are, the harder your core has to work to stabilize your body. "As you do the lunge, focus on moving your torso only up and down, not pushing it forward," says Craig Rasmussen, a fitness coach at Results Fitness in Santa Clarita, California. This keeps your weight balanced evenly through your front foot, allowing you to press into the floor with your heel, which tones more lower-body muscle.

279

Medicine Ball Workout 2

Decline Toss

A

- Set an adjustable abs bench at a 45-degree angle. Lie down on it with your head toward the floor and hook your feet under the padded support bar. Hold a medicine ball at your chest as you lower yourself.

B

- As you curl up, chest-pass the ball straight up.
- Catch it at the top of the curl, then lower yourself and repeat.

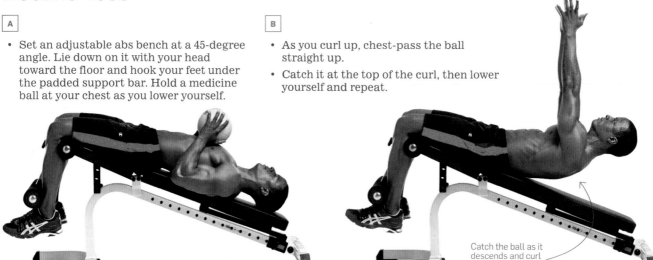

Catch the ball as it descends and curl your back down to the bench.

REPS: Do 15 to 20.

Suitcase Crunch

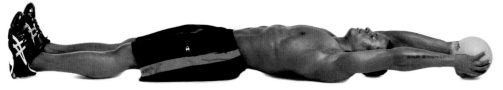

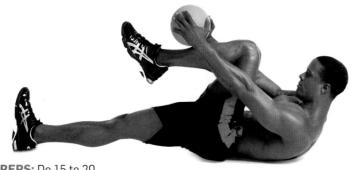

A

- Lie on your back with your legs straight. Use both hands to hold the ball above your head and barely off the floor.

B

- Simultaneously raise your arms and shoulders and bend your left knee toward your chest, as you bring the ball over your knee and toward your foot. Reverse the move.
- Repeat with your right knee. That's 1 rep.

REPS: Do 15 to 20.

Ditch Digger

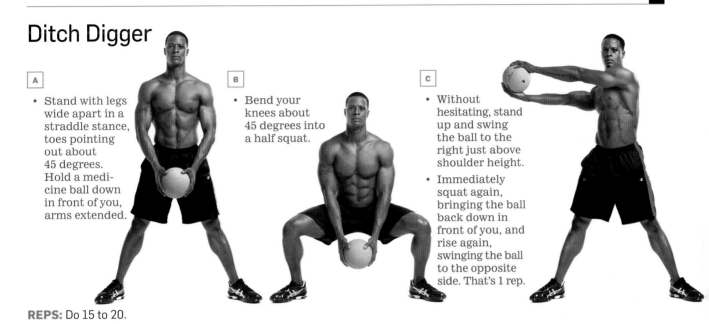

A

- Stand with legs wide apart in a straddle stance, toes pointing out about 45 degrees. Hold a medicine ball down in front of you, arms extended.

B

- Bend your knees about 45 degrees into a half squat.

C

- Without hesitating, stand up and swing the ball to the right just above shoulder height.
- Immediately squat again, bringing the ball back down in front of you, and rise again, swinging the ball to the opposite side. That's 1 rep.

REPS: Do 15 to 20.

Inchworm

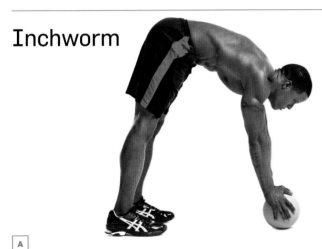

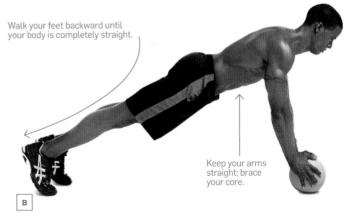

Walk your feet backward until your body is completely straight.

Keep your arms straight; brace your core.

A

- Stand with your feet shoulder-width apart and lean forward, knees slightly bent, to place both hands on a medicine ball on the floor.

REPS: Do 10.

B

- Slowly walk your feet (a few inches with each step) away from your hands until your body is in a straight line from head to heels.
- Hold for 1 second, then walk your feet back to the starting position. That's 1 rep.

Stability Ball Workout 1

These large inflated balls (also known as Swiss balls) are terrific for abs exercises. Their rocking, rolling instability cranks up the effectiveness of crunches and other core moves by forcing your muscles to work harder. In fact, stability ball moves work better than any crunch. In a California State University study of men and women, researchers found that just doing pushups on a stability ball worked the abs and obliques as well as situps and crunches, plus the exercise toned the chest, shoulders, and arms as well.

For these routines, be sure to use a ball that "fits" you properly and isn't too small or too large. As a rule of thumb, when you sit on top of the ball, your hips and legs should be bent to 90 degrees. On the following pages, you'll find two stability ball workouts that will work your core like it never has been before.

START HERE:

Move from one exercise to the next without resting. When you've finished the last exercise in the circuit, take a 60-second break, and then do the circuit again.

Rollout

A

- Kneel in front of a stability ball.
- Place your hands, clenched in loose fists, palms facing each other, on top of the ball.
- Cross your ankles and lift your feet off the floor.
- Lean forward slightly.

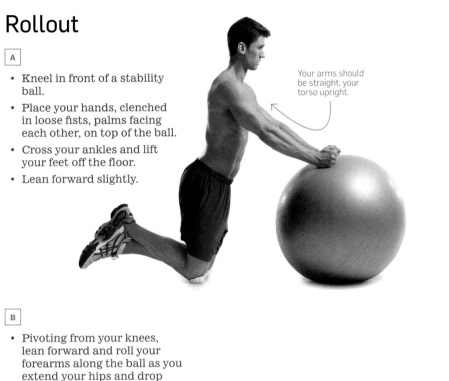

Your arms should be straight, your torso upright.

B

- Pivoting from your knees, lean forward and roll your forearms along the ball as you extend your hips and drop your chest toward the ball.
- Stop when your body forms a straight diagonal line from your shoulders to knees.
- Contract your abs, and pull the ball back to the starting position.

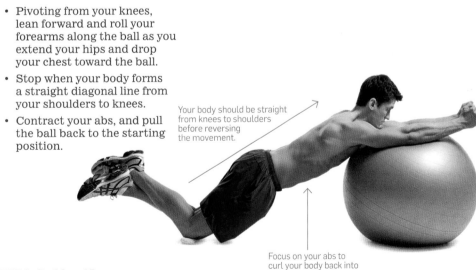

Your body should be straight from knees to shoulders before reversing the movement.

Focus on your abs to curl your body back into the upright position.

REPS: Do 10 to 15.

Stability Ball Workout 1

Pike

A

- Lie facedown on a stability ball with both hands on the floor.
- Walk your hands out, allowing the ball to roll beneath your body until it is under your shins.
- Your hands should be directly below your shoulders, so it looks like you're ready to do a pushup.
- Your body should form a straight line from your heels to your head.

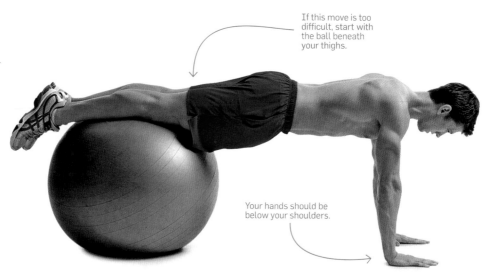

If this move is too difficult, start with the ball beneath your thighs.

Your hands should be below your shoulders.

B

- Keeping your legs straight, tighten your abs, exhale, and lift your hips toward the ceiling while you pull the ball toward your hands as far as it is comfortably possible.
- Hold for a second. Then lower back to the starting position.

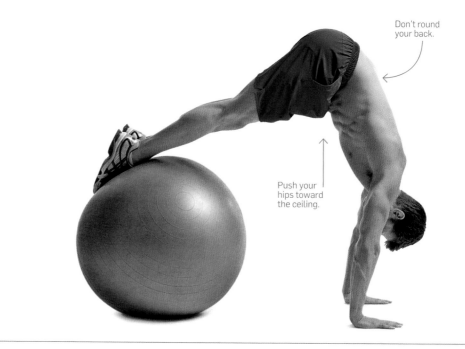

Don't round your back.

Push your hips toward the ceiling.

REPS: Do 10.

Skier

A

- Lie facedown on a stability ball with both hands on the floor.
- Walk your hands out, allowing the ball to roll beneath your body until the ball is under your shins.
- Position your hands slightly wider than shoulder-width apart.

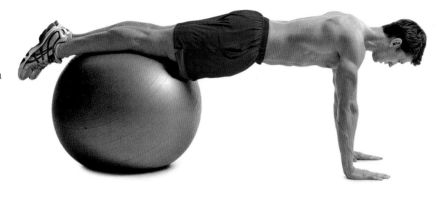

B

- Bend your knees, drawing them forward until your feet are on top of the ball and your hips are pointed toward the ceiling.

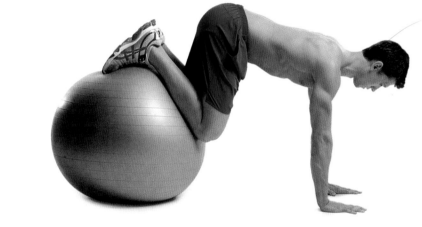

C

- Slowly drop your hips to the left side and your knees to the right, allowing the ball to roll to the right. Immediately pull your hips back to the starting position and drop them to the right. That's 1 rep.
- As you become more comfortable with the move, perform it at a slightly faster pace.

REPS: Do 10 to 15.

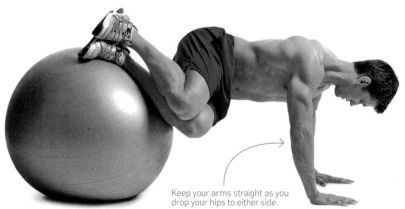

Keep your arms straight as you drop your hips to either side.

Stability Ball Workout 1

Rear Lateral Raise

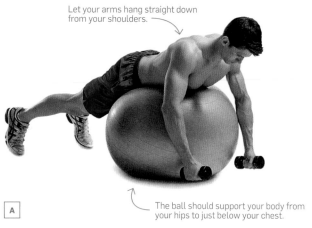

Let your arms hang straight down from your shoulders.

The ball should support your body from your hips to just below your chest.

A

- Lie facedown on a stability ball and hold a pair of light dumbbells (no more than 5 pounds) with your arms hanging down to the floor, palms facing inward.

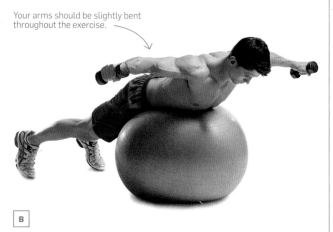

Your arms should be slightly bent throughout the exercise.

B

- Raise your arms back until they're in line with your body, and pull your shoulder blades down and together.
- Hold for 2 to 3 seconds, then lower the weights.

REPS: Do 10 to 15.

Decline Pushup

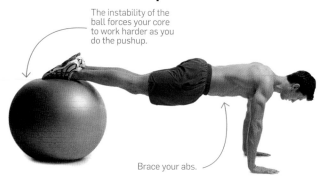

The instability of the ball forces your core to work harder as you do the pushup.

Brace your abs.

A

- Lie facedown on a stability ball with both hands on the floor.
- Walk your hands out, allowing the ball to roll beneath your body until it is under your shins.
- Your hands should be directly below your shoulders, so it looks like you're ready to do a pushup.

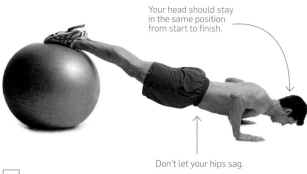

Your head should stay in the same position from start to finish.

Don't let your hips sag.

B

- Keeping your torso straight and abs contracted, bend your elbows and lower your chest toward the floor.
- Stop when your upper arms are parallel to the floor. Pause, and return to the starting position.

REPS: Do 10 to 15.

Leg Curl

> **TRAINER'S TIP:**
> *Make the move harder by doing it one leg at a time.*

Lift your hips so your body forms a straight line from ankles to shoulders.

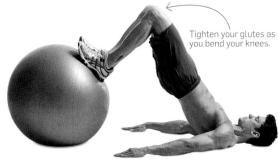

A

- Lie on the floor with your arms at your sides and place your heels on the ball.
- Press up, so that your hips are in the air and your torso forms a straight line.

Tighten your glutes as you bend your knees.

B

- Next, pull the ball toward you, squeezing your hamstrings, and then roll it back out without dropping your hips.

REPS: Do 10 to 15.

Stretch Lunge

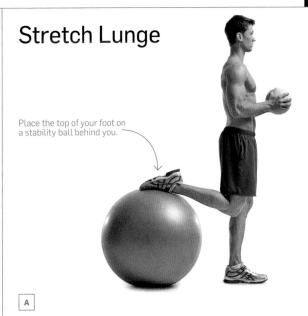

Place the top of your foot on a stability ball behind you.

A

- Hold a medicine ball in both hands.
- Place the top of your right foot on top of a stability ball. Keep your left foot flat on the floor.

Emphasize the stretch in your hips and quads.

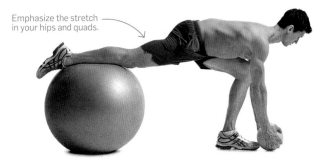

B

- Bend your left knee and lower your hips.
- Straighten your right leg out behind you and bend forward to touch the medicine ball to the floor.
- Return to the starting position and repeat for all reps. Then do the move with your left leg on the ball.

REPS: Do 8 to 10 with each leg.

Stability Ball Workout 2

You can do dozens of different moves on a stability ball. Here are some more that target your core, hips, and hamstrings. Alternate between workouts 1 and 2 during the week.

START HERE: ▮

Go from one exercise to the next without resting. When you've finished the last move, take a 60-second break, and then do the circuit again.

Walk-Up Crunch

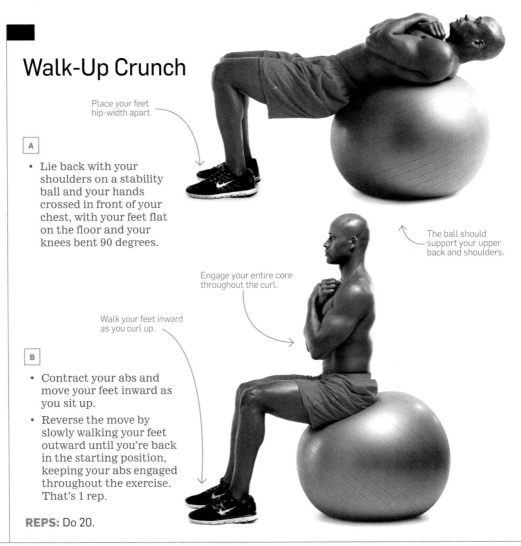

Place your feet hip-width apart.

A

- Lie back with your shoulders on a stability ball and your hands crossed in front of your chest, with your feet flat on the floor and your knees bent 90 degrees.

The ball should support your upper back and shoulders.

Engage your entire core throughout the curl.

Walk your feet inward as you curl up.

B

- Contract your abs and move your feet inward as you sit up.
- Reverse the move by slowly walking your feet outward until you're back in the starting position, keeping your abs engaged throughout the exercise. That's 1 rep.

REPS: Do 20.

Hand Walk

> **TRAINER'S TIP:** *Try to walk as far out as you can; the farther you go, the harder it is.*

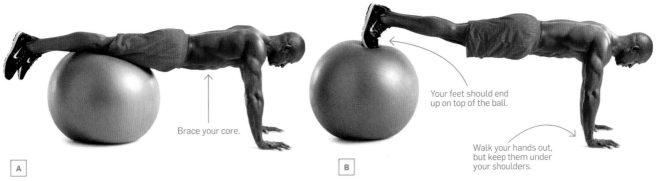

Brace your core.

Your feet should end up on top of the ball.

Walk your hands out, but keep them under your shoulders.

A

- Lie facedown with your torso on the ball, place your hands on the floor, raise your legs, and walk your hands out until just your thighs are on the ball.

REPS: Do 10 to 15.

B

- Squeeze your glutes and walk out until you're in the plank position, with just your feet on the ball.
- Pull your abs in tight to keep your body stable.
- Hold for 5 seconds, then walk your hands back to the starting position. That's 1 rep.

Leg Raise

Raise your leg until it is at least parallel with the floor.

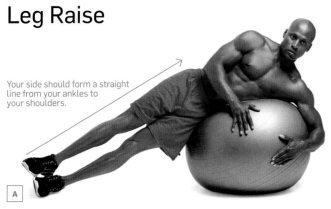

Your side should form a straight line from your ankles to your shoulders.

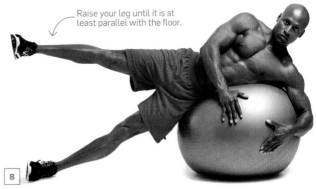

A

- Lie on your left side on the stability ball, legs extended straight out and feet stacked.
- Position your left hand in a comfortable spot on the ball, and lift your hips so that your body forms a straight line.

B

- Keeping your body in that position, slowly raise your right leg. Pause, then slowly return to the starting position.

REPS: Do as many as you can in 60 seconds, then repeat on the other side.

289

Stability Ball Workout 2

Row Combination

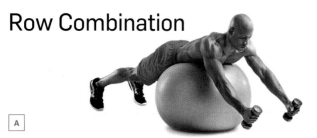

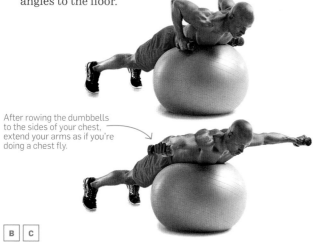

A

- Lie facedown on a stability ball and hold a pair of light dumbbells (no more than 5 pounds), thumbs up, with your arms hanging down and forward at 45-degree angles to the floor.

After rowing the dumbbells to the sides of your chest, extend your arms as if you're doing a chest fly.

B **C**

- Pull the weights to your chest, then lift them out to your sides.

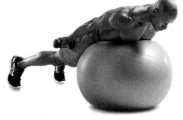

D

- Pull the weights back to the sides of your butt.
- Return the weights to the starting position. That's 1 rep.

REPS: Do 10 to 15.

Jackknife

TRAINER'S TIP: *To make it harder, perform the move with your hands on a step or bench.*

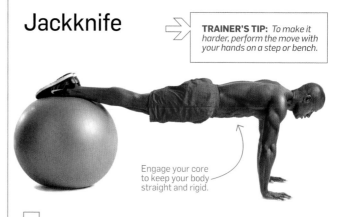

Engage your core to keep your body straight and rigid.

A

- Lie facedown on a stability ball with both hands on the floor.
- Walk your hands out, allowing the ball to roll beneath your body until it is under your shins.
- Your hands should be directly below your shoulders, so it looks like you're ready to do a pushup.

Keep your back flat.

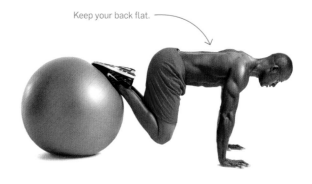

B

- Tighten your abs and bend your knees, drawing them forward, so you bring your legs and the ball closer your torso. Hold for a second.
- Straighten your legs and uncoil as you press back to the starting position.

REPS: Do 10 to 15.

Single-Leg Balance Bridge

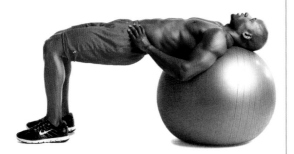

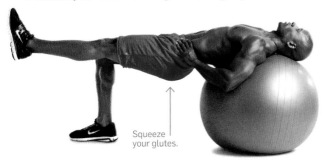

A

- Lie faceup on a stability ball with your legs bent, hips raised, and feet flat on the floor so you're in a tabletop position.
- Extend your arms out to the sides and down toward the floor.
- Walk your feet out until you are balanced with the ball between your shoulder blades.
- Position your feet close together, thighs parallel.

Squeeze your glutes.

B

- Contract your glutes and slowly raise your left foot, extending your left leg.
- Hold for a count of 10. Repeat to the other side.

REPS: Do 5 to 6, alternating legs.

Balancing Bicycle

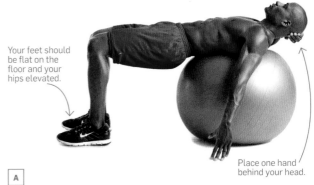

Your feet should be flat on the floor and your hips elevated.

Place one hand behind your head.

A

- Lie faceup on a stability ball with your legs bent and your feet flat on the floor.
- Place your right hand behind your head and extend your left arm to the side and down, placing your fingertips on the floor for balance.

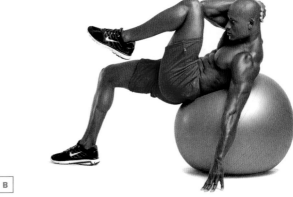

B

- Contract your abs and simultaneously lift your right shoulder up and to the left while drawing your left knee toward your right elbow. Return to the starting position.

REPS: Do 10, then switch sides.

Sandbag Workout 1

As you might imagine, an NFL weight room sparkles with state-of-the-art fitness equipment. But players don't spend all their off-season training in these gleaming, air-conditioned facilities. They're outside in the heat shouldering, flipping, and dragging sandbags. The ever-shifting sand constantly alters the shape of a sandbag, making it nearly impossible for you to settle into a lifting groove like you do with free weights or machines. So every workout is unique and challenging. The following two sandbag workouts prepare your muscles for real-life tasks in which the weight isn't conveniently packaged in a dumbbell. They're total-body workouts that target your abdominal and spinal muscles.

Start one of these head-to-toe workouts at the home-improvement store by carrying a 50-pound bag of playground sand to the cashier; then to your car; then unload it at home. Tougher than you thought, right?

START HERE:
Perform this workout as a circuit—doing one exercise after another without stopping. Rest 90 to 120 seconds between circuits. Do three circuits.

Rotational Put-Back

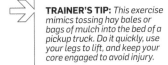

TRAINER'S TIP: *This exercise mimics tossing hay bales or bags of mulch into the bed of a pickup truck. Do it quickly, use your legs to lift, and keep your core engaged to avoid injury.*

A

- Stand with your feet shoulder-width apart and your left side toward the front of your workbench (not pictured), or the bed of a pickup, or any sturdy ledge that's about hip height.
- Place the sandbag on the ground to the right of your right foot.
- Squat while reaching across your body with both hands to grab the bag on its short sides.

B

- Lift the bag across your body and place it on the workbench by straightening your legs and twisting your upper body to the left to place the bag on the workbench.
- Without letting go of the bag, rest it there for a second or just hold it elevated, and then reverse the move, lowering the sandbag to the starting position.

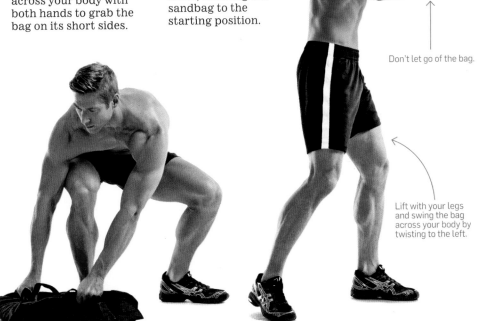

Don't let go of the bag.

Lift with your legs and swing the bag across your body by twisting to the left.

REPS: Do 10, then repeat with the bag starting outside your left foot.

293

Sandbag Workout 1

Clean and Press

A

- Squat over a sandbag with your feet shoulder-width apart.
- Grab the bag on its short sides, shrug your shoulders, and rise up on your toes to pull it to your chest.

B

- When the bag reaches chest level, bend your knees, rotate your forearms under it, and bend your wrists so you "catch" the bag on the fronts of your shoulders.

C

- Explosively straighten your knees and press the bag overhead.
- Lower it to your shoulders, then rotate your arms and wrists back to their starting positions as you lower the bag to the floor.

Press the bag directly over your shoulders.

Bend your knees to dip your body under the bag and catch it. This also puts you in position for the next step: a push press.

Pull the sandbag up explosively.

REPS: Do 6 to 8.

Zercher Traveling Lunge

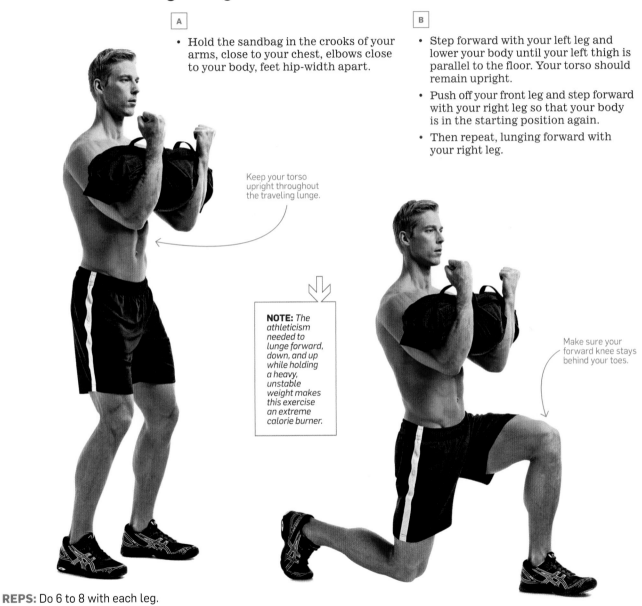

A

- Hold the sandbag in the crooks of your arms, close to your chest, elbows close to your body, feet hip-width apart.

Keep your torso upright throughout the traveling lunge.

B

- Step forward with your left leg and lower your body until your left thigh is parallel to the floor. Your torso should remain upright.
- Push off your front leg and step forward with your right leg so that your body is in the starting position again.
- Then repeat, lunging forward with your right leg.

NOTE: *The athleticism needed to lunge forward, down, and up while holding a heavy, unstable weight makes this exercise an extreme calorie burner.*

Make sure your forward knee stays behind your toes.

REPS: Do 6 to 8 with each leg.

Sandbag Workout 2

Shoulder the Load

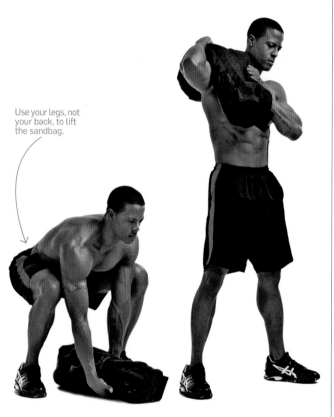

Use your legs, not your back, to lift the sandbag.

A

- Place a heavy sandbag on the floor in front of you.
- Stand with your feet shoulder-width apart, bend your knees, and reach down to grab the sandbag.

REPS: Do 8 to 10.

B

- Using your legs, press up explosively to lift the bag and allow its momentum to help you sling it over your shoulder.
- Reverse the motion and repeat over the opposite shoulder. That's 1 rep.

Bear Hug Walk

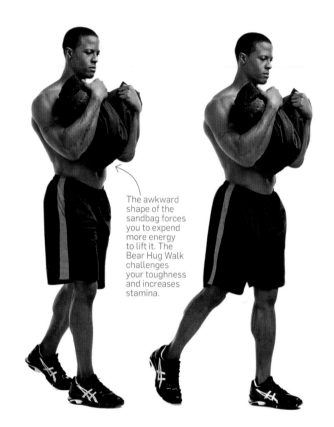

The awkward shape of the sandbag forces you to expend more energy to lift it. The Bear Hug Walk challenges your toughness and increases stamina.

A B

- Wrap your arms around a sandbag and walk for 20 yards while maintaining perfect posture—that is, standing tall with your abs braced, chest up, and shoulder blades pulled back and down.

 TRAINER'S TIP: *To make it harder, hold the sandbag over your head with straight arms as you walk.*

REPS: Do three 20-yard walks.

Grip, Row, and Grow

Maintain the natural arch in your lower back.

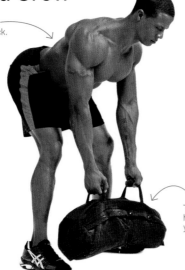
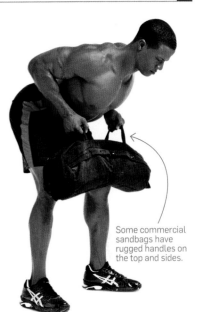

A

- Grab the sandbag with both hands and stand with your knees slightly bent.
- Bend forward at your waist until your upper body is almost parallel to the floor, your arms hanging straight down under the weight of the bag.

REPS: Do 8 to 10.

The bag should hang straight from your shoulders.

B

- Without moving your torso, pull the bag as close to your lower rib cage as possible.
- Pause, lower the bag, and row again.

Some commercial sandbags have rugged handles on the top and sides.

Sandbag Get-Up

A

- Kneel on the floor and hold a 30- to 60-pound sandbag in both arms.
- Your arms should be underneath, palms facing up and around the front of the bag.
- Pull the bag to your chest.

B

- Lift your right leg and place the right foot on the floor to start standing up.

C

- Push through your heel to stand and bring your left foot next to your right to stand completely straight up.

REPS: Do 8 to 10 with each leg.

D

- Squat by bending both knees, then move your right knee to the floor, then the left knee until you are once again kneeling.
- Repeat, starting with your left foot and pushing through your heel to stand up.

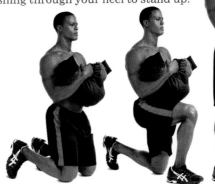
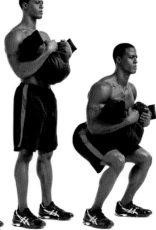

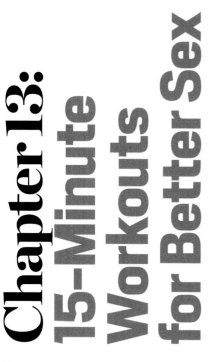

Chapter 13: 15-Minute Workouts for Better Sex

Build Endurance, Flexibility, and Strength for Longer, More Sensational Sessions in the Sack.

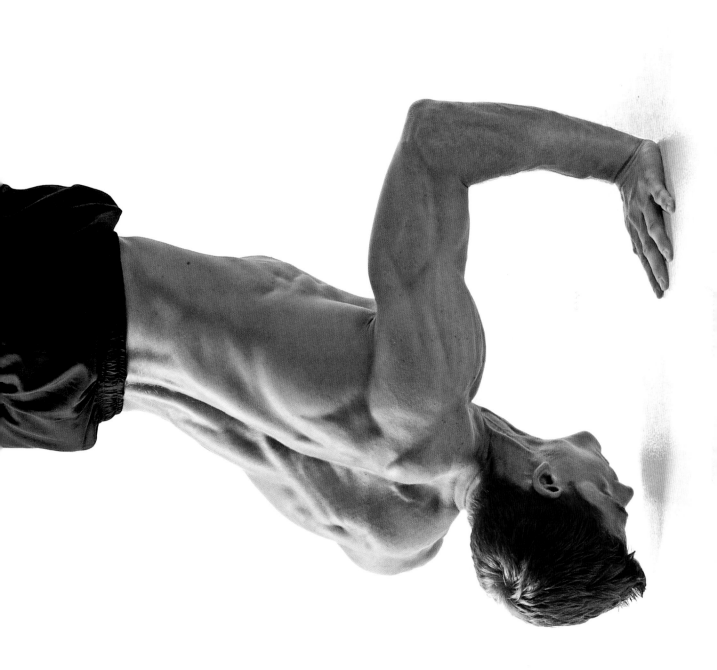

Superfast Better-Sex Workouts

Great sex is an athletic performance. It engages your arms, legs, chest, back, abs, glutes, and a whole mess of tiny muscles that you don't see in the mirror—muscles that you don't use every day. To be able to deftly maneuver into new positions, move your hips just right (without throwing out your back), and delay the inevitable, it helps to have a body that's not just in shape, but also in shape for sex. The following workouts are designed to build flexibility for challenging positions, upper-body strength to support her body weight, core power for thrusting motions, and aerobic stamina for greater endurance. But only you need to know that. These routines resemble any good exercise program, so no one will recognize your ulterior motives.

The Sex Exercise You Can Do Anywhere

It takes just 5 minutes. No one will know you're doing it, and it could make your orgasms more intense! We're talking about Kegels. Named for Arnold Kegel, MD, these exercises strengthen the pubococcygeus or PC muscle, the one you tighten to stop the flow of urine. These simple exercises may also be useful for improving ejaculatory control and enhancing sexual pleasure by making ejaculations stronger and orgasms more enjoyable. Here's how to do them: Without using your butt muscles, contract those pee-stopping muscles for 15 seconds, then release and repeat. Do three sets of 10 reps. Over time, work up to longer holds of 30 seconds or a minute. Nobody will ever know that you are doing these exercises, so you can tap a Kegel anytime, anywhere.

Find It Quick: Your 15-Minute Workouts for Better Sex

IS THAT A CANARY IN YOUR TROUSERS?

The strength of your erection is a key measure of your heart and artery health—a "canary in a coal mine" that can warn of impending danger when there's still time to take preventive action. That's because a penile artery is much narrower than a coronary artery. If a buildup of arterial plaque is starting to occur, it'll probably show up first as softer erections. Take that as a sign that your doctor should check a more critical organ.

The Stamina Workout

The average sex session lasts about 15 to 20 minutes. (Don't worry; that includes foreplay). Depending on how aggressive it is, how many positions are attempted, and the complexity of those contortions, that could be quite an aerobic workout in itself. Make sure you don't tucker out just as she's getting warmed up by training with this endurance-building routine that uses pyramid repetitions.

START HERE:
How to do pyramid reps: First, warm up using the first pair of exercises. Then do 1 rep of exercise pair 2, then 2 reps, then 3, then 4, then work back down to 1 rep. Follow the same pattern with exercise pair 3. That's one full round. Do as many rounds as you can in fit into 15 minutes.

PAIR 1

Boxer's Punch and Dumbbell Squat (warmup)

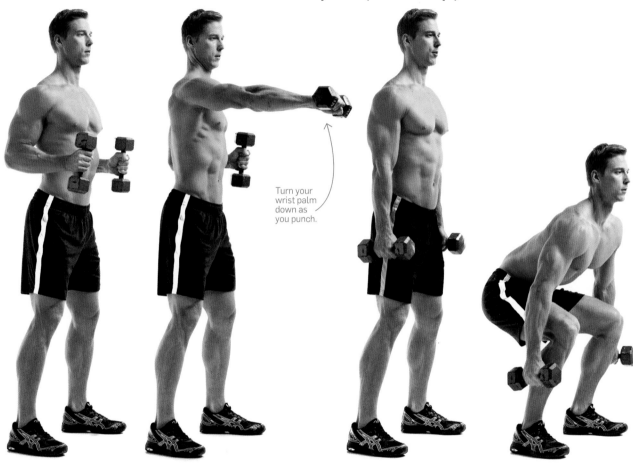

Turn your wrist palm down as you punch.

| A | B | | C | | D |

- With a 5-pound dumbbell in each hand, throw 32 punches, alternating lefts and rights.

- Let your arms hang loosely at your sides and place your feet slightly wider than hip-width apart.

- Bend at the hips and knees to lower your body until your thighs are parallel to the floor, and then press back up.

- Complete 16 squats. Repeat the sequence once more.

REPS: Do 32 punches and 16 squats.

The Stamina Workout

Pushup and Prone Row

A

- Place two hexagonal dumbbells on the floor and grip them, palms facing each other, while assuming a pushup stance.

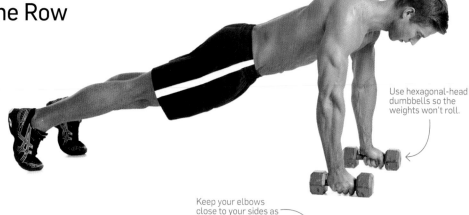

Use hexagonal-head dumbbells so the weights won't roll.

B

- Take 2 seconds to lower your body until your chest is about 2 inches above the floor.
- Push yourself up explosively.

Keep your elbows close to your sides as you lower your body.

C

- In the up position of the pushup (still holding onto the dumbbells), bring your right-hand weight up to your armpit and squeeze your shoulder blade back while balancing on the left-hand dumbbell.
- Lower the weight and repeat the move with your left arm. (Take 1 second to raise the weight and 2 seconds to lower it.)

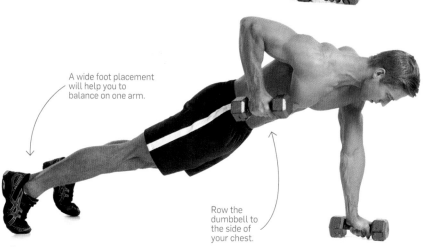

A wide foot placement will help you to balance on one arm.

Row the dumbbell to the side of your chest.

REPS: Do pyramids; see "Start Here."

PAIR 3
Jump Squat and Curl

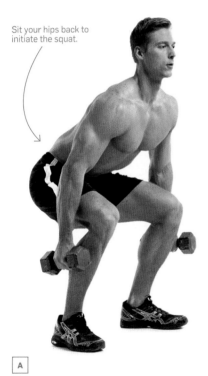

Sit your hips back to initiate the squat.

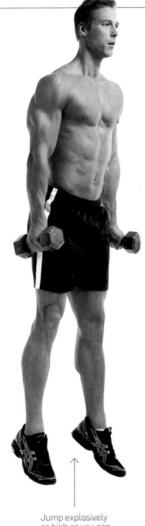

Jump explosively as high as you can.

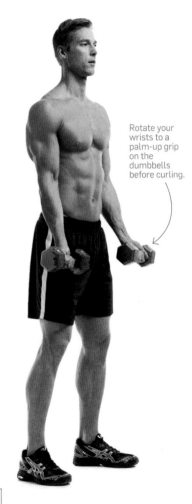

Rotate your wrists to a palm-up grip on the dumbbells before curling.

A

- Assume a squat position as you hold dumbbells at your sides, your feet slightly wider than hip-width apart.

REPS: Do pyramids; see "Start Here."

B

- Press through your heels to explode up quickly. Then land softly on the balls of your feet and sink back onto your heels.

C

- After landing, let the dumbbells hang at your sides.
- Without moving your upper arms, curl the weights up. (Take 1 second to raise them and 2 seconds to lower.)

Over-the-Top Workout

This quick cardio routine is called a "finisher" when used at the end of a longer exercise session, but it makes a terrific 15-minute workout by itself when you do the circuit three times. It's especially effective at melting fat off your body so you won't carry extra baggage into bed.

START HERE: Do these moves one after another with no rest in between. Then repeat the circuit for a total of three times.

Bodyweight Jump Squat

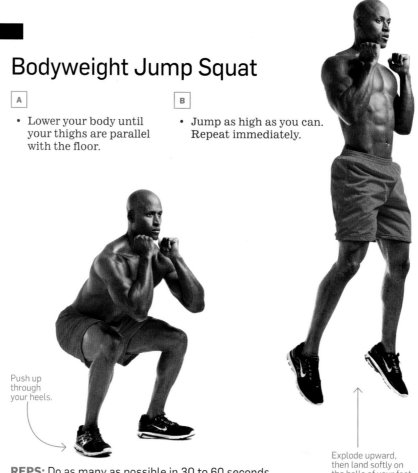

A
- Lower your body until your thighs are parallel with the floor.

B
- Jump as high as you can. Repeat immediately.

Push up through your heels.

REPS: Do as many as possible in 30 to 60 seconds.

Explode upward, then land softly on the balls of your feet.

Isometric Squat

Place your hands behind your head throughout the hold.

Contract your core and glutes as you hold this position.

Angle your feet outward slightly.

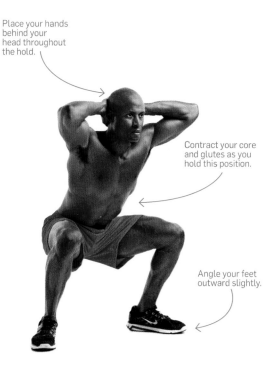

A

- Lower your body until your thighs are parallel to the floor, and pause. Hold the position for 30 to 60 seconds.
- Press up to the starting position to complete.

REPS: DO 1.

Single-Arm Dumbbell Swing

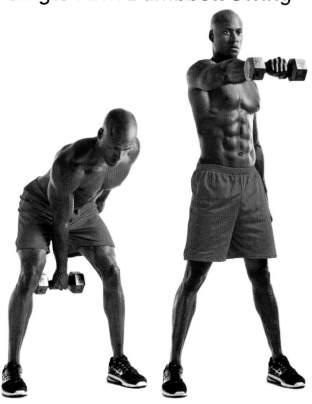

A

- Using an overhand grip, hold a dumbbell at arm's length in front of your waist.
- Bend at your hips and knees and lower your torso until it's at a 45-degree angle to the floor.
- Swing the dumbbell between your legs.

B

- Thrust your hips forward and swing the dumbbell up to chest level as you stand. Reverse the move, and repeat.
- Halfway through, switch arms.

REPS: Do as many as you can for 30 to 60 seconds.

Over-the-Top Workout

Squat Thrust

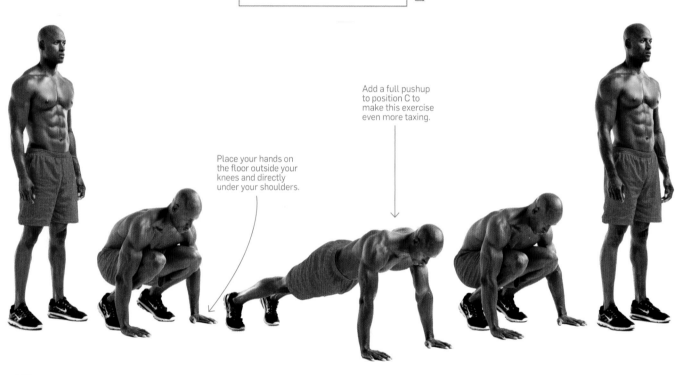

TRAINER'S TIP: *Also known as burpees, the squat thrust is one of the most athletically challenging moves in the book—a terrific calorie burner.*

Add a full pushup to position C to make this exercise even more taxing.

Place your hands on the floor outside your knees and directly under your shoulders.

A
- Stand with your feet shoulder-width apart and your arms at your sides.

B
- Push your hips back, bend your knees, and lower your body as deep as you can into a squat.

C
- Kick your legs backward so that you're in a pushup position.

D
- Quickly bring your legs back to the squat.

E
- Stand up quickly and repeat the entire series of moves.

REPS: Do as many as possible in 30 to 60 seconds.

Explosive Pushup

A

- Assume a pushup position, your hands slightly beyond shoulder-width apart.

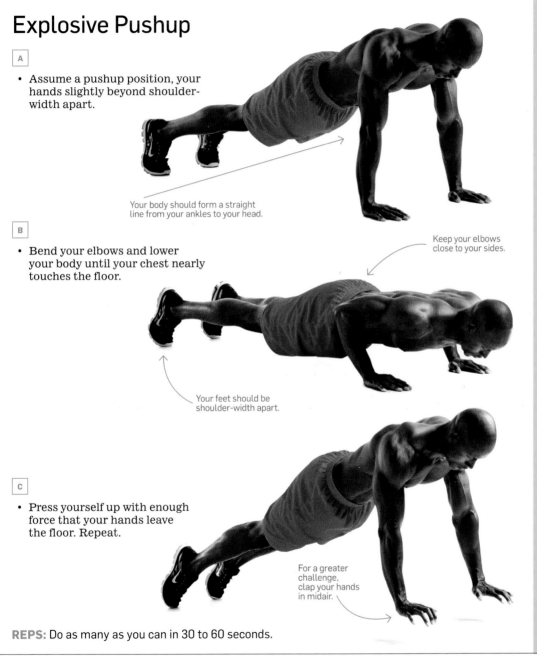

Your body should form a straight line from your ankles to your head.

B

- Bend your elbows and lower your body until your chest nearly touches the floor.

Keep your elbows close to your sides.

Your feet should be shoulder-width apart.

C

- Press yourself up with enough force that your hands leave the floor. Repeat.

For a greater challenge, clap your hands in midair.

REPS: Do as many as you can in 30 to 60 seconds.

ERECTION SETS

Daily strolls can keep the lead in your pencil, according to a study of 31,000 men by Harvard scientists. The researchers found that men who walked briskly for 2 miles a day or did the equivalent in other aerobic activity reduced their risk of erection problems by 30 percent. You can even get a good walking workout in just 15 minutes by doing it interval style: Alternate between a moderate pace, a brisk walk, and speed walking at 1½- to 3-minute intervals. After you build endurance, toss running into the interval mix.

309

Man-On-a-Mission Workout

Even if you're a studied pupil of the *Kama Sutra*, chances are the sex position you use most often is the missionary. So, make it last longer and produce more pleasure for both of you with this routine that improves strength in your arms and chest for stamina and in your glutes and lower back for strong, steady thrusting.

START HERE:
Do these exercises as a circuit, one after another, with no rest in between. Rest for 60 seconds after completing the circuit. Do a total of three circuits.

Hinge

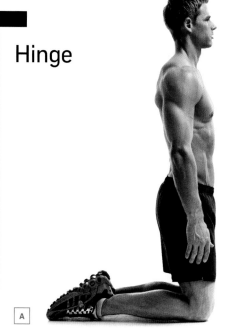

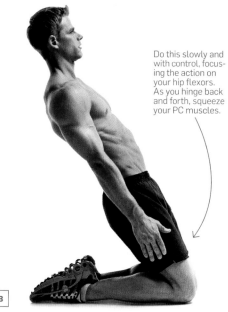

Do this slowly and with control, focusing the action on your hip flexors. As you hinge back and forth, squeeze your PC muscles.

A
- Kneel on the floor with your hands at your sides.
- Resist the urge to sit back and rest your weight on your heels.
- Your back should be straight and your knees bent at 90-degree angles.

REPS: Do 10 to 12.

B
- Keeping your head and back in a straight line with your thighs at all times, slowly lean back a few inches.
- Hold this position for 2 to 3 seconds, then slowly return to the starting position.

Stability-Ball Decline Pushup

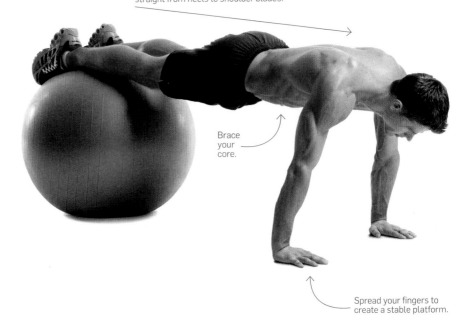

Your back should be ironing-board straight from heels to shoulder blades.

Brace your core.

Spread your fingers to create a stable platform.

- Kneel with a stability ball behind you and place your hands flat on the floor, shoulder-width apart.
- Place your shins on the ball and get into the standard pushup position—arms straight, hands directly under your shoulders.
- Your back should be flat and your abs drawn in.

B

- Tuck your chin and, leading with your chest, lower your body to the floor.
- Push yourself back up and repeat.

Maintain a straight back while you lower your body until your nose barely touches the floor.

The instability of the ball forces you to recruit more muscles to maintain balance.

REPS: Do 15 to 20.

Man-On-a-Mission Workout

Lying Gluteal Bridge

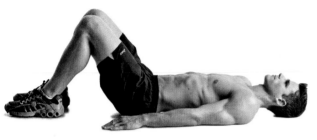

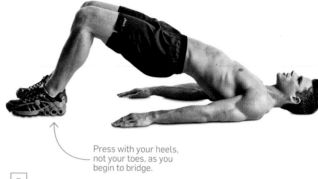

Press with your heels, not your toes, as you begin to bridge.

A

- Lie on your back with your knees bent and your feet flat on the floor.
- Place your arms at your sides, palms facing down.

REPS: Do 10 to 12.

B

- Squeeze your glutes and slowly raise your butt off the floor until your body forms a straight line from your knees to your shoulders.
- Hold this position for 3 to 5 seconds, then slowly lower yourself back to the floor.

Sock Slide

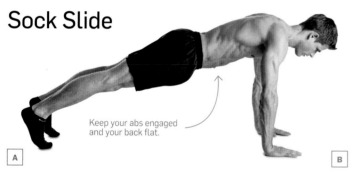

Keep your abs engaged and your back flat.

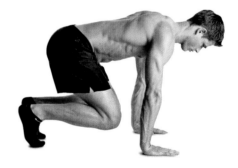

A

- For this move, you need to wear socks on a slippery floor surface.
- Assume the pushup position, with your hands flat on the floor, shoulder-width apart, your arms and legs straight, and your feet together.
- Keeping your hands in place, slowly slide your body back and down until your nose is pointing down at the space between your hands.

REPS: Do 10 to 15.

B

- Slowly slide your feet forward by bending your knees and contracting your abs. That's 1 rep.

Kneeling Leg Crossover

- Kneel and place your hands on the floor. Your knees and hands should both be shoulder-width apart. Look down at the floor.
- Straighten your right leg out behind you.

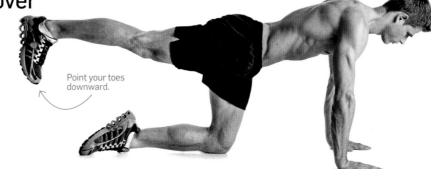

Point your toes downward.

- Cross your right leg over your left foot and drop it down until your toes touch the floor.
- Keep your leg straight throughout the motion. Return to the starting position with your leg extended behind you off the floor.

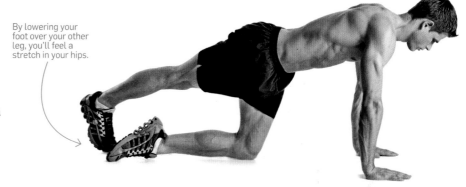

By lowering your foot over your other leg, you'll feel a stretch in your hips.

C

- Extend your right leg out to the right and lower it until the toes touch the ground. That's 1 rep. Complete all reps, then repeat the moves using your left leg.

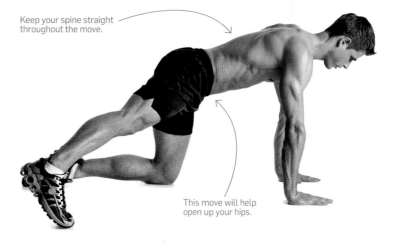

Keep your spine straight throughout the move.

This move will help open up your hips.

REPS: Do 10 with each leg.

Pretzel-Position Workout

It's not easy to work your way into The Spider sex position or lift her into Ballet Dancer if your sacroiliac is sore and your hamstrings tight. Your body needs to flex for great sex. The following workout stretches and strengthens all the key thrusting, twisting, turning muscles so you can go all night long without twinging your schwing.

START HERE: Do these moves one after another with no rest in between. Then repeat the circuit two to three times.

Standing Hip Thrust

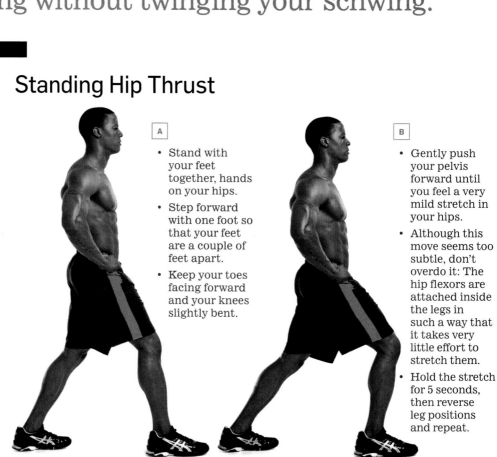

A
- Stand with your feet together, hands on your hips.
- Step forward with one foot so that your feet are a couple of feet apart.
- Keep your toes facing forward and your knees slightly bent.

B
- Gently push your pelvis forward until you feel a very mild stretch in your hips.
- Although this move seems too subtle, don't overdo it: The hip flexors are attached inside the legs in such a way that it takes very little effort to stretch them.
- Hold the stretch for 5 seconds, then reverse leg positions and repeat.

REPS: Do 3 with each leg forward.

Lower-Back Lie-Down

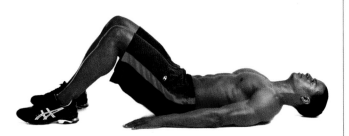

A

- Lie flat on your back with your legs bent, feet flat on the floor, and arms at your sides.

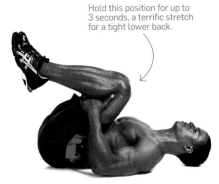

Hold this position for up to 3 seconds, a terrific stretch for a tight lower back.

B

- Draw your knees up to your chest and gently grab your legs just behind the knees.
- Slowly pull both knees toward your chest as far as you comfortably can, keeping your back flat on the floor at all times.
- Hold the stretch for 2 to 3 seconds, then slowly lower your legs.

REPS: Do 12 to 15.

Stability Ball Hip Extension

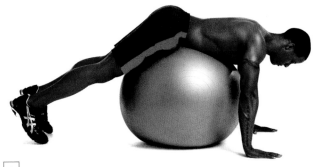

A

- Lie facedown over a stability ball, with your hips at the apex of the ball.
- Place your hands flat on the floor directly beneath your shoulders.
- Extend your legs so you're balanced on your toes, feet hip-width apart.

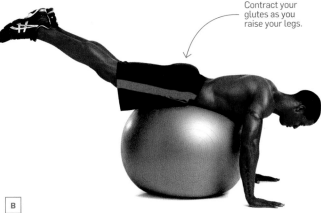

Contract your glutes as you raise your legs.

B

- Contract your glutes and raise your legs so they're in line with (or above) your torso.
- Return to the starting position. That's 1 rep.

REPS: Do 12 to 15.

315

Pretzel-Position Workout

Low Side-to-Side Lunge

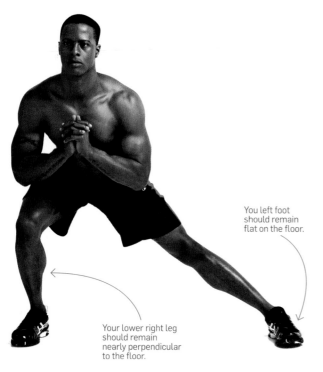

Your lower right leg should remain nearly perpendicular to the floor.

You left foot should remain flat on the floor.

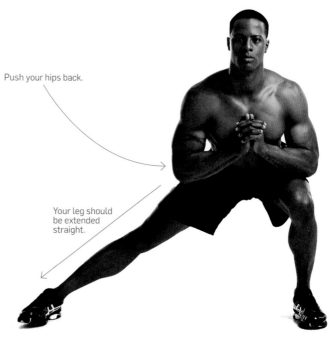

Push your hips back.

Your leg should be extended straight.

A

- Stand with your feet spread wide, about twice shoulder-width apart, your feet pointing straight ahead.
- Bend slightly at the waist and clasp your hands in front of your chest.
- Shift your weight to your right leg as you push your hips backward and lower your body by dropping your hips and bending your right knee.
- Without pausing, reverse the movement to a standing position.

REPS: Do 10 to 20 on each side.

B

- Repeat the move to the left side. Remember to keep your right foot on the floor as you shift your weight over the left foot.
- Alternate back and forth, pausing only briefly when you raise yourself back to a standing position.

Corkscrew Pushup

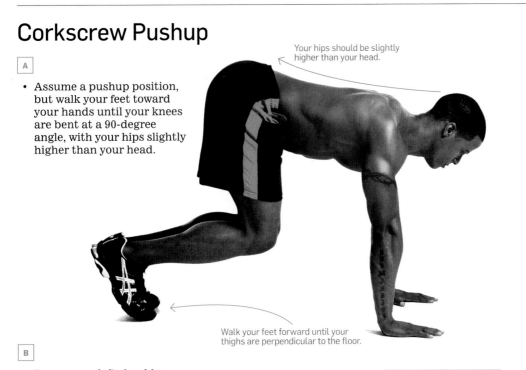

A

- Assume a pushup position, but walk your feet toward your hands until your knees are bent at a 90-degree angle, with your hips slightly higher than your head.

Your hips should be slightly higher than your head.

Walk your feet forward until your thighs are perpendicular to the floor.

B

- Lower your left shoulder close to the floor by rotating your body right and bending your elbows.
- Pause, then rise slightly and rotate your right side to the floor.
- Pause again, then push up to the starting position with your arms straight. That's 1 rep.

TRAINER'S TIP: *This move works your quads, calves, core, and all the upper-body muscles.*

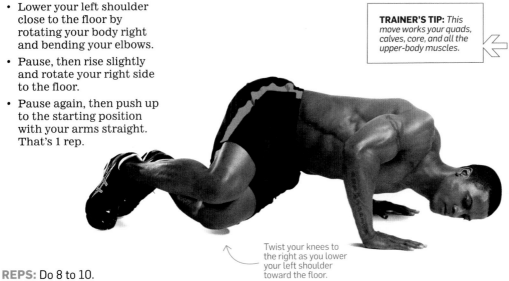

Twist your knees to the right as you lower your left shoulder toward the floor.

REPS: Do 8 to 10.

LESS WEIGHT, GREATER PLEASURE

Being overweight can depress anyone's sex life. Researchers studying 1,210 people at Duke University Medical Center say obese people are 25 times more likely to report dissatisfaction with sex as people who are at a healthy weight. The good news is that good sex can be achieved without a huge change in body composition. Other studies report that people can significantly improve their sexual satisfaction with just a 10 percent reduction in body weight.

Four-on-the-Floor Workout

The Four-on-the-Floor moves are composed of three highly athletic exercises and an excellent stretch for opening your hips and flexing your piriformis muscle. Both the Renegade Row and Inchworm challenge your core, back, and chest for greater endurance in you-on-top positions, while the Sandbag Standup builds leg and arm strength for sex moves requiring you to lift and hold your partner. And all are great general exercises for performing better beyond the bedroom.

START HERE:
Do these exercises and stretches as a circuit, one after another, with no rest between them. Rest for 60 seconds after completing the circuit. Do a total of three circuits.

Lying Crossover Stretch

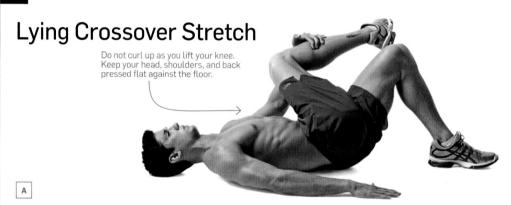

Do not curl up as you lift your knee. Keep your head, shoulders, and back pressed flat against the floor.

A

- Lie on your back with your knees bent, feet flat on the floor, and hands at your sides, palms down.
- Slowly draw your right knee up to your chest.
- Grab the outside of the knee with your left hand and gently pull it toward your left shoulder as far as is comfortable.
- Hold for 20 seconds, then lower the leg to the starting position.
- Repeat the move, this time raising your left knee and pulling it toward your right shoulder. That's 1 rep.

REPS: Do 2.

Inchworm

A

- Stand with your legs straight and feet hip-width apart.

TRAINER'S TIP:
The Inchworm is also a superb warmup exercise that loosens your thigh, hip, and oblique muscles.

B

- Bend at the waist and place your hands on the floor.

Bend your knees slightly if you can't keep them straight.

C

- Keeping your legs straight, walk your hands forward while keeping your abs and lower back braced.

Walk your hands out as far as you can without allowing your hips to sag.

D

- Take tiny steps to walk your feet back to your hands. That's 1 rep. Repeat walking your hands out and feet in.

Walk your feet back toward your hands.

Keep your core engaged.

REPS: Do 6.

Four-on-the-Floor Workout

Renegade Row

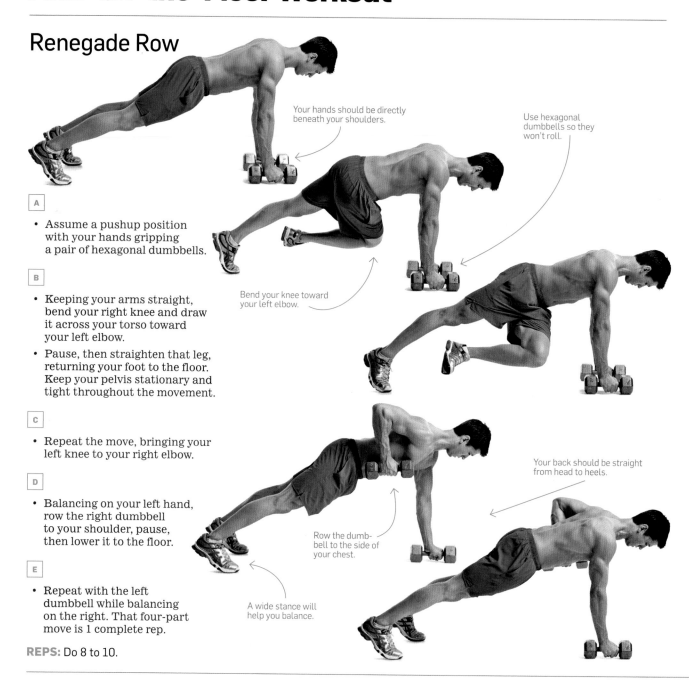

Your hands should be directly beneath your shoulders.

Use hexagonal dumbbells so they won't roll.

Bend your knee toward your left elbow.

Your back should be straight from head to heels.

Row the dumbbell to the side of your chest.

A wide stance will help you balance.

A

- Assume a pushup position with your hands gripping a pair of hexagonal dumbbells.

B

- Keeping your arms straight, bend your right knee and draw it across your torso toward your left elbow.
- Pause, then straighten that leg, returning your foot to the floor. Keep your pelvis stationary and tight throughout the movement.

C

- Repeat the move, bringing your left knee to your right elbow.

D

- Balancing on your left hand, row the right dumbbell to your shoulder, pause, then lower it to the floor.

E

- Repeat with the left dumbbell while balancing on the right. That four-part move is 1 complete rep.

REPS: Do 8 to 10.

Sandbag Standup

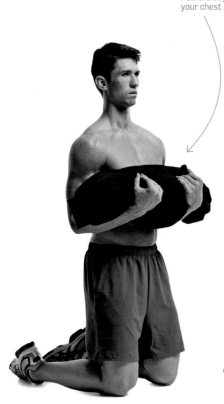

Pull the bag to your chest.

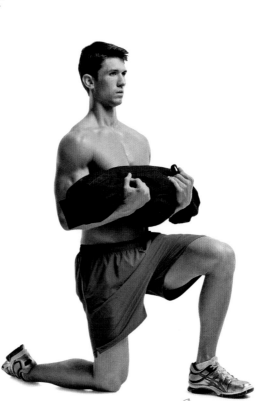

Push through your heel to rise up.

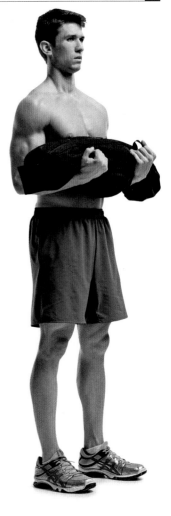

A

- Kneel on the floor while holding a heavy sandbag in both arms.
- Your arms should be underneath the bag, your palms facing up, and your hands around the front of the bag.

REPS: Do 8 to 10 with each leg.

B

- Lift your left knee and place your left foot flat on the floor to start standing up.

C

- Push through your heel to stand and bring your right foot next to your left.
- Squat down and place your left knee on the floor, then the right knee so you are kneeling again. Repeat, starting with your right foot and pushing through the heel to stand up.

Chapter 14:
15-Minute Healing Workouts

Who Needs Ibuprofen When You Have Endorphins?
Open This Chapter When Pain Threatens
to Derail Your Workout. It's Exercise for What Ails You.

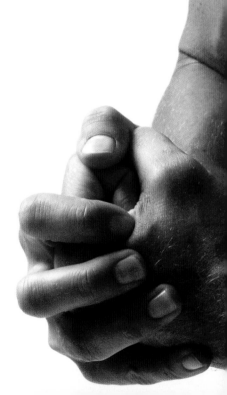

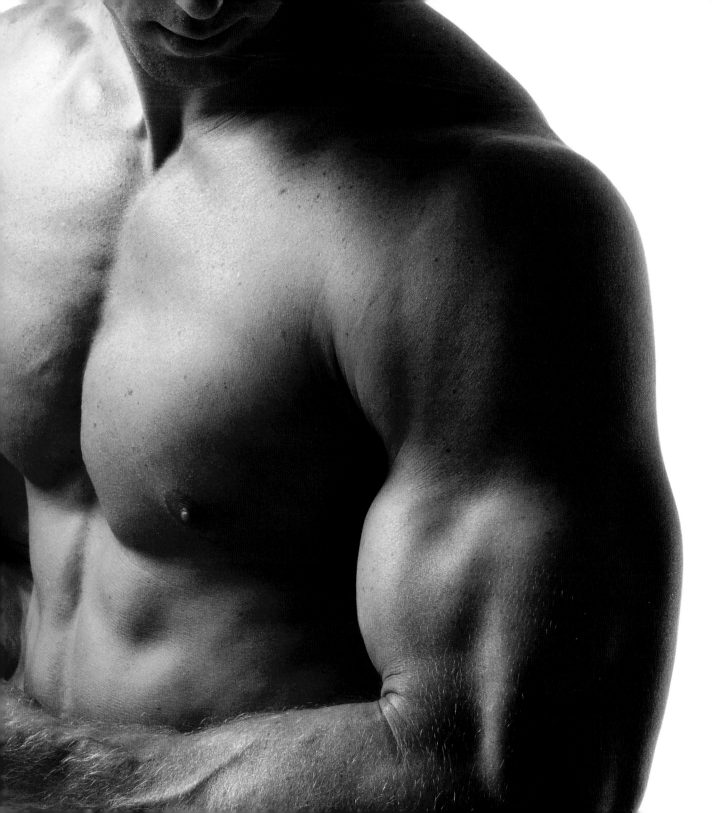

Superfast Workouts That Heal

"The best defense is a good offense." Legendary Green Bay Packers coach Vince Lombardi was talking about football, but his famous quote could also apply to the human body: Being proactive—on the offense—is the best way to defend against pain, illness, and even the passage of time. That's where exercise comes in; studies have shown that people who exercise regularly, eat nutrient-rich foods, and limit stress have stronger immune systems. So use the workouts in this chapter not only to treat what ails you, but also to prevent health problems from slowing you down. One 15-minute workout that everyone should try to build into their monthly fitness program is ideal for doing just that: the Age Eraser workout starting on page 340. It uses a special exercise technique called plyometrics—high-energy hops, agility drills, and other jumping exercises—to strengthen the fast-twitch muscle fibers that tend to decline with age.

Find It Quick: Your 15-Minute Healing Circuit Plans

DO SOME MORE IF YOU'RE SORE

We recommend taking a rest day between tough workouts, but when you are very sore, a round or two of calisthenics or other light exercise may help. Australian researchers found that men who lifted light weights the day after a hard workout reported a 40 percent decrease in muscle soreness compared with those who didn't exercise. By increasing bloodflow to the damaged muscles tissue, light exercise may speed recovery. Two sets of 10 pushups the day after a grueling chest workout or bodyweight squats the day after an intense leg session should do it.

Shoulder Stretch and Strengthen

The shoulders' amazing range of motion allows you to shoot baskets, cast delicate trout flies, and scratch your back. But all of its complexity also leads to instability. Making matters worse, these joints tend to be abused and misused, especially if you work a desk job. The average human head weighs 8 pounds. And if your chin moves forward just 3 inches—as it tends to when you work at a computer—the muscles of your neck, shoulders, and upper back must support the equivalent of 11 pounds. That's a weight-bearing increase of 38 percent—often for hours at a time. Left untreated, the effect of chronic desk slump is a postural dysfunction that physical therapists call upper-cross syndrome; you know it as rounded shoulders. Reverse this forward-slumping trend with this shoulder-fixing routine.

START HERE: Do these moves one after another with no rest between them. Then repeat the circuit for a total of two times.

Shoulder-Adductor Stretch

A

- Lie on the floor with your knees bent and your arms straight up in the air.

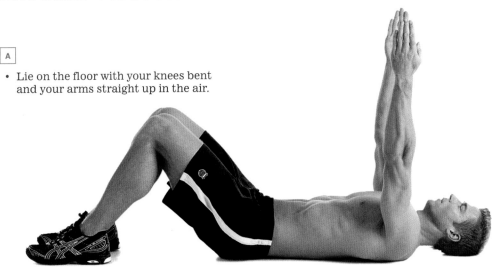

B

- With your back flat, slowly move your arms back and down toward the floor, keeping them straight and close to the sides of your head. Hold this position for 20 seconds.

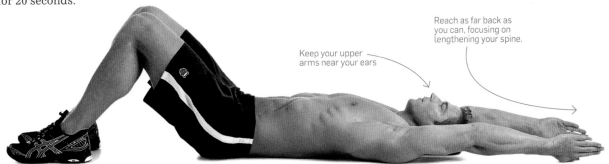

Reach as far back as you can, focusing on lengthening your spine.

Keep your upper arms near your ears

REPS: Do 12.

Shoulder Stretch and Strengthen

Peel

TRAINER'S TIP:
After you've gained enough flexibility to perform the stretch with your body and arm perpendicular against the wall, move your arm up to 2 o'clock, then progress to 1 o'clock.

 A

- Stand facing a wall and place your right arm against it, fingers pointing to 3 o'clock.
- Keeping your shoulder and arm flush against the wall, rotate your body to the left by moving your feet.
- When you feel a stretch along your chest, hold that position for 20 to 30 seconds.

REPS: Do 6 with each arm.

Stability Ball T

A

- Grab a pair of 2- or 5-pound dumbbells and lie facedown on a stability ball.
- Start with your back flat, your chest off the ball, and your arms hanging down, palms forward.

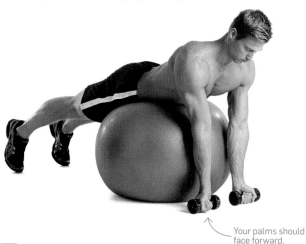

Your palms should face forward.

B

- Squeeze your shoulder blades down and together as you extend your arms to the sides, forming a T with your body.
- Pause, then return to the starting position.

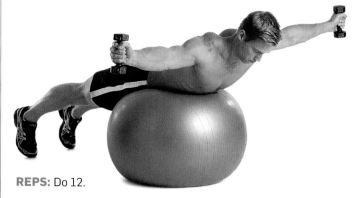

REPS: Do 12.

Kneeling Lat Stretch

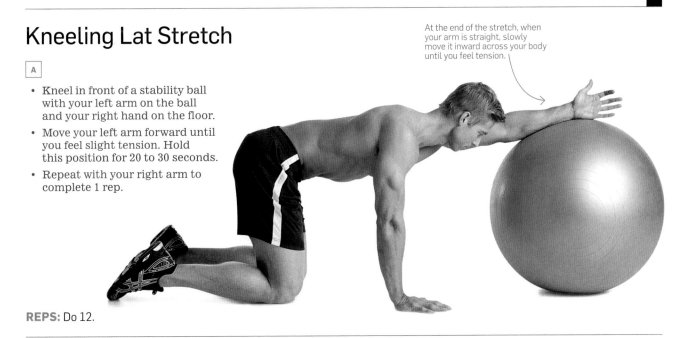

A

- Kneel in front of a stability ball with your left arm on the ball and your right hand on the floor.
- Move your left arm forward until you feel slight tension. Hold this position for 20 to 30 seconds.
- Repeat with your right arm to complete 1 rep.

At the end of the stretch, when your arm is straight, slowly move it inward across your body until you feel tension.

REPS: Do 12.

Incline Dumbbell V Raise

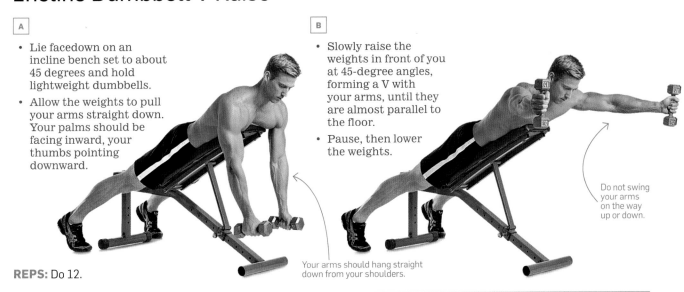

A

- Lie facedown on an incline bench set to about 45 degrees and hold lightweight dumbbells.
- Allow the weights to pull your arms straight down. Your palms should be facing inward, your thumbs pointing downward.

B

- Slowly raise the weights in front of you at 45-degree angles, forming a V with your arms, until they are almost parallel to the floor.
- Pause, then lower the weights.

Do not swing your arms on the way up or down.

Your arms should hang straight down from your shoulders.

REPS: Do 12.

329

Shoulder Stretch and Strengthen

Shoulder PNF

TRAINER'S TIP: *PNF stands for "proprioceptive neuromuscular facilitation," a type of active stretching used by physical therapists in rehab training. Its purpose is to treat and prevent overuse injuries by flexing muscles and limbs through a wide range of motion, in this case a diagonal pattern for good shoulder biomechanics.*

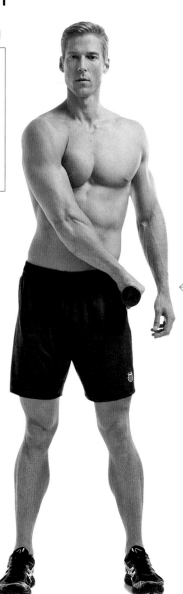

Raise the dumbbell diagonally above your head to the right, and rotate your hand so that your knuckles point toward the ceiling.

Your knuckles should be facing the floor.

A

- Hold a lightweight dumbbell in your right hand next to your left-side hip bone.

B

- Pull the dumbbell diagonally across your body while rotating your thumb to the right so that at the top of the move, your arm is straight and to the right of your shoulder.

- Reverse the move to the starting position and finish the set before repeating with your other arm.

REPS: Do 12 with each arm.

Standing Cable Reverse Fly

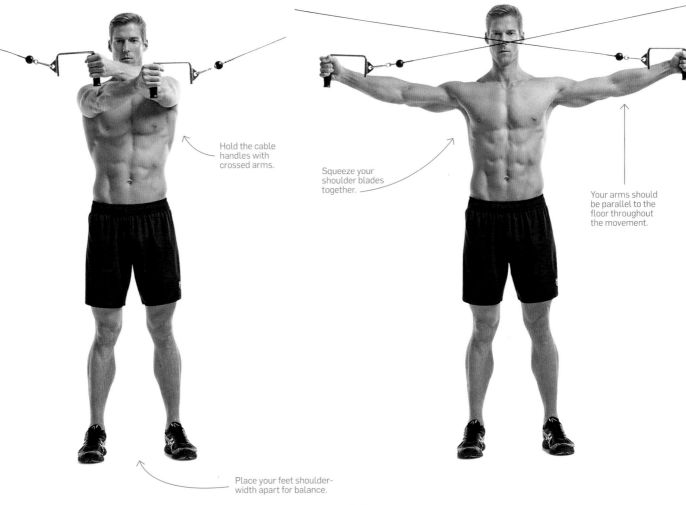

Hold the cable handles with crossed arms.

Squeeze your shoulder blades together.

Your arms should be parallel to the floor throughout the movement.

Place your feet shoulder-width apart for balance.

A

- Stand with your feet shoulder-width apart and grab the left handle of a cable-crossover system with your right hand and the right handle with your left.

REPS: Do 12.

B

- Lean back slightly and spread your arms to the sides (forming a T with your body) while squeezing your shoulder blades together.
- Pause, then return to the starting position.

Knee Saver

One possible reason Mr. Miyagi (Pat Morita) of Karate Kid fame was indestructible: Kicks decrease your risk of a knee injury, concluded a recent study in the *Journal of Strength and Conditioning Research*. How? By strengthening the hamstrings, which support and stabilize the knee while stepping, running, and bearing loads. In the study, martial arts athletes were found to have about 20 percent greater hamstring strength when compared with a fit control group. All those kicks the athletes do during drills clearly builds hamstring strength, which is why we've included some in the workout that follows.

START HERE: Do these moves one after another with no rest in between. Then repeat the circuit for a total of three times.

Lunge and Front Kick

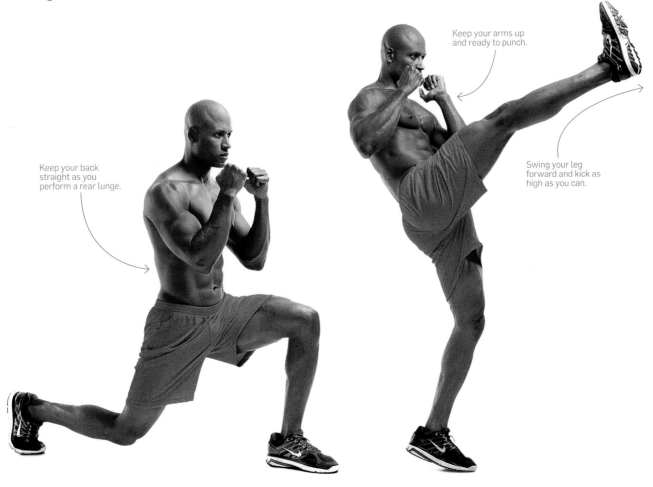

Keep your back straight as you perform a rear lunge.

Keep your arms up and ready to punch.

Swing your leg forward and kick as high as you can.

- Step back into a deep lunge with your right leg, so that your right knee almost touches the floor.
- Keep your back straight.

REPS: Do 12 with each leg.

- With your left foot firmly planted on the floor, rise and kick your right foot in front of you as high as you can.
- Return to the standing position and repeat, stepping back and kicking with your left leg.

333

Knee Saver

Head Crusher

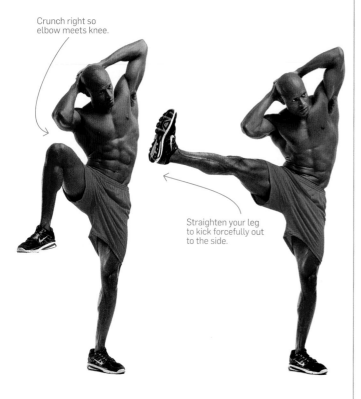

Crunch right so elbow meets knee.

Straighten your leg to kick forcefully out to the side.

A

- Stand with your hands behind your head.
- Bring your right knee up to meet your elbow as you crunch your obliques to the right.

B

- Kick your right foot out to the side, then snap it back.
- Return to the starting position and repeat the move with your left knee and elbow and kicking with your left foot.

REPS: Do 12 on each leg.

Offset Squat

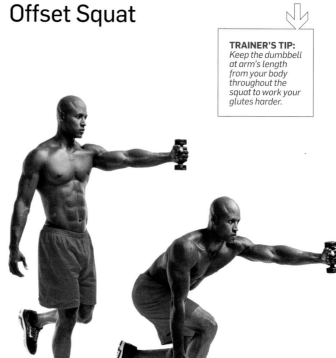

> **TRAINER'S TIP:**
> *Keep the dumbbell at arm's length from your body throughout the squat to work your glutes harder.*

A

- Grab a 5- to 8-pound dumbbell in your left hand and raise it straight out in front of you until your arm is parallel with the floor.
- Lift your left leg behind you and balance on your right.

B

- Bend your right knee to squat down until your thigh is as close to parallel to the floor as possible.
- Pause for a second and then push back up to the starting position.

REPS: Do 8 to 10 with each arm and leg.

Single-Leg Plank

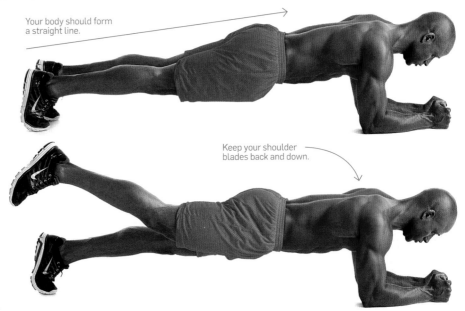

Your body should form a straight line.

Keep your shoulder blades back and down.

 A

- Assume a plank position with your toes flexed underneath you and your forearms on the floor, elbows directly under your shoulders.

B

- Brace your abs and lift your right leg up about 10 inches
- Balance your weight on your forearms and the stabilizing leg. Hold for up to 60 seconds.

REPS: Do 1 with each leg elevated.

Side-to-Side Leg Swing

A

- Stand and grab a sturdy object in front of you with both hands.
- Swing your right leg out to the right as high as you can, then swing it back down and across your left leg. That's 1 rep.

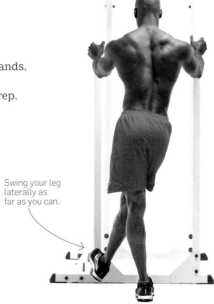

Swing your leg laterally as far as you can.

REPS: Do 12 to 20, then switch legs and repeat.

Lower-Back Booster

Protect your back by strengthening your entire core—your obliques and abdominals—and you'll also be able to endure any long-lasting activity without fatiguing. The best way to prepare is with sustained isometric contractions. The workout below uses "iso moves" to boost the endurance of all of your spine-supporting muscles.

START HERE:
Do two sets of each move, resting for 30 seconds between moves.

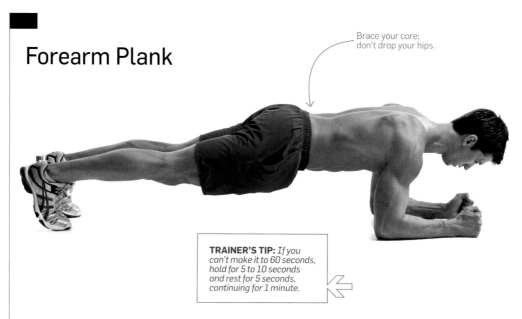

Forearm Plank

Brace your core; don't drop your hips.

TRAINER'S TIP: *If you can't make it to 60 seconds, hold for 5 to 10 seconds and rest for 5 seconds, continuing for 1 minute.*

A

- Starting at the top of a pushup position, bend your elbows and lower yourself down until you can shift your weight from your hands to your forearms.
- Your body should form a straight line; don't drop your hips or raise your butt.
- Brace your abs (imagine that someone is about to punch you in the gut) and hold for 60 seconds.

REPS: Do 1 for 60 seconds.

Side Forearm Plank

- Lie on your left side with your legs straight and your feet stacked.
- Prop yourself up with your left forearm so your torso forms a diagonal line. Rest your right hand on your hip.

Stack your feet.

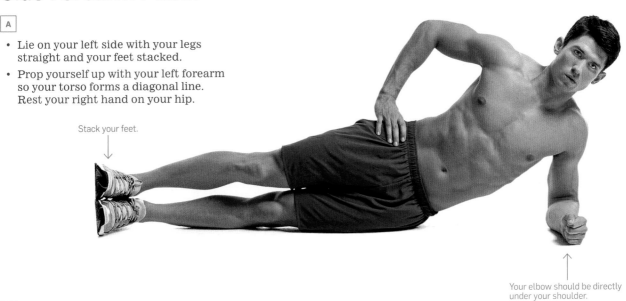

Your elbow should be directly under your shoulder.

B

- Brace your abs, lift your hips from the floor, and hold for 60 seconds.
- If you can't make it to 60 seconds, hold for 5 to 10 seconds and rest for 5; continue for 1 minute. Repeat on the opposite side.

Keep your hips and knees off the floor.

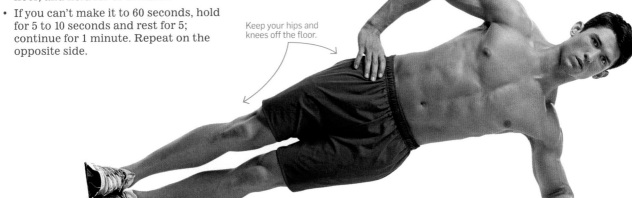

REPS: Do 1 for 60 seconds.

Lower-Back Booster

Forearm Plank with Arm Raise

A

- Assume a plank position (toes and forearms on the floor, body lifted).
- Your body should form a straight line.

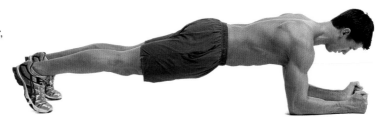

B

- Brace your abs and carefully shift your weight to your left forearm.
- Extend your right arm in front of you and hold for 3 to 10 seconds.
- Slowly bring your arm back in.
- Repeat with the left arm. That's 1 rep.

REPS: Do 5 to 10.

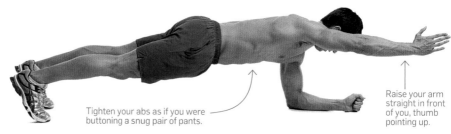

Tighten your abs as if you were buttoning a snug pair of pants.

Raise your arm straight in front of you, thumb pointing up.

Flat-Back Position with Knees Slightly Bent

A

- From a standing position, bend your knees slightly and fold at the waist until your back is parallel to the floor.
- Hold your arms out to the sides to give your back some strength resistance.
- Imagine that you are holding an orange under your chin and draw your abdomen up toward your spine to flatten your back as much as possible. Hold for 10 to 20 seconds.
- Come back to standing with straight legs.

REPS: Do 5.

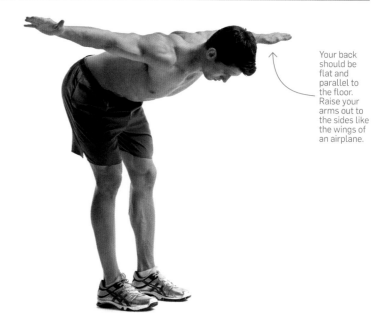

Your back should be flat and parallel to the floor. Raise your arms out to the sides like the wings of an airplane.

Superman

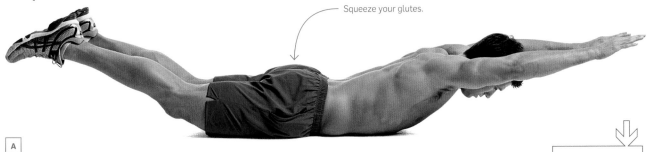

Squeeze your glutes.

A

- Lying facedown, extend and lift your arms out in front of you and lift your legs behind you as if you were the Man of Steel soaring over Metropolis.
- Hold that position for 3 seconds, then relax to the floor.
- Lift only your right arm and your left leg; hold for 3 seconds. Then lift your left arm and right leg. Hold for 3 seconds. That's 1 rep.

TRAINER'S TIP:
For the second part of the move, extend through the arm and back through the leg to create a deep diagonal stretch.

REPS: Do 10.

Cobra

A

- Lying facedown with your hands underneath your shoulders, inhale and lift your head and torso up off the floor into a cobra backbend.
- Keep your elbows in at your waist and your shoulders down. Hold for 5 breaths.
- As you exhale, lower back down until your forehead touches the floor.

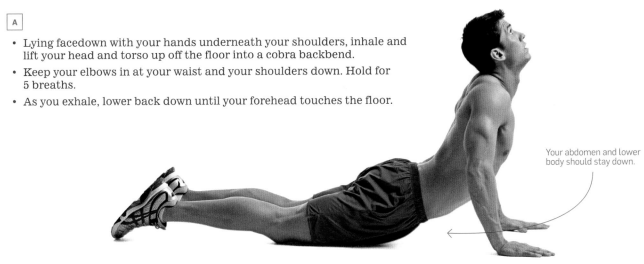

Your abdomen and lower body should stay down.

REPS: Do 5.

The Age Eraser Workout

The best workouts to combat aging make use of plyometrics—high-energy jumping, hopping, and otherwise explosive exercises that tap into fast-twitch muscle fibers most effectively. Bonus: Stressing your skeleton with explosive movements also triggers bone growth. And all that bounding and leaping builds metabolism-boosting muscle.

START HERE:
Do all of the moves without resting in between, and then take a 60 second break. Repeat for a total of three circuits.

Power Skaters

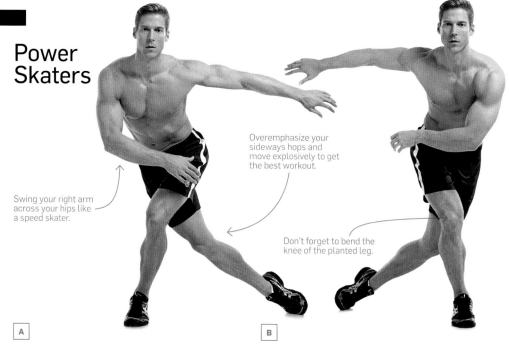

Swing your right arm across your hips like a speed skater.

Overemphasize your sideways hops and move explosively to get the best workout.

Don't forget to bend the knee of the planted leg.

A

- Stand with your feet shoulder-width apart, then jump left, crossing your right leg behind your left leg as you bend your left knee into a half-squat position.

REPS: Do 10.

B

- Hop a few feet directly to the right, switching the positions of your legs and arms. That's 1 rep.
- Continue hopping from side to side without pausing or resetting your feet.

Seal Jacks

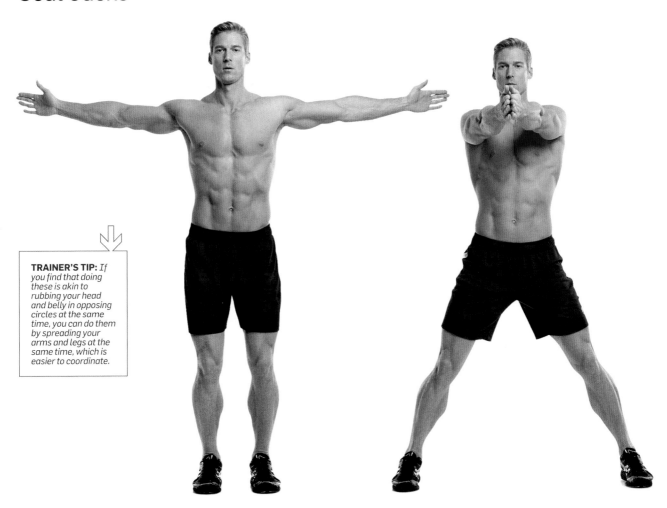

TRAINER'S TIP: *If you find that doing these is akin to rubbing your head and belly in opposing circles at the same time, you can do them by spreading your arms and legs at the same time, which is easier to coordinate.*

A

- Start with your feet about hip-width apart, arms straight out to the sides at shoulder height.

REPS: Do 20 as quickly as you can with control.

B

- Jump just high enough to spread your feet wide while simultaneously clapping your hands in front of your chest.
- Without pausing, quickly return to the starting position and repeat.

The Age Eraser Workout

Clock Walk

 A B

- Assume a standard pushup position with your feet hip-width apart and your hands on the floor directly under your shoulders.
- Instead of bending your arms to lower yourself, step your right hand out to the side to create a wide upper-body stance. Follow with your left hand to return to a shoulder-width stance.

C D

- Continue this pattern to complete 1 full rotation leading with your right arm. Then do 1 full rotation counterclockwise, leading with your left arm.

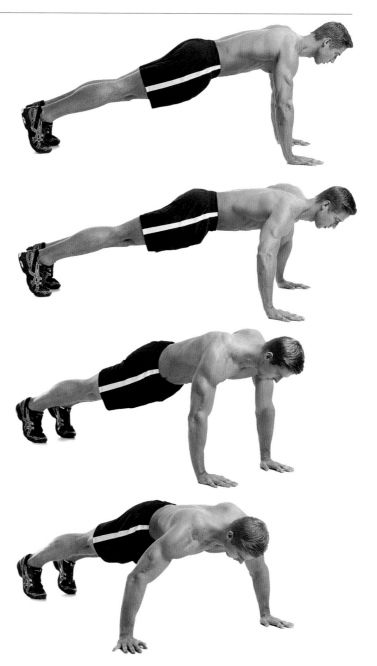

REPS: Do 1 complete circle in each direction.

Low-Step Lateral Shuffle

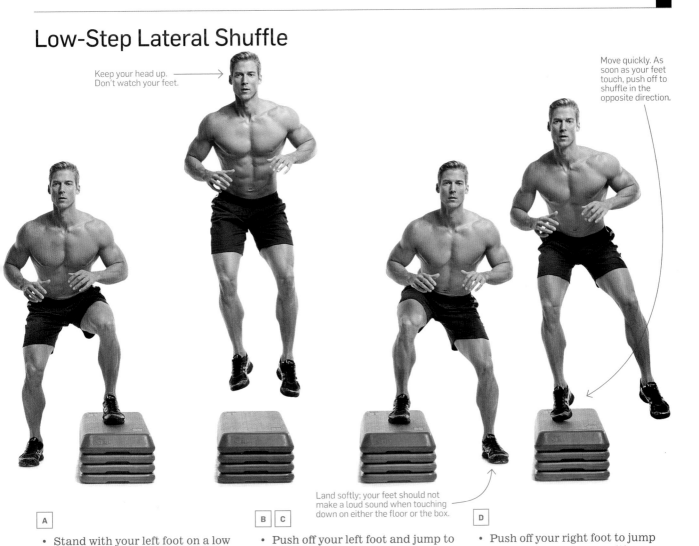

Keep your head up. Don't watch your feet.

Move quickly. As soon as your feet touch, push off to shuffle in the opposite direction.

Land softly; your feet should not make a loud sound when touching down on either the floor or the box.

A

- Stand with your left foot on a low box (or step) and your right foot on the floor about 1 foot to the right of the box.
- Bend your knees slightly, keep your chest up, and bend your arms 90 degrees in an athletic stance.

REPS: Do 10.

B **C**

- Push off your left foot and jump to your left, landing with your right foot on the box and your left foot on the floor, knees bent.

D

- Push off your right foot to jump back to the starting position. That's 1 rep.

Foam Roller Workout

If you work out long enough, eventually you're going to get stuck—literally. Your muscles will develop adhesions, knots that make you stiff and sore. Foam rollers can untie those knots— they're like a massage you give to yourself. They break the adhesions, stretch muscles, and give you instant relief (and they are a lot cheaper than a session with a masseuse because a foam roller only costs a quarter of the price of a professional massage). Tip: If a spot feels extra tender, try this: Start below the area, work up to it, and hold for a few seconds, then roll through it.

START HERE: Follow these directions, rolling each body part over the foam roller 5 to 10 times. Complete all reps with each limb before moving to the next massage.

Calf Massage

A

- Sit on the floor with your legs straight out and your hands on the floor behind you supporting your weight.
- Place the roller under your calves, then cross your left leg over your right.

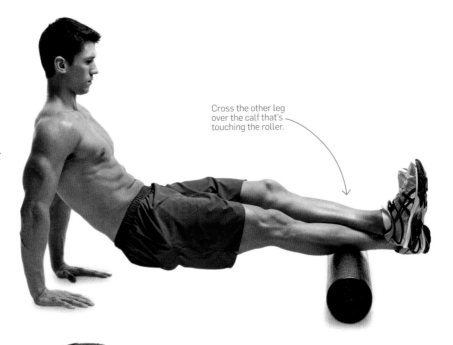

Cross the other leg over the calf that's touching the roller.

B

- Slowly roll up and down along the back of your right leg from your knee to your ankle. Complete all the reps, then repeat with the right leg crossed over your left.

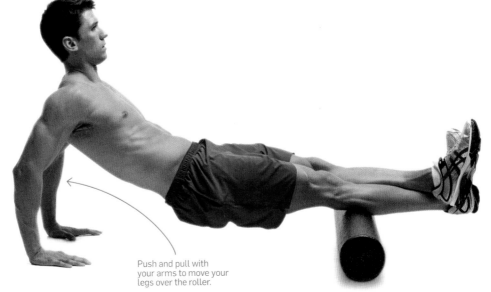

Push and pull with your arms to move your legs over the roller.

REPS: Do 5 to 10.

Foam Roller Workout

Hamstrings Massage

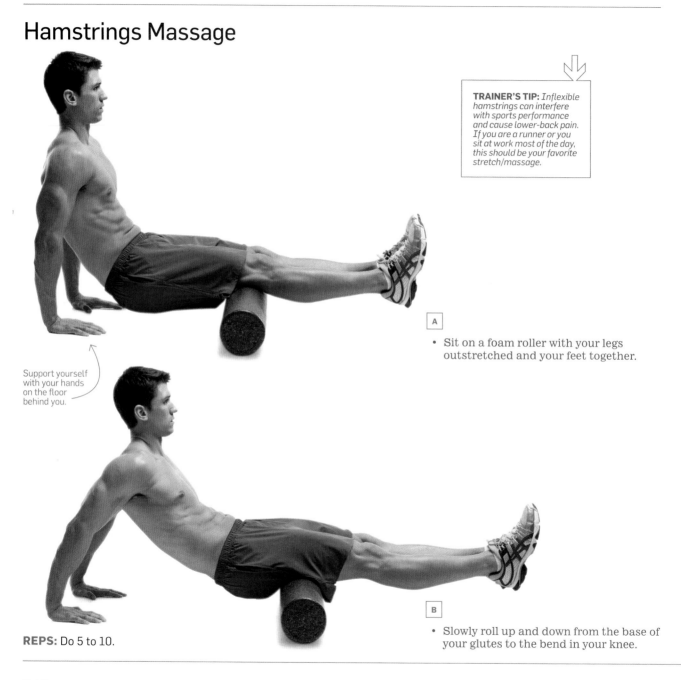

TRAINER'S TIP: *Inflexible hamstrings can interfere with sports performance and cause lower-back pain. If you are a runner or you sit at work most of the day, this should be your favorite stretch/massage.*

- Sit on a foam roller with your legs outstretched and your feet together.

Support yourself with your hands on the floor behind you.

- Slowly roll up and down from the base of your glutes to the bend in your knee.

REPS: Do 5 to 10.

Quads Massage

A

- Lie facedown on the floor and place the roller under your hips.
- Lean on your right leg.
- Roll up and down from your hip to your knee. Switch to the left leg.

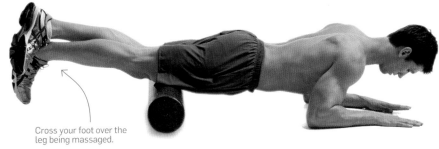

Cross your foot over the leg being massaged.

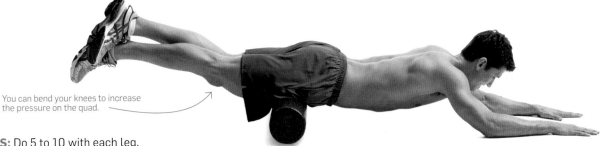

You can bend your knees to increase the pressure on the quad.

REPS: Do 5 to 10 with each leg.

Butt (Piriformis) Massage

A

- Sitting on the foam roller, cross your right leg over your left knee and lean toward the your hip, putting your weight on the right butt cheek.
- Place your right hand behind you for support.
- Roll back and forth over the piriformis, then switch sides.

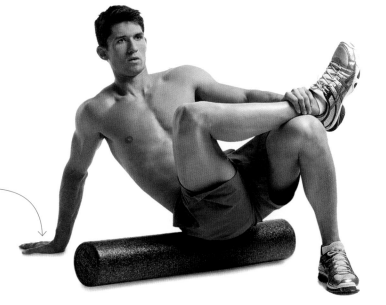

Place your right hand behind you for support.

REPS: Do 5 to 10 on each side.

Foam Roller Workout

Back Massage

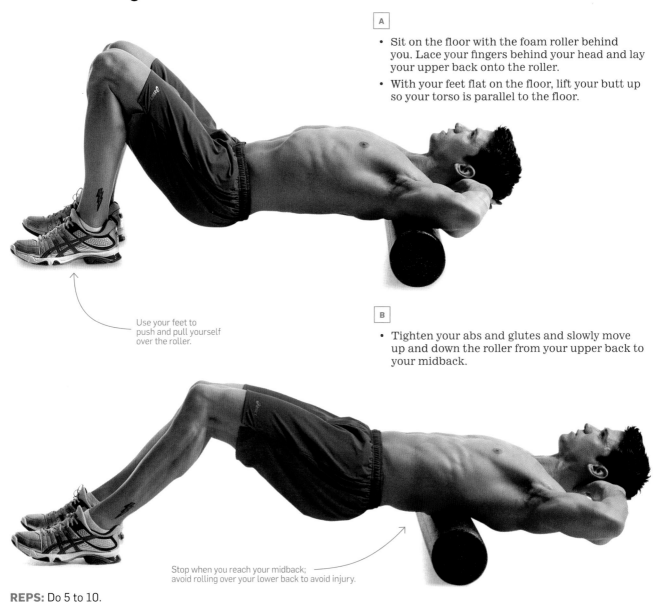

- Sit on the floor with the foam roller behind you. Lace your fingers behind your head and lay your upper back onto the roller.
- With your feet flat on the floor, lift your butt up so your torso is parallel to the floor.

Use your feet to push and pull yourself over the roller.

B

- Tighten your abs and glutes and slowly move up and down the roller from your upper back to your midback.

Stop when you reach your midback; avoid rolling over your lower back to avoid injury.

REPS: Do 5 to 10.

348

Outer Hip and Thigh Massage

A

- Lie on your left side with the roller under your left hip.
- Cross your right leg over your outstretched left leg, bending the knee and placing your foot flat on the floor.

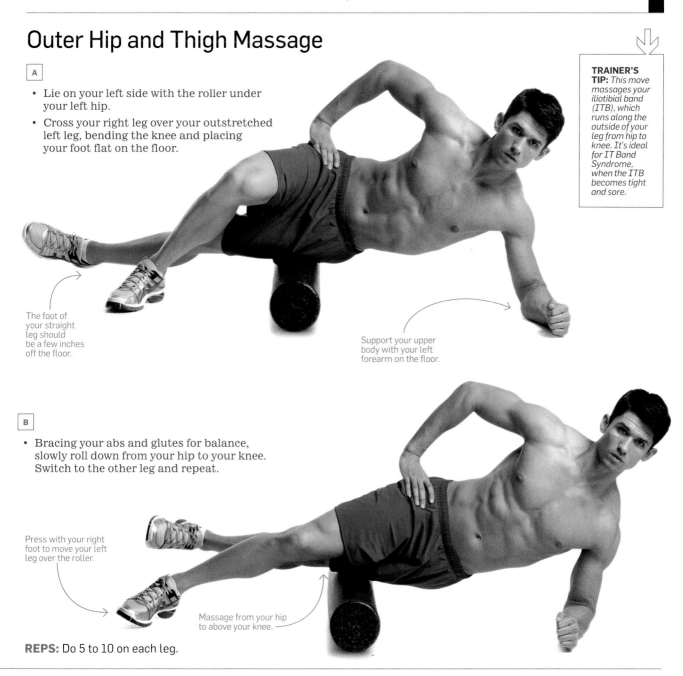

TRAINER'S TIP: *This move massages your iliotibial band (ITB), which runs along the outside of your leg from hip to knee. It's ideal for IT Band Syndrome, when the ITB becomes tight and sore.*

The foot of your straight leg should be a few inches off the floor.

Support your upper body with your left forearm on the floor.

B

- Bracing your abs and glutes for balance, slowly roll down from your hip to your knee. Switch to the other leg and repeat.

Press with your right foot to move your left leg over the roller.

Massage from your hip to above your knee.

REPS: Do 5 to 10 on each leg.

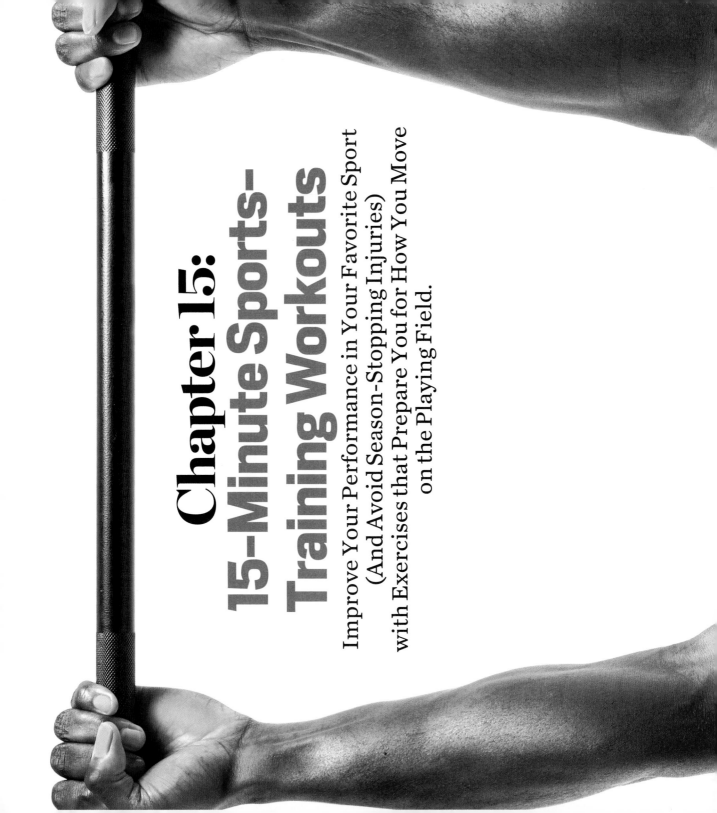

Chapter 15:
15-Minute Sports-Training Workouts

Improve Your Performance in Your Favorite Sport
(And Avoid Season-Stopping Injuries)
with Exercises that Prepare You for How You Move
on the Playing Field.

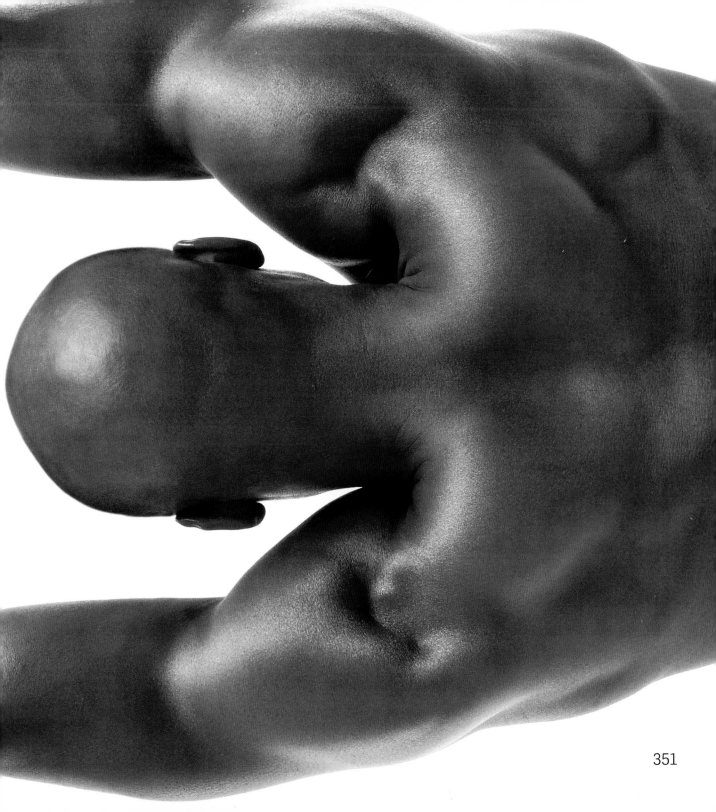

Superfast Workouts for Sports

When you have a busy life, it's easy to forget that your performance in your chosen sport comes down to repeatedly executing a few basic fundamentals. They're basics, they're rote, you've done them thousands of times, and so you don't practice them. And that's why your first golf outing of the season is so embarrassing—and often painful. Sports is all about muscle memory and muscle preparation. That's why we've put together this chapter of routines that specifically target the muscles you use for different sports—and re-create the way you need to use them. They won't replace practicing your short game or reverse layup, but they will strengthen your muscles in the ways you'll use them in the game.

Find It Quick: Your Superfast Sports Training Circuits

BUILD YOUR ATHLETICISM

Great athletes—especially those who play tennis, basketball, lacrosse, and volleyball—are defined by their ability to change speed and direction quickly. Improving agility can benefit anyone in any sport, which is why we recommend adding an old-school agility drill to the end of your workouts. It'll build speed and endurance, and hone your catlike reflexes. Try the T-drill.

Set it up: Form a large T with four cones. Place three in a line 8 feet apart (the top of the T) and a fourth 16 feet away from the middle cone (the bottom of the T).

How to do it: Sprint from that bottom T cone to the middle cone. Then immediately shuffle left to the side cone. (Shuffle your feet with short, quick strides and don't cross them. Then shuffle right, passing the middle cone, to the right cone. Bend down and touch each cone as you pass it. Shuffle as quickly as possible to the middle cone and then run backward to the starting cone. Repeat.

The Golf Workout

Even a leisurely round of golf requires you to twist and turn and generate significant force with your hips and obliques—muscles that go largely unused in normal daily life. The following moves target those core muscles, as well as your hamstrings and shoulders, to put more power in every drive and stroke.

START HERE:
Do the routine as a circuit, performing the prescribed number of each move and then immediately moving to the next. Rest for 60 seconds after completing the circuit, then repeat the circuit. Go through the entire routine three times.

Lawn Mower

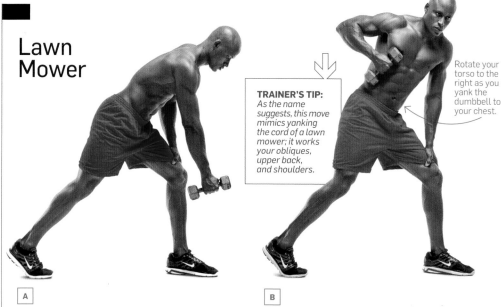

TRAINER'S TIP:
As the name suggests, this move mimics yanking the cord of a lawn mower; it works your obliques, upper back, and shoulders.

Rotate your torso to the right as you yank the dumbbell to your chest.

A

- Grab a 10- to 20-pound dumbbell in your right hand and let it hang at your side, palm facing inward.
- Lunge forward with your left leg until your right leg is straight. Bend forward at the waist.
- Place your left hand on your left knee.

B

- Bend your right arm to pull the weight up toward your ribs as you rotate your torso to the right.
- Lower the weight and return to the lunge position with your left leg bent and your right leg straight. That's 1 rep.

REPS: Do 12, then repeat the move with the dumbbell in your left hand and your right foot forward.

Windmill

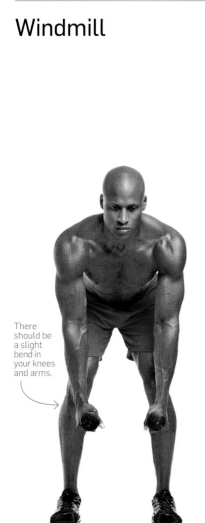

There should be a slight bend in your knees and arms.

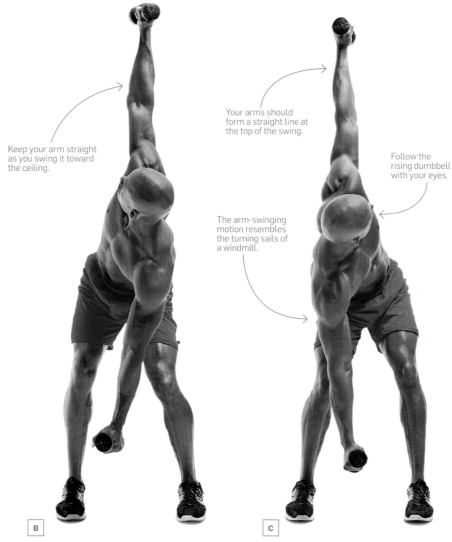

Keep your arm straight as you swing it toward the ceiling.

Your arms should form a straight line at the top of the swing.

Follow the rising dumbbell with your eyes.

The arm-swinging motion resembles the turning sails of a windmill.

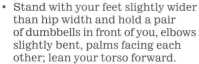

A
- Stand with your feet slightly wider than hip width and hold a pair of dumbbells in front of you, elbows slightly bent, palms facing each other; lean your torso forward.

REPS: Do 20 total, alternating sides.

B
- Rotate to the right as you raise your right arm toward the ceiling.
- Pause before returning the dumbbell to the starting position.

C
- Rotate to the left as you swing the dumbbell in your left hand toward the ceiling.
- Continue alternating arm swings.

Leaning Hamstring Curl

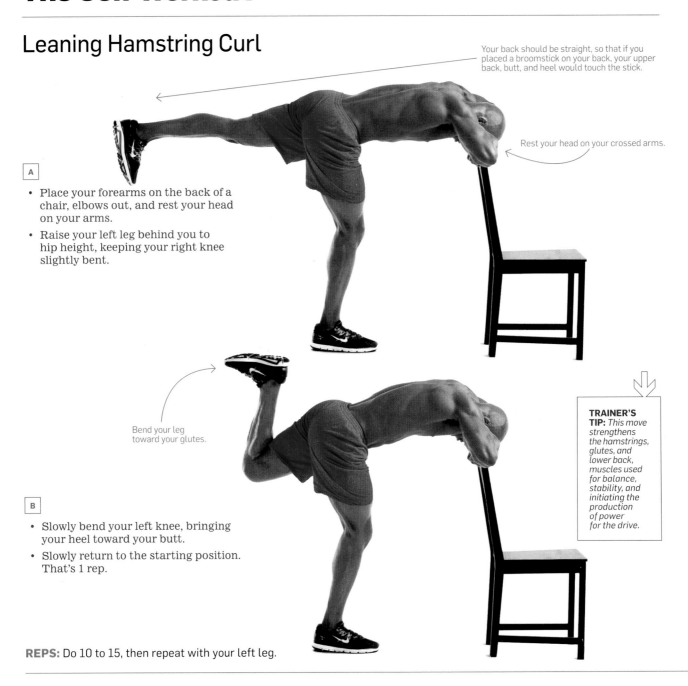

Your back should be straight, so that if you placed a broomstick on your back, your upper back, butt, and heel would touch the stick.

Rest your head on your crossed arms.

A

- Place your forearms on the back of a chair, elbows out, and rest your head on your arms.
- Raise your left leg behind you to hip height, keeping your right knee slightly bent.

Bend your leg toward your glutes.

TRAINER'S TIP: *This move strengthens the hamstrings, glutes, and lower back, muscles used for balance, stability, and initiating the production of power for the drive.*

B

- Slowly bend your left knee, bringing your heel toward your butt.
- Slowly return to the starting position. That's 1 rep.

REPS: Do 10 to 15, then repeat with your left leg.

Medicine Ball Transfer

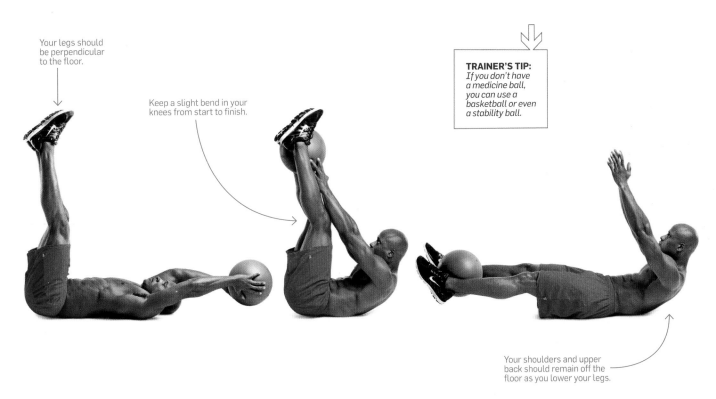

Your legs should be perpendicular to the floor.

Keep a slight bend in your knees from start to finish.

TRAINER'S TIP:
If you don't have a medicine ball, you can use a basketball or even a stability ball.

Your shoulders and upper back should remain off the floor as you lower your legs.

A

- Lie on your back on the floor holding a medicine ball between your hands above your head so that your arms are straight in line with your torso.
- Lift your legs toward the ceiling to form a 90-degree angle with your upper body.

REPS: Do 10 to 15.

B

- Curl your upper body so that your head and shoulders rise off the floor.
- Place the medicine ball between your feet.

C

- Lower your legs with the ball between your feet to just a few inches above the ground. Keep your shoulders curled and your arms up.
- Pause, then raise your feet to meet your arms and transfer the ball back to your hands.
- Lower your shoulders and arms to the starting position.

The Tennis Workout

In tennis, speed and agility can make up for some of what you may lack in racquet talent. Shoulder strength can help, too. This workout is designed to quicken your reflexes and improve your ability to dash from side to side to reach the ball, which is half the battle. It builds power, flexibility, and agility through your legs, hips, shoulders, and core.

START HERE:
Do these moves as a circuit with no rest in between exercises. After completing the circuit, rest for 60 seconds, then do two more rounds.

Power Lunge and Pull

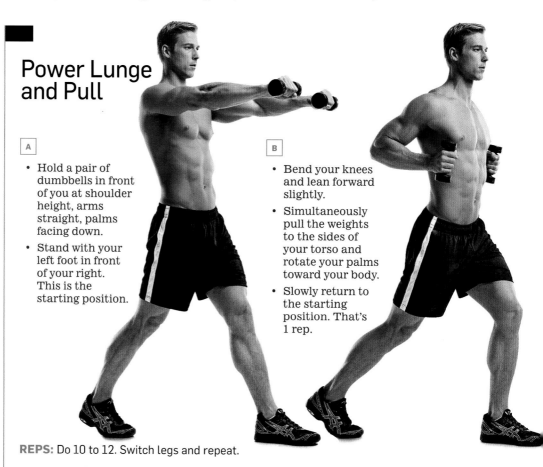

A
- Hold a pair of dumbbells in front of you at shoulder height, arms straight, palms facing down.
- Stand with your left foot in front of your right. This is the starting position.

B
- Bend your knees and lean forward slightly.
- Simultaneously pull the weights to the sides of your torso and rotate your palms toward your body.
- Slowly return to the starting position. That's 1 rep.

REPS: Do 10 to 12. Switch legs and repeat.

Calf Raise

A

- Hold a dumbbell in each hand at your sides and stand with the ball of each foot on a low riser that's about 2 inches high.

B

- Rise up on your toes as high as you can.
- Pause, then slowly lower back to the starting position.

Stand as tall as you can.

Lift your heels as high as possible.

If you don't have an exercise riser, use a 25-pound weight plate under each foot.

Your heels should be touching the floor.

REPS: Do 10 to 12.

The Tennis Workout

Rotation Swing

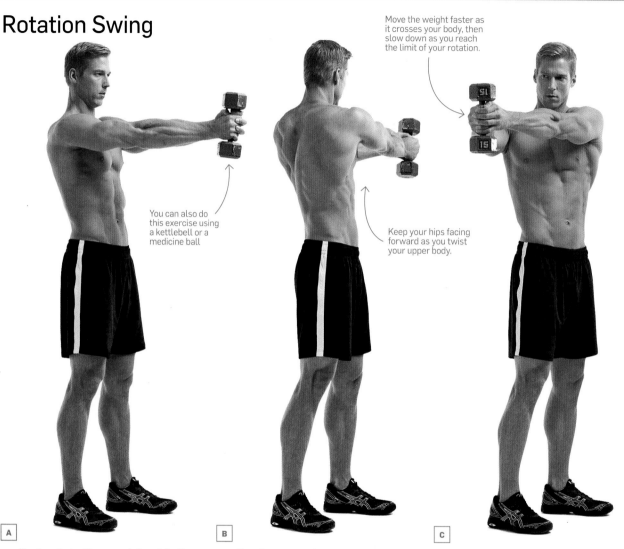

Move the weight faster as it crosses your body, then slow down as you reach the limit of your rotation.

You can also do this exercise using a kettlebell or a medicine ball

Keep your hips facing forward as you twist your upper body.

A

- Grab a 5- to 10-pound dumbbell with both hands and stand with your feet shoulder-width apart.
- Extend the dumbbell straight out in front of you at shoulder height.

B

- Keeping your hips square and your arms straight, rotate your torso and arms to the left as far as you can.

C

- Swing the dumbbell as far to the right as possible.
- Accelerate the weight across the front of your body, then slow it down as it reaches your side. That's 1 rep.

REPS: Do 10, then switch the side you start on and do another 10.

Lateral Leap with Reach

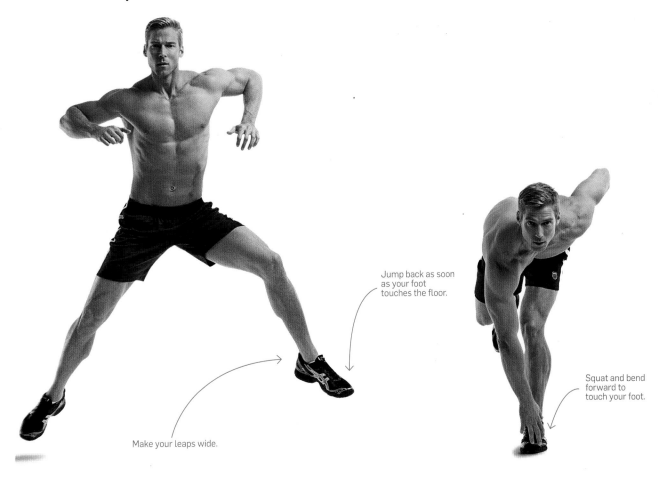

Jump back as soon as your foot touches the floor.

Make your leaps wide.

Squat and bend forward to touch your foot.

A

- Stand with your feet together, your knees slightly bent, your elbows bent to 90 degrees, and your hands in front of you.
- Jump to the left, landing on your left foot, then jump to the right, landing on your right foot. Repeat 5 times.

REPS: Do 5, then switch the side you started on and do another 5.

B

- Next, jump back onto your left foot and squat until you can touch the top of your left foot with your right hand.
- Jump back to the right and touch your right foot with your left hand. That's 1 rep.

The Ski and Snowboard Workout

Anyone who's ever experienced rubbery legs after a day on the slopes knows that snow sports demand leg power like almost nothing else. Those legs act as shock absorbers, working with your core as you carve down the mountain. Whether you board or ski, this workout will help you stay in control through the day's last run.

START HERE:
Do the routine as a circuit, performing the prescribed number of each move and then immediately moving to the next. Rest for 60 seconds, then repeat the circuit again. Do a total of three full circuits.

Bosu Jumps

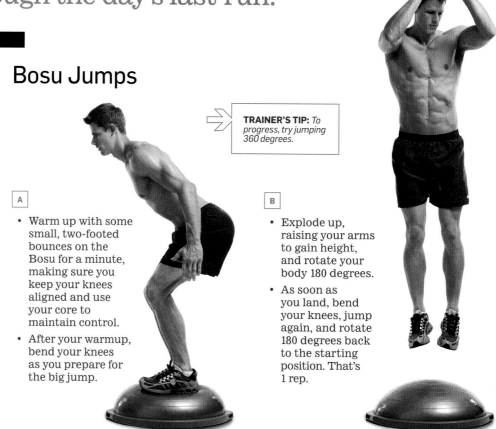

TRAINER'S TIP: *To progress, try jumping 360 degrees.*

A

- Warm up with some small, two-footed bounces on the Bosu for a minute, making sure you keep your knees aligned and use your core to maintain control.
- After your warmup, bend your knees as you prepare for the big jump.

B

- Explode up, raising your arms to gain height, and rotate your body 180 degrees.
- As soon as you land, bend your knees, jump again, and rotate 180 degrees back to the starting position. That's 1 rep.

REPS: Do 10.

Ski Hops

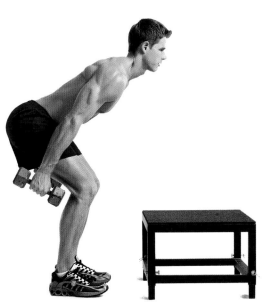

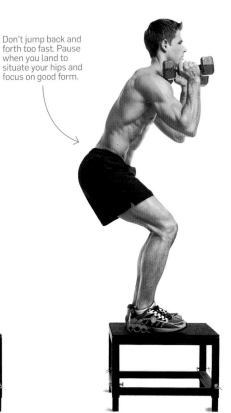

Don't jump back and forth too fast. Pause when you land to situate your hips and focus on good form.

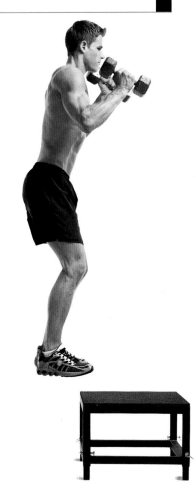

A

- Hold a 10-pound dumbbell in each hand at your sides, palms facing your legs.
- Stand with your feet hip-width apart in front of a sturdy box or step that's about 18 inches high.
- Bend your knees and lean forward as you prepare to jump.

REPS: Do 20.

B

- Press your feet into the floor to explode up in a jump.
- Simultaneously bend your elbows to raise the weights to your shoulders as you leap onto the box.
- Land softly on the balls of your feet and immediately bend your knees to jump again.

C

- Push down with your feet and straighten your legs to jump backward off the box and back into the starting position.
- Again, land softly, bend your knees to absorb the impact, and lower the weights to your sides. That's 1 rep.

The Ski and Snowboard Workout

Lateral Medicine Ball Hops

A

- Stand holding a medicine ball in front of your chest, feet together.
- Bound laterally to your right.

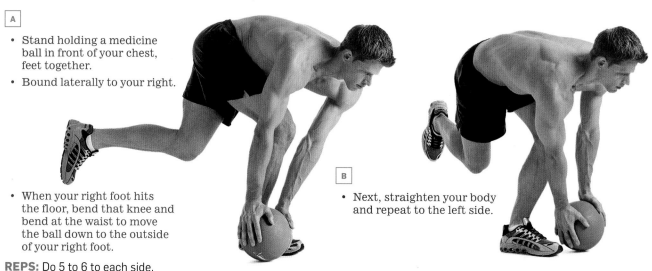

- When your right foot hits the floor, bend that knee and bend at the waist to move the ball down to the outside of your right foot.

B

- Next, straighten your body and repeat to the left side.

REPS: Do 5 to 6 to each side.

Drop Lunge

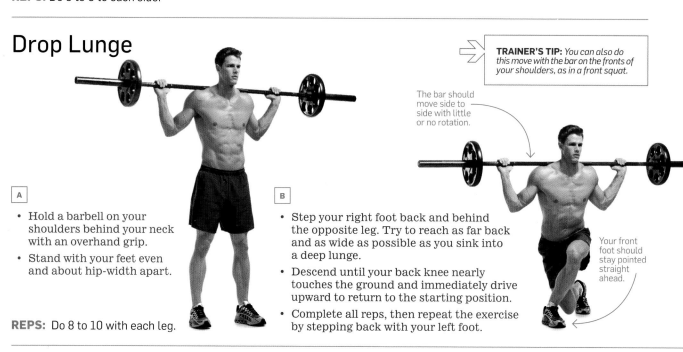

TRAINER'S TIP: *You can also do this move with the bar on the fronts of your shoulders, as in a front squat.*

The bar should move side to side with little or no rotation.

A

- Hold a barbell on your shoulders behind your neck with an overhand grip.
- Stand with your feet even and about hip-width apart.

REPS: Do 8 to 10 with each leg.

B

- Step your right foot back and behind the opposite leg. Try to reach as far back and as wide as possible as you sink into a deep lunge.
- Descend until your back knee nearly touches the ground and immediately drive upward to return to the starting position.
- Complete all reps, then repeat the exercise by stepping back with your left foot.

Your front foot should stay pointed straight ahead.

Bosu Medicine Ball Twist

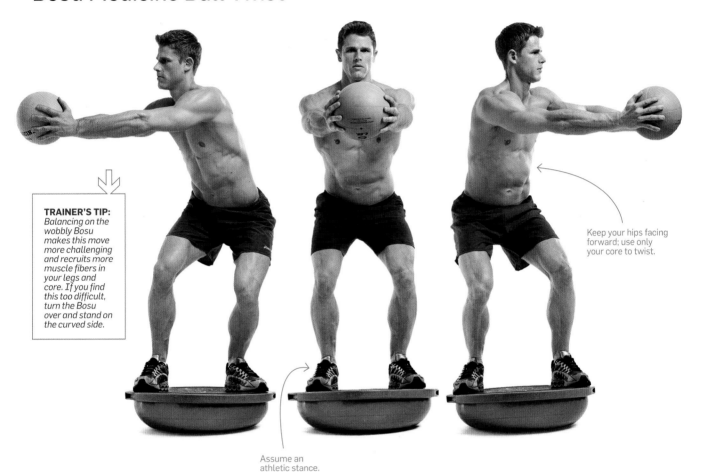

TRAINER'S TIP:
Balancing on the wobbly Bosu makes this move more challenging and recruits more muscle fibers in your legs and core. If you find this too difficult, turn the Bosu over and stand on the curved side.

Keep your hips facing forward; use only your core to twist.

Assume an athletic stance.

A

- Stand on the flat side of a Bosu in an athletic stance with a slight bend in your knees and hips.
- Hold a medicine ball with straight arms at chest level (center).

REPS: Do 5 to 8.

B

- Keeping your hips forward, rotate your upper body as far as possible to the right using only your core.

C

- Return to the center position, then rotate your upper body as far as possible to the left. That's 1 rep.

The Running Race Workout

Running involves way more than your legs. You need strong abs, obliques, and back muscles to keep from collapsing forward as you start to fatigue. Even your shoulders are star players because a strong arm swing is key to a powerful stride. This workout bolsters all those muscles.

START HERE: Do the routine as a circuit, performing the prescribed number of each move and then immediately moving to the next. Rest for 60 seconds, then repeat the circuit again. Go through the entire routine three times.

Jump Squat

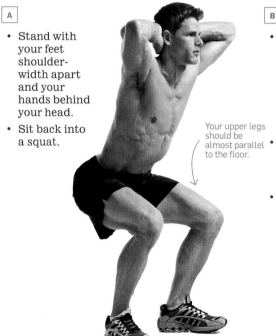

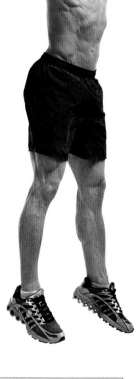

A
- Stand with your feet shoulder-width apart and your hands behind your head.
- Sit back into a squat.

Your upper legs should be almost parallel to the floor.

B
- Drive your heels into the floor to straighten your legs and jump explosively as high as you can.
- Land with your knees soft to absorb the impact.
- Immediately jump again.

TRAINER'S TIP: *To get greater height, hold your arms at your sides, then swing them up and reach toward the ceiling.*

REPS: Do as many as possible in 60 seconds.

Standing Leg Lift

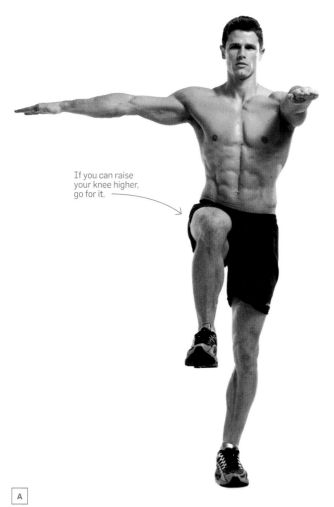

If you can raise your knee higher, go for it.

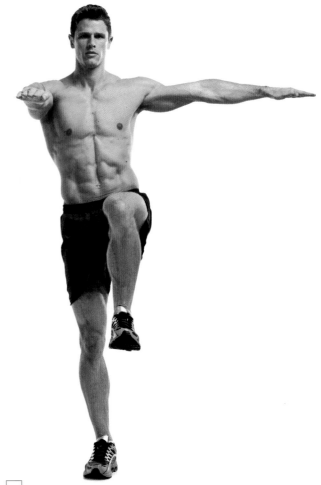

A

- Stand with your feet shoulder-width apart and your arms extended to your sides at shoulder height.
- Lift your right knee as high as you can and swing your left arm forward until it's parallel to the floor.

REPS: Do as many as possible in 60 seconds.

B

- Return to the starting position and repeat with your left knee and right arm.
- Continue alternating sides with good form.

The Running Race Workout

Bulgarian Split Squat

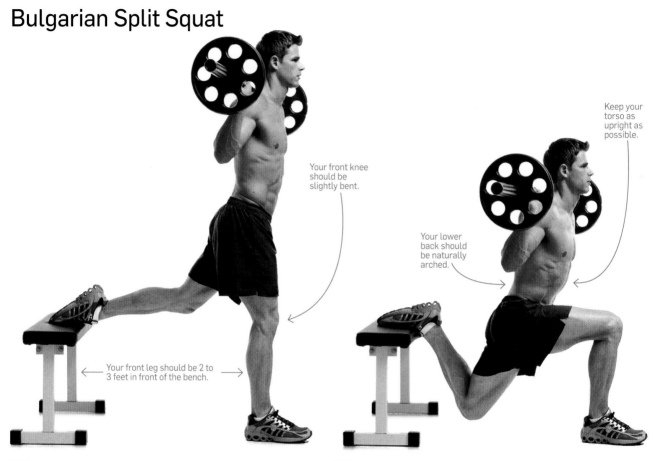

Your front knee should be slightly bent.

Keep your torso as upright as possible.

Your lower back should be naturally arched.

Your front leg should be 2 to 3 feet in front of the bench.

A

- Hold a barbell across your upper back with an overhand grip.
- Stand about 2 to 3 feet in front of a bench. Place one foot behind you on the bench, supporting most of your weight on the front leg.
- Brace your core.
- Pull your shoulders back so the bar rests comfortably on the shelf created by your shoulder blades.

REPS: Do 8 to 10 with each leg.

B

- Slowly lower your body until your front thigh is about parallel to the ground.
- Pause, then use your forward leg to push yourself back to the starting position explosively.
- Complete all repetitions, then do the same number with your left leg forward and right foot on the bench.

Hip Hike

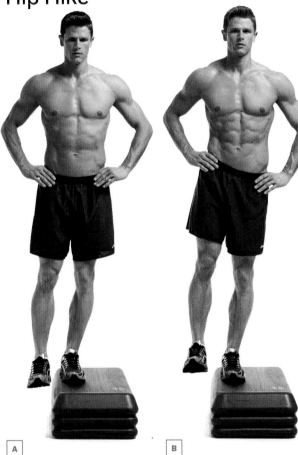

A

B

- Stand sideways on a step or box with your left foot planted on the step and your right hanging off the edge in the air.

- Place your hands on your hips.

- Keeping your shoulders level, hips pointed forward, and both legs straight, use your glutes to raise your right hip.

- Then lower the leg.

- Return to the starting position. That's 1 rep.

REPS: Do 12 to 15 on each leg.

Plate Push

 TRAINER'S TIP: *Drive one knee into your chest while pushing back with the opposite leg as hard as you can. Push the plate as fast as you can. Avoid lifting your head to eliminate strain on your neck and back.*

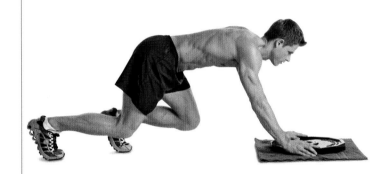

A

- Place a 45-pound plate on a towel on a smooth floor.

- Assume a bear-crawl position with your back parallel to the floor, your hands on the top of the plate, and the balls of your feet on the floor ready to push.

- Drive your feet into the floor to push the plate forward. Push it about 30 yards, keeping your hips straight and your head in a neutral position. Rest for 30 seconds, then push it back to the starting point. That's 1 rep.

REPS: Do 1 to 2.

The Triathlon Workout

True to its design, the triathlon—swimming, biking, and running—puts every muscle to the test. This routine does it all with explosive moves to develop power for your run, core-stabilizing moves to hold yourself strong on the bike, and full-body strength and stretching moves to keep you slicing long and strong through the water.

START HERE:
Do the routine as a circuit, performing the prescribed number of each exercise and then immediately moving to the next. Rest for 60 seconds, then repeat the circuit again. Do three full circuits.

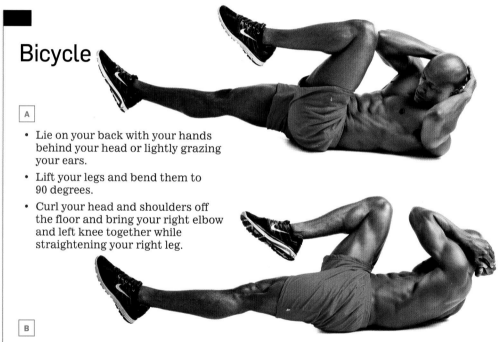

Bicycle

A

- Lie on your back with your hands behind your head or lightly grazing your ears.
- Lift your legs and bend them to 90 degrees.
- Curl your head and shoulders off the floor and bring your right elbow and left knee together while straightening your right leg.

B

- As you straighten your left leg, bend your right knee toward your chest.
- Simultaneously twist your upper body to bring your left elbow toward your right knee. That sequence is 1 rep.
- Continue alternating this way; the motion of your legs should be like pedaling a bicycle, thus the name of the exercise.

REPS: Do 10 to 20.

Hindu Pushup

A

- Start in a pushup position, with your back flat and your arms straight.
- Lift your hips and allow your head to drop so your head and back are in line with your arms. This is similar to yoga's downward-facing dog pose. Your legs should be locked straight.
- Press your heels into the floor if you can.

B

- Drop your hips toward the floor as you simultaneously sweep your torso forward and up, raising your chest and shifting your weight forward into a cobra-like pose.
- Reverse the movement to return to the starting position. That's 1 rep.

REPS: Do 10.

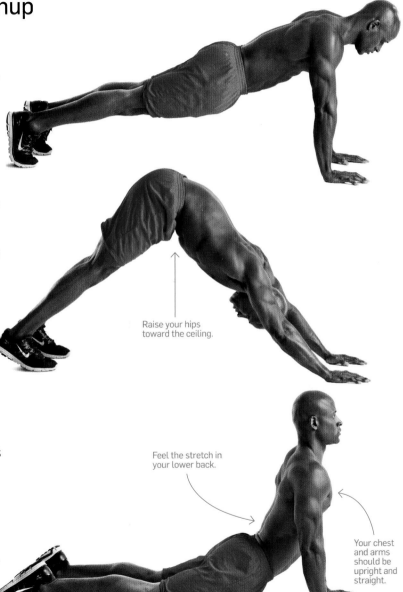

Raise your hips toward the ceiling.

Feel the stretch in your lower back.

Your chest and arms should be upright and straight.

THE 15-MINUTE TRIATHLON

Give yourself a mini-triathlon and get a swimmer's cut shoulders, a cyclist's toned legs, and a runner's lean physique, says Karl Scott, a trainer at The Sports Club/LA in New York City.

HOW TO DO IT: Pedal a bike at a moderate pace—an effort level of 5 or 6 (you're working hard but can still carry on a conversation)—for 5 minutes. Next, run either outside or on a treadmill for 5 minutes, again at an effort level of 5 or 6. Last, head to the pool or a rowing machine, which approximates the upper-body demands of swimming, and put in 5 minutes at the same effort level.

371

The Triathlon Workout

Switch Lunge

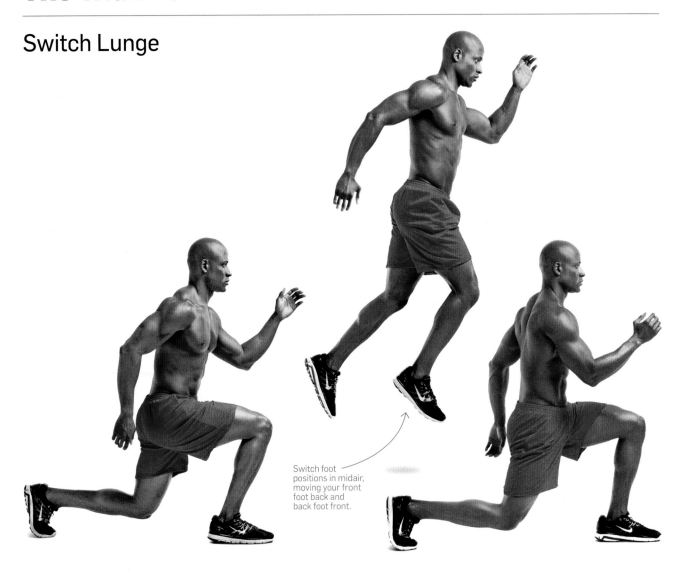

Switch foot positions in midair, moving your front foot back and back foot front.

A

- Lunge forward with your right thigh parallel to the floor.

REPS: Do 12 to 15.

B

- Swinging your arms for balance and momentum, jump up and switch arms and legs in midair.

C

- Land softly in a lunge with your left foot forward.
- Repeat to return to the right-leg-forward position. That's 1 rep.

Hyperextension with Rotation

A

- Position yourself on a hyper-extension station with your calves tucked under the padded bars and your hips and upper thighs resting on the flat pad.
- Place your hands behind your head and bend your upper body toward the floor.

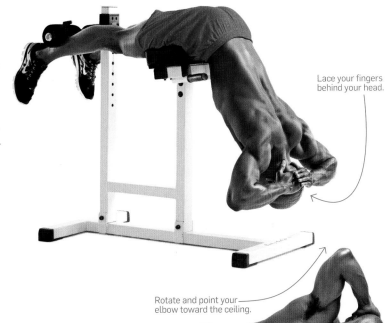

Lace your fingers behind your head.

Rotate and point your elbow toward the ceiling.

B

- Lift your upper body until it's parallel with the floor while simultaneously rotating your torso to the right.
- Lower to the starting position and then rise and rotate to the left. That's 1 rep.

REPS: Do 10.

SWIM YOURSELF SLIM

If you have time to get to a pool, there's nothing like a swimming workout for slimming down. The body-shaping benefits of swimming come from muscle recruitment and calorie burn. An easy swim burns about 500 calories an hour, while a vigorous effort can torch about 700. Because water is nearly 800 times denser than air, each kick of the legs and pull of the arms is like a resistance workout for your core, hips, arms, legs, shoulders and glutes. So in addition to blasting calories as you swim, you build lean muscle, which ignites your metabolism so you burn more calories once you've showered and dried off.

The Cycling Workout

Your legs might seem like the only things moving when you ride, but cycling is a full-body event. With each revolution, your upper body acts as a platform for your legs to push off of. Your arms and shoulders help you leverage power going uphill, and your hips keep you stable in the saddle. This routine hits the whole cast of characters.

START HERE:
Do the routine as a circuit, performing the prescribed number of each move and then immediately going to the next. Rest for 60 seconds, then repeat the circuit twice more for a total of three.

Spider

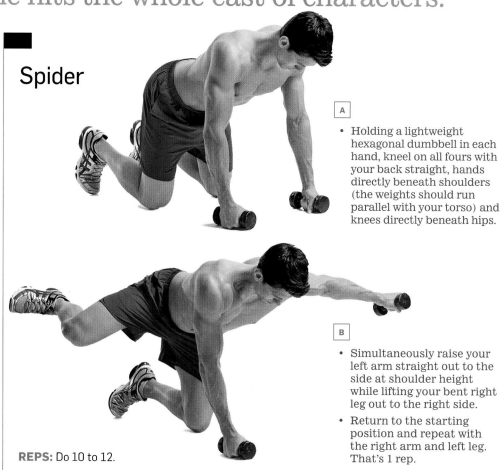

A
• Holding a lightweight hexagonal dumbbell in each hand, kneel on all fours with your back straight, hands directly beneath shoulders (the weights should run parallel with your torso) and knees directly beneath hips.

B
• Simultaneously raise your left arm straight out to the side at shoulder height while lifting your bent right leg out to the right side.
• Return to the starting position and repeat with the right arm and left leg. That's 1 rep.

REPS: Do 10 to 12.

Scoop Squat

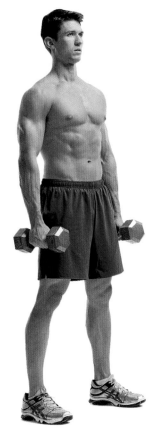

When prepping to curl, keep your palms facing inward, in a hammer-curl position.

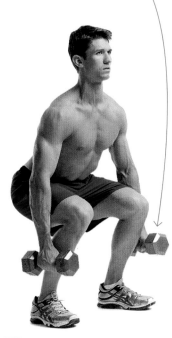

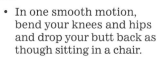

GO FAST, FRY MORE FAT

Forget about steady state cardio. "It's a simple fact: The faster you go, the more calories you burn and the more weight you will lose," says exercise physiologist Tom Holland, author of *The Marathon Method.* Holland recommends that half of your workout be near your anaerobic threshold, or AT, which is what you'll get with our superfast fat-burning workouts. "That's the point where we begin to have trouble breathing and our bodies can no longer clear lactic acid from our bloodstream," Holland says. "Runners call this a tempo workout—which means increasing your speed until you hit and sustain a 'comfortably hard' pace for a set period of time."

A

- Holding 20- to 35-pound dumbbells at your sides, palms inward, stand with your feet hip- to shoulder-width apart.

REPS: Do 12 to 15.

B

- In one smooth motion, bend your knees and hips and drop your butt back as though sitting in a chair.
- Immediately push back to stand while bending your elbows and curling the weights to your shoulders as you do.

C

- When you reach the standing position, immediately press the weights overhead, again, keeping your palms facing in.
- Lower the weights back to your sides. That's 1 rep.

The Cycling Workout

Balance, Dip, Extend

14

Hours a cyclist's metabolism may stay elevated after a high-intensity riding workout.

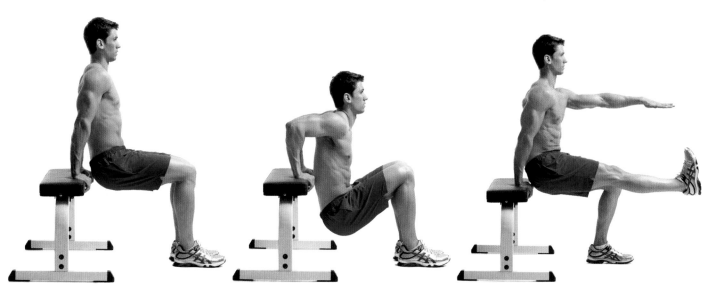

A

- Sit on the edge of a chair, hands grasping the seat to either side of your hips.
- Keep your knees bent and your feet flat on the floor. Scoot your butt off the chair seat.

REPS: Do 10 to 12.

B

- Bend your elbows and lower your hips toward the floor until your upper arms are parallel to the floor.

C

- Straighten your arms to raise yourself, then extend your left arm to the front at shoulder height, palm down, while simultaneously extending your right leg with the foot flexed.
- Pause, then bring the arm and leg back to the starting position.
- Repeat the entire sequence with the other arm and leg. That's 1 rep.

Single-Leg Stepdown

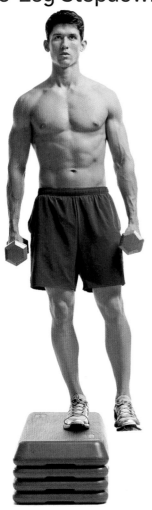

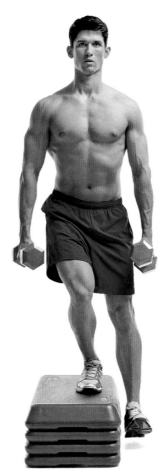

A

- Holding relatively heavy dumbbells (35 pounds or more), stand sideways on an 18-inch-high step with only the right foot on the step, allowing the left leg to hang in the air.

REPS: Do 10 to 12 with each leg.

B

- Pull your navel toward your spine and, keeping your chest lifted, bend your knee to slowly step down with the left foot and gently tap the left heel on the floor.
- Keeping the right heel firmly planted on the step, return to the starting position.
- Complete a full set, then switch legs.

GET YOUR HEAD IN THE GAME

Brain training is an essential part of any sports warmup. "Preparing your central nervous system for activity is just as important as preparing your muscles," says Vern Gambetta, former director of conditioning for the Chicago White Sox. That's because your central nervous system tells your muscles when to contract. Try standing on one leg while you squat down and touch the floor in front of it with your opposite hand. Do two sets of 10 to 12 reps with each leg.

The Basketball Workout

To skitter all over the court in the classic low defensive stance, you need to improve leg endurance and your ability to change directions quickly. We developed these basketball-specific weight exercises with help from Greg Brittenham, CSCS, an assistant coach for the New York Knicks.

START HERE: Do this workout as straight sets. Complete all repetitions in a set, then rest for 30 seconds before repeating. Do three sets of each exercise, then rest for at least 60 seconds before moving on to the next exercise.

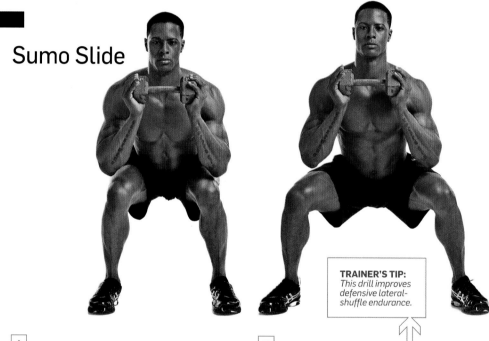

Sumo Slide

A
- Grab a dumbbell with both hands and hold it by cradling your fingers around the ends of the weight.
- Stand with your feet wider than shoulder-width apart, and then lower your body until your thighs are parallel to the floor.

REPS: Do 4 to 8.

B
- Slide 2 steps to the left, as if you are performing a defensive shuffle.
- Stop and press back to a standing position.
- Repeat in the opposite direction. That's 1 rep.

TRAINER'S TIP:
This drill improves defensive lateral-shuffle endurance.

Two Down and One Back

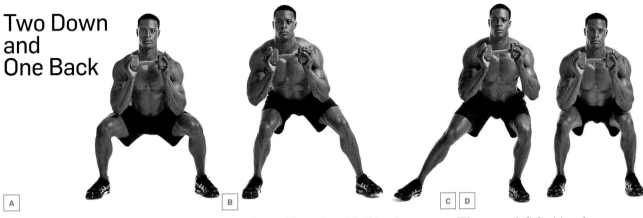

A

- Start in the down position of the Sumo Slide with your thighs parallel to the floor and a dumbbell in your hands, using the same grip as in the Sumo Slide.

REPS: Do 8 to 10 stepping left and 8 to 10 stepping right.

B

- Take 2 wide and rapid slide-steps to your left.

C **D**

- When your left foot touches the floor on your second step, immediately take one slide-step back to your right.
- Repeat until you've done 8 to 10. Then do the exercise sliding right first. That's one set.

Dumbbell Power Clean

A

- Squat over a pair of dumbbells as if you are going to deadlift them.
- Grasp them with an overhand grip, your palms facing you.

B

- Explosively stand and pull the dumbbells straight up.
- When you're upright, lift the weights in an arc over your upper arms, to the tops of your shoulders.
- Your upper arms should be parallel to the floor, your elbows pointing forward, palms facing inward.
- Reverse the movement to return the dumbbells to the floor. That's 1 rep.

REPS: Do 5.

TRAINER'S TIP: *This move builds explosiveness and agility.*

Push through your heels as you stand explosively. This move will improve your vertical leap.

Index

Boldface page references indicate photographs. Underscored references indicate boxed text.

E